YOGA SPARKS

108 Easy Practices for
Stress Relief in a Minute or Less

CAROL KRUCOFF, E-RYT

NEW HARBINGER PUBLICATIONS, INC.

Distributed in Canada by Raincoast Books

Copyright © 2013 by Carol Krucoff
New Harbinger Publications, Inc.
5674 Shattuck Avenue
Oakland, CA 94609
www.newharbinger.com

Acknowledgments for the use of copyrighted material appear on pages 232, which constitute an extension of the copyright page.

Cover design by Amy Shoup; Text design by Michele Waters-Kermes; Acquired by Jess O'Brien; Edited by Jasmine Star

All Rights Reserved

Library of Congress Cataloging-in-Publication Data

Krucoff, Carol.
  Yoga sparks : 108 easy practices for stress relief in a minute or less / Carol Krucoff, E-RYT.
     pages cm
  Includes bibliographical references.
  ISBN 978-1-60882-700-8 (pbk. : alk. paper) -- ISBN 978-1-60882-701-5 (pdf e-book) -- ISBN 978-1-60882-702-2 (epub) 1. Stress management. 2. Relaxation. 3. Yoga--Therapeutic use. I. Title.
  RA785.K78 2013
  613.7'046--dc23
                                                            2013014405

Printed in the United States of America

15   14   13

10   9   8   7   6   5   4   3   2   1   First printing

To my teachers, on whose shoulders I stand,
And to my students, who have taught me so much

The *Gita* sums up [what] this means in one word—yoga… This ancient word is pressed by the *Gita* into service to mean the entire gamut of human endeavor to storm the gates of Heaven. It is derived from the verb *yuj*…which has numerous meanings: to join, to attach, to yoke; to direct, to concentrate one's attention on; to use, to apply, to employ. In the *Yoga Sutras* it is used to mean discipline or control. It thus means the yoking of all the powers of the body and the mind and soul to God; it means the discipline of the intellect, the mind, the emotions, the will, which such a yoking presupposes; it means a poise of the soul which enables one to look at life in all its aspects and evenly.

—*The Gita According to Gandhi*, by Mahadev Desai

CONTENTS

Meditation Sparks

Principle Sparks

Posture Sparks

• 4 • ON THE GO PRACTICES 167

·5· PRACTICES WITH OTHERS **199**

EPILOGUE **221**

REFERENCES **224**

FOREWORD

When it comes to yoga, meditation, or anything you know is good for you, you might feel as though you don't have enough time to truly get anything out of it. Maybe you feel overwhelmed by just thinking about how to fit it into an already busy schedule. We live in a world where the message is "If a little bit is good, a lot is better." Yet there never seems to be enough time in the day to do "a lot."

Here's some good news: Sometimes a little bit *is* enough. Sometimes a small dose can even be the most healing. This is true for yoga and all of its benefits. A single moment can provide relief, and a small taste can trigger profound transformation. The benefits of small doses is the premise of Carol Krucoff's book *Yoga Sparks*, which can help you find health, happiness, and meaning in less time than it will take to read this foreword. As radical a promise as this may seem, the latest science supports it.

Research has shown that you can shift the state of your brain with as little as a minute of meditation or mindful breathing. Changing your physical posture—say, from slumped to standing tall—can transform your mood. A brief burst of movement can do more to relieve stress than a longer workout. A short reflection on gratitude can improve your relationships. Choosing to engage in these sorts of brief practices—what Carol calls micropractices or Yoga Sparks—throughout the day is a powerful way to create lasting change. And it's a much more effective way to create joy and well-being than trying to squeeze in a practice you don't have time for.

Carol is a trustworthy guide in this journey. I first met her years ago at a conference for yoga therapists. Even among professionals dedicated to teaching yoga, Carol stood out as a fierce advocate of the idea that yoga is for everyone. She has been a pioneer is the field, demonstrating that simple practices can have profound effects. She honors the idea that each person's body is different, and she teaches other instructors how to make yoga safe. She has also helped demonstrate the healing effects of yoga by bringing it into medical settings. As yoga fads come and go, Carol has always communicated the wisdom of the tradition through its most timeless practices.

Whatever drew you to this book, I hope you will trust that part of yourself—the part of you that wants to do this for you, that values your health, that wants to find great happiness and meaning in life. As Carol writes, yoga is the process of discovering and becoming this version of yourself. Each time you practice one of the Yoga Sparks in this book, you strengthen your self-compassion, courage, and wisdom. May you give yourself this gift every day and truly make these practices a part of your life.

—Kelly McGonigal, PhD
Health Psychologist, Stanford University
Author of *Yoga for Pain Relief*

ACKNOWLEDGMENTS

I am grateful for the support, wisdom, and kindness of many wonderful people who have contributed to this book. In particular, I offer heartfelt thanks to Stanford University health psychologist Kelly McGonigal, PhD, for her generous and inspiring foreword. An extraordinary yogini of many talents—researcher, author, lecturer, and dancer—her intellect is matched by a compassionate spirit and loving heart.

Numerous master teachers have given me permission to share their wisdom in these pages, and I offer admiration and gratitude to them: Mary Brantley, Jim and Kimberly Carson, Steven Cope, Nischala Joy Devi, Roshi Joan Halifax, Tesilya Hanauer, Kate Holcombe, Sally Kempton, Thich Nhat Hanh, Sarah Powers, M. J. Ryan, Erich Schiffmann, Martin Seligman, and the estates of Mahadev Desai and Eknath Easwaran. I'm also grateful to the many yoga teachers I've studied with over more than thirty years—in particular my mentor Esther Myers, her teacher Vanda Scaravelli, and her teacher T. K. V. Desikachar.

Thanks to the excellent editorial team at New Harbinger, particularly Jess O'Brien for initiating the conversation that resulted in this book, Jess Beebe for her insightful guidance, and Jasmine Star for her careful copyediting.

My outstanding colleagues at Duke Integrative Medicine are a living example of how medical care can go beyond treating disease to help people actively cultivate and optimize their health. Working with this incredibly talented group of healers is an ongoing inspiration.

Special thanks to Tracy Bogart, Phil Botjer, and Danielle Koppel of Triangle Yoga in Chapel Hill for modeling the postures so expertly, and to Lynn Shwadchuck for turning their photos into wonderful illustrations.

I offer deep gratitude to my family and friends for their love and healing energy, which supports and nourishes me. I'm blessed to be the mother of two amazingly accomplished adult children, Max and Rae, whose light illuminates my world.

And I'm eternally grateful to the love of my life, my remarkable husband Mitchell, for gracing this book with an epilogue and for much more than I can possibly say.

INTRODUCTION

Have a minute? In sixty seconds—or even less—you can practice yoga and gain significant and lasting benefits. This book is filled with quick, simple micropractices designed to help you integrate powerful yogic teachings into your daily life. And they are accessible to virtually anyone, regardless of age or fitness level. If you can breathe, you can do Yoga Sparks.

There's no need for a yoga mat or special clothing. Despite the common misconception that yoga is primarily a form of physical exercise, this ancient discipline is actually a practice of awareness designed to quiet your mind and help you connect with your true self. That's why each Yoga Spark is geared toward enhancing your awareness—bringing you into the present moment and helping you find ease in your body, mind, and spirit.

You'll find Yoga Sparks that focus on four main aspects of yoga practice:

- **Postures:** yoga poses, also known as *asanas*
- **Breathing:** also called *pranayama*, which means extension and control of *prana*, the yogic term for breath, vital energy, or life force
- **Meditation:** a process of focusing attention and stilling the chatter of the mind
- **Principles:** guidelines for ethical conduct, including honesty, contentment, and greedlessness

Some Yoga Sparks primarily impact muscles and bones, others address behaviors and breathing, and still others center on thoughts and attitudes. Over time, these micropractices can have major effects—relieving pain and stress, stretching and strengthening your body, calming your mind, and lifting your spirits. And because they're so easy and quick, you can fit them into activities you're already doing, such as showering, cooking, or driving, to help cultivate ease, joy, and well-being.

In the midst of our busy, stressful lives, Yoga Sparks can become transformative moments. It is my sincere hope that you'll find these practices so useful that they become welcome habits, igniting the myriad benefits of the profoundly healing discipline of yoga into your life.

Why Yoga Sparks?

Yoga Sparks arose through my own practice—studying yoga for more than thirty-five years—as well as my work with hundreds of yoga students and yoga therapy clients. Frequently, people tell me they're intrigued by yoga or have even tried it but were discouraged because it was too difficult or time-consuming. Micropractices offer an easy, practical way for people to step their toes into the yoga waters. This is often so helpful that people are inspired to make time for a longer practice.

Similarly, many dedicated yoga students who rarely miss a yoga class confess that they never practice at home. For various reasons (commonly "no time," "not sure what to do," or "lack of discipline") they only practice yoga in class. Yet many are eager for suggestions on how to expand their practice. Yoga Sparks are simple, effective tools to help initiate or deepen a home yoga practice and take the benefits off the mat and into daily life.

In my own experience, I've found that interweaving micropractices into my day can be transformative, turning ordinary activities into sacred rituals and bringing awareness to the precious gifts of body and breath. In this book I share many of the Yoga Sparks I practice regularly, such as taking a mindful breath before answering the phone, standing in Mountain Pose while cooking dinner, and being careful to park inside the lines. In addition, I'm honored to share some practices taught by great teachers, including Zen master Thich Nhat Hanh, Nobel laureate Mother Teresa, psychotherapist and yoga expert Stephen Cope, and His Holiness the Dalai Lama.

The notion of integrating yoga into daily life wasn't part of my early experience with yoga, nor was recognition that attitudes like contentment and behaviors like sharing can be yoga practices. Like many people, I thought yoga was a form of exercise and started taking a weekly yoga class largely for the physical benefits. I was in my early twenties, working as a reporter for the *Washington Post* and running several miles every morning. Yoga helped bring flexibility to my tight runner's legs and offered profound relief from the chronic neck pain I'd developed writing newspaper articles on deadline. (I describe how to use the tools of yoga to relieve this common problem in my book *Healing Yoga for Neck and Shoulder Pain*.)

Over time, however, I began to realize that yoga offered much more than stress reduction and physical flexibility. I discovered that yoga was a journey of self-discovery and found that the lessons I'd learned while tackling challenging postures on the yoga mat helped me navigate more skillfully through challenging situations at work and at home. In addition to relieving my neck pain and stretching my hamstrings, yoga helped me become happier, healthier, and better able to welcome whatever arose in my life.

As my physical body has changed with age—through two pregnancies in my early thirties, earning a second-degree black belt in karate in my forties, and facing some health crises in my fifties—my practice has changed as well. A serious bout of hyponatremia, brought on by drinking too much water during a marathon in Jamaica in 2003, landed me in a four-day coma and gave me a new appreciation for the deeper practices of yoga. Waking up in the neurointensive care unit at Duke University Medical Center, with no idea how I'd gotten there, was a humbling experience. I couldn't do the vigorous postures of my typical yoga practice. But I could do breathing practices, meditation, relaxation, and simple movements, and

I found this profoundly healing. My near-death experience taught me something I'd known intellectually yet never truly understood: yoga's true power lies in its ability to harness the mind for healing and spiritual development.

Then, in 2008, I had open-heart surgery to replace a congenitally abnormal heart valve and repair a resulting aneurysm in my aorta. My yoga practice proved extremely powerful in preparing for and recovering from my surgery, and I adapted it to fit my needs. Some days it was dynamic and energizing, other days calming and restorative. I discovered that I could even practice yoga in the intensive care unit—although the only posture I could do was Savasana, the Corpse Pose: lying still and surrendering completely. Meditation, prayer, listening to chanting on my iPod, and visualizing a positive outcome were all useful yoga practices that helped me through this difficult experience and restored me to full health.

I've also been privileged to create yoga practices for other people facing a broad array of health challenges, from cancer and chronic pain to heart failure, osteoporosis, post-traumatic stress disorder, and blindness. This work has inspired a deep respect for individual differences and helped me discover safe and effective ways to guide people in cultivating self-awareness and using yoga's versatile tools to relieve physical and emotional suffering.

Yoga 101

Yoga is a powerful form of mind-body medicine that approaches health in a holistic manner, recognizing that physical ailments also have emotional and spiritual components. At its heart, yoga is a comprehensive system for self-development and transformation.

In Western cultures, however, the word "yoga" is often used to mean "posture," and progress is mistakenly measured by the ability to perform complex poses. This just shows that people misunderstand the purpose of yoga, a view renowned Indian yoga master T. K. V. Desikachar shared with me in 2006, when I had the opportunity to interview him for a *Yoga Journal* article about the healing power of meditation. He explained, "Yoga is definitely not just posture. A lot of people are doing postures, but are they happy? They can do a beautiful posture, but their life is a big headache." Mastery of yoga is really measured, he said, by "how it influences our day-to-day living, how it enhances our relationships, how it promotes clarity and peace of mind" (Krucoff 2007, 111).

Despite, or perhaps because of, yoga's booming popularity, misconceptions abound about this ancient practice, which originated more than five thousand years ago in India. The word "yoga" comes from the Sanskrit word *yuj*, which means to "yoke" or "unite," and the practice is designed to unify many things. At the most basic level, yoga helps unite body and mind. At a deeper level, yoga unites the individual with the universal.

When people in the West say "yoga," they're commonly referring to *hatha yoga*, one branch of this ancient discipline that focuses on physical postures, breathing practices, and meditation. There are six other main branches of yoga, all seeking the same goal— enlightenment—but through different routes. For example, *karma yoga*, the yoga of action, focuses on doing good works unselfishly, without attachment, and *jnana yoga*, the yoga of wisdom, centers on using the mind to reach higher states of consciousness.

Hatha yoga, the yoga of physical discipline, considers the body a precious vessel that must be healthy and strong enough to support its essential nature, which is a state of unchanging awareness—what some might term an undying spirit or soul. Virtually all Western yoga classes—and all of the practices in this book—are based on hatha yoga.

Hatha yoga was designed to enhance health because the ancient yogis considered disease to be an obstacle on the path to enlightenment. After all, it's difficult to sit still in meditation and unite with the divine if you have a pounding headache or a sore back. Likewise, if illness or sedentary habits have left you too weak and inflexible to sit comfortably, yoga postures and breathing practices can help you become healthy and strong enough to sit quietly and meditate. Yoga helps you de-stress and nourish the vehicle of your body, like taking your car to the garage for a tune-up or currying your horse after a vigorous ride. You learn how to relax and release tension, strengthen weak muscles, and stretch tight ones. Yoga helps balance and integrate mind, body, and spirit to enhance energy flow and stimulate your body's own natural healing processes. The practice provides an opportunity for all aspects of your being to come into compassionate and friendly connection—to realign, refresh, and unite.

In recent years, an increasing number of scientific studies have been conducted to measure yoga's effectiveness as a treatment for various ailments. A growing body of research suggests that yoga offers a wide range of health benefits, including improving blood pressure, relieving pain, enhancing sleep, and boosting mood (Wang 2009). These days when I ask new students why they've come to yoga, more and more of them tell me that it's just what their doctor ordered. In fact, nearly fourteen million Americans say their doctor or therapist has recommended yoga to them, according to a 2008 study on yoga in America. Almost half of current practitioners took up yoga to improve their overall health, the study found, and 4.1 percent of nonpractitioners—about 9.4 million people—said they will definitely try yoga within the next year (Macy 2008).

Yoga is powerful medicine, and it is most potent when taken regularly, over time. Igniting Yoga Sparks throughout your day will help you find the healthy alignment of your body, the peaceful potential of your mind, and the joyous nature of your spirit. Breath by breath, moment by moment, you can move with compassion and diligence in the direction of health.

How Yoga Works

Yoga is based on a holistic approach to health that takes into account much more than just our physical bodies. It also embraces the subtle energies of our lives that can have profound impact on our well-being. A central tenet is the concept of prana, an intangible vital energy or life force that animates all human beings. While there's no one word in English that encompasses this concept, it's known as *chi* in traditional Chinese medicine (as in tai chi). Traditional Indian medicine, called ayurveda and considered a sister science to yoga, maintains that the proper flow of prana is essential to health and that disease is related to a blockage or other problem with the movement of this vital energy. Yoga practices are designed to enhance the healthy flow of prana throughout all the pathways of the body and mind. Similar to traditional Chinese medicine's concept of meridians, these subtle energy channels are called *nadis*, and there are said to be about seventy-two thousand in each person. Like water through a hose, energy flows through these nadis to sustain life. But just as a kink in a hose will block the steady flow of water, blockage in a nadi—for example, from physical or emotional tension—is said to impede the flow of prana, which can lead to pain and disease.

Yogic teachings view human beings as comprised of multilayered gross and subtle bodies—called *koshas*, or sheaths—and consider body and mind different but interrelated expressions of energy. This perspective recognizes that virtually everything in our lives, including our thoughts, behaviors, and relationships, can impact our health. That's why yoga's tool kit for cultivating a smooth flow of vital energy throughout the entire system includes physical postures, breathing practices, mental focus, and moral disciplines—represented in this book as four different types of Yoga Sparks.

Posture Sparks

A famous line from James Joyce's classic collection of stories entitled *Dubliners* describes Mr. Duffy, a man who "lived at a little distance from his body" (2006, 86). Like the fictional Mr. Duffy, many of us in our hurried, worried culture are often not really present in our bodies. Living in our heads, we seldom pay attention to what's going on below the neck until there's a major breakdown. Sometimes mind and body are at odds—even at war—as we complain of betrayal by a "bad" back or "bum" knee.

Posture Sparks are designed to help you reconnect your mind and body, find proper physical alignment, and enhance your health. Some focus on helping you stretch and strengthen your muscles, others help release tension and relieve pain, and a few cultivate qualities such as better balance and improved physical function. They all encourage you to befriend your body and treat it with compassion and respect.

Breathing Sparks

Breathing is the only physiologic function that you can do either consciously or unconsciously, as it's controlled by two different sets of nerves and muscles: voluntary and involuntary. You don't need to think about breathing; your body will breathe automatically. But you can also take control of your breath, which provides a unique doorway into the autonomic nervous system—the control center that revs you up for fight or flight when you perceive danger and calms you down to "rest and digest" when the emergency is over.

As a link between the conscious and unconscious mind, breathing practices can help change our physiology and our emotional state. For example, deep abdominal breathing can slow the heart rate, lower blood pressure, ease anxiety, and relieve stress. Yoga master B. K. S. Iyengar explains the relationship this way in his classic guide *Light on Yoga*: "Regulate the breathing, and thereby control the mind" (1979, 21).

This connection between the breath and the spirit is apparent in the Sanskrit language, which uses the same word, *prana*, to mean "breath" and "vital energy" or "life force." Other ancient languages also have one word that means both breath and spirit: the Latin *spiritus*, the Hebrew *ruach*, and the Greek *pneuma*. English gives a brief nod to this concept in the word "respiration." Breathing Sparks can help you cultivate this connection, inviting the breath to nourish your spirit and become a powerful tool to enhance your health.

Meditation Sparks

Yoga postures and breathing practices are traditionally considered a warm-up for the higher practice of meditation. Moving the body and breathing can help prepare you to sit or lie still and focus the mind, which is at the heart of meditation practice.

Despite the common misperception that meditation requires *emptying* the mind, meditation actually involves *filling* the mind with an object of focus, such as a candle flame, picture, deity, sound, or virtually anything. Typically, the object of meditation is something positive, appealing, and healing, because whatever happens in the mind happens in the entire system. For example, if you're anxious, your body is likely to be on high alert, with a racing heart and tense muscles, even if you're safe in your own bed.

Meditation helps harness the mind-body connection, transforming mental and physical agitation into peacefulness. A growing body of research suggests that meditation may help relieve varied medical conditions, particularly those exacerbated by stress, including allergies, anxiety disorders, asthma, cancer, depression, heart disease, hypertension, pain, sleep problems, and substance abuse (Mayo Clinic Staff 2011).

Principle Sparks

In the West, arguably the least well-known of yoga's tools are the yogic principles for ethical and moral conduct. They are part of the Eightfold Path designed to lead to enlightenment outlined in the classic text on yoga, the Yoga Sutras of Patanjali. Sometimes called the Ten Commandments of Yoga, these principles align with the ethical precepts of the world's great religions. They include five guidelines for moral conduct with others, called *yamas*, and five guidelines for self-restraint or personal discipline, called *niyamas*. Practicing these ethical behaviors can improve our relationship with ourselves and with others. In fact, scientific evidence suggests that stronger relationships support health and that loneliness is a risk factor for morbidity and mortality (Luo et al. 2012).

The five yamas governing social responsibilities and relationships are as follows:

1. *Ahimsa*, or nonharming. This refers to refraining from physical violence and also to avoiding emotional violence through unkind words, criticism, and judgment.

2. *Satya*, or truthfulness. We are encouraged to be honest with ourselves and others and to speak our truth in a loving way when appropriate.

3. *Asteya*, or nonstealing. In addition to not taking or coveting someone else's possessions, the notion of nonstealing includes not taking credit for someone else's ideas.

4. *Brahmacharya*, or sexual continence. Traditionally said to mean chastity or celibacy, today this yama is generally considered to mean keeping sexual behavior moderate and appropriate.

5. *Aparigraha*, or nonhoarding. Translated as "greedlessness" or "nonpossessiveness," this involves not taking more than we need.

The five niyamas regarding personal discipline are as follows:

1. *Saucha*, or purity. This relates both to the internal practice of keeping our minds and our hearts pure and to the external practice of good hygiene.

It also involves keeping our environment neat and clean.

2. *Santosha*, or contentment. Rather than yearning for something else, we are encouraged to be grateful for what we have.

3. *Tapas*, or austerity. The literal translation of *tapas* is "heat," and traditionally this principle included demanding practices designed to test willpower, such as fasting. Today it's often viewed as self-discipline or a burning effort to pursue our goals.

4. *Svadhyaya*, or study. This refers both to study of sacred texts and to self-study, which is a vehicle for self-understanding and, ultimately, transformation.

5. *Ishvara-pranidhana*, or surrender to the divine. This practice encourages us to let go of our ego's attachment to the outcome of our actions and to dedicate our efforts to something greater than ourselves.

In addition to these ten main precepts, other key values from the yoga tradition, such as *kshama* (patience or forbearance) and *daya* (compassion or sympathy), are also highlighted as Principle Sparks.

It's important to recognize that, while yoga is a spiritual practice, it's not a religion. You don't need to believe in any specific deity or even to believe in God at all to practice yoga. People of all faiths, as well as agnostics and atheists, practice yoga regularly. It's also fine to embrace the aspects of the practice that appeal to you and ignore the rest. Feel free to modify any aspect of the practice to suit your needs, interests, and beliefs.

How to Practice

Yoga teaches that it's not just *what* you do, but also *how* you do it that matters. In contrast to the Western approach, which encourages striving and pushing ourselves to do more, yoga invites us to find an appropriate balance—to challenge ourselves but avoid strain. Indeed, the very name of the practice, hatha yoga, reflects this focus on balance, being rooted in two Sanskrit words that describe opposing energies: *ha* for sun and *tha* for moon. In the words of my mentor, the late Esther Myers, "Hatha yoga is a balance and integration of opposites: positive and negative, active and passive, left and right" (1997, 15).

That's why it's important when practicing yoga—and the Yoga Sparks in this book—to be mindful of balancing these contrasting qualities:

- Effort and surrender
- Courage and caution
- Doing and undoing

Although yoga practice is about learning to find your own personal balance between these opposites in each pose, it can also be helpful to recognize and balance your own natural tendencies. For example, if you generally have an assertive personality, be particularly mindful to cultivate the quality of surrender in your practice. If you're naturally laid-back, be sure to energize and activate your practice.

When practicing yoga postures, apply the ethical principles (yamas and niyamas) in your approach to each pose, including nonviolence, honesty, and self-study. Noncompetitiveness and self-acceptance are essential parts of the practice, so please keep the following points in mind:

Start where you are. Don't be concerned with where you think you *should* be in a pose or where anyone else is. Be where you are and breathe. This means letting go of ambition. Striving to "achieve" a particular pose is inadvisable and may lead to injury.

Be patient. Yoga practice isn't about getting somewhere. It's about being where you are, right now, fully and completely. Yoga is not a race or a test. It is a moment-by-moment practice of awareness. Take your time, do your best, and enjoy your breath.

Focus on being steady and comfortable. The Yoga Sutras say that a yoga posture should be "steady and comfortable"—or according to some translations, "stable and sweet," "firm but happy," or "alert and relaxed." If you're gasping and shaking in your posture, you're doing gymnastics or calisthenics, not practicing yoga. But just because a pose is steady and comfortable doesn't mean that it should be so easy that you derive no benefit. In other words, don't be lazy, but don't be pushy either.

Many yogis call this place of optimal yoga practice "the edge." Yoga practice teaches us to approach our edge in each pose while keeping focused and centered, with the breath steady throughout. If you can't keep breathing evenly in a posture, it's probably a signal that you're straining and may need to back off to a simpler version of the pose, modify with props, or take a rest.

Have fun. Approach your practice as a welcome play break or recess and have gratitude for what you *can* do. Rather than agonizing over what's wrong, pay attention to what's right. Instead of working at a posture, play with it.

Yoga encourages cultivating an attitude of honesty, openness, curiosity, and compassion. This can teach you a great deal about your strengths and weaknesses and help you find a healthy balance in your life.

How to Use this Book

The practices in this book are organized by setting, or where you might typically practice each Yoga Spark: at home, at work, on the go (in a car, plane, boat, subway, and so on), with others, or anywhere. Consider beginning with the Anywhere Practices of chapter 1, which teach the basic skills of healthy alignment and breathing. In particular, Mountain Pose (Yoga Spark 2), Seated Mountain Pose (Yoga Spark 3), and Relaxed Abdominal Breath (Yoga Spark 10) offer a foundation for many of the other practices. Once you're familiar with these practices, feel free to flip through the book and play with the Yoga Sparks that seem most relevant to you. Over time, consider adding a few more so that eventually you try them all. Then, make those that are most rewarding to you a regular part of your life.

Why 108 Yoga Sparks

The number 108 is considered auspicious by many traditions. Buddhist and Hindu *malas*, or prayer beads—used for keeping count while reciting mantras or prayers—typically have 108 beads. Hebrew letters have numerical values, and the word *chai*, which means "life," has a value of 18. As a result, 18 and its multiples, including 108 (18 x 6), are considered good luck. It's a Jewish custom to donate money in multiples of chai to signify a gift of life.

Mathematically, if you multiply 1 to the first power (1) times 2 to the second power (4) times 3 to the third power (27), the result is 108 (1 x 4 x 27 = 108). In addition, 108 is a *harshad* number, which means it's a positive integer divisible by the sum of its digits. The word *harshad* comes from the Sanskrit and means "bringer of joy."

Astrology identifies 12 zodiac signs and 9 planets, and 9 x 12 equals 108. The diameter of the sun (1,390,000 km) divided by the diameter of the earth (12,756 km) equals approximately 108.

The individual numbers in 108 also have special significance: the numeral 1 represents "one thing," the numeral 0 represents "nothing," and the numeral 8 represents "everything" or "infinity."

Inner Wisdom

The guidelines in this introduction are just that: suggestions for your practice. Each person is unique, and the best teacher for you is your own inner wisdom. So please listen to the messages from your body, mind, and spirit and trust this inner teacher. The key is to quiet down enough—physically, mentally, and emotionally—to hear the still, small voice of your heart.

The ability to access this inner knowing is one of the most important teachings of yoga. Awareness is at the heart of this practice, and the Yoga Sparks in this book are designed to help you pay attention and move mindfully through your life.

• 1 •

ANYWHERE
PRACTICES

As a practice of awareness that connects you with your innermost self, yoga can be done at any time, in any place. Yoga's primary tool, the breath, is always right under your nose. Wherever you are—a classroom or an athletic field, a mansion or a prison cell, outer space or intensive care—yoga is available. If you're alive and conscious, you can practice yoga.

Of course, not all practices are suitable for all occasions. If you're a brain surgeon in the middle of a procedure, balancing on one leg in Tree Pose is probably inadvisable. However, taking a relaxed, abdominal breath might be quite useful, as could softening tension in your face or speaking kindly to an associate.

The Yoga Sparks in this chapter are portable, versatile practices in basic skills—of posture, breath, meditation, and principles—that can be done in virtually any location. No matter where you are, they offer a brief, precious opportunity to pause, pay attention, and come into the present moment while aligning your body, easing your breath, and nurturing your spirit.

POSTURE SPARKS

1. Freeze, Ground, Breath, Spine

Freeze: Stay exactly as you are and don't move. Notice your posture, with a particular focus on the following:

- Where is your head in relation to your shoulders? Is it forward or balanced over your shoulder girdle?

- What shape is your spine? Is it slumped or elongated? Does it have its natural curves?

- What's happening with your jaw, shoulders, hands, face, and feet? Are they tense or relaxed?

This quick freeze practice can help you become aware of your posture and shine a light on unhealthy habits, and then the following focus on ground, breath, and spine can help you find proper alignment. My mentor, Esther Myers, based her approach to yoga on this simple, elegant technique.

Ground: Bring your awareness to the support underneath you. If you're standing, place both feet firmly on the ground, hip-width apart. If you're sitting, root yourself through your sit bones, located at the base of your pelvis, and place your feet on the floor or a footstool. Establish a secure and stable foundation.

Breath: Bring your awareness to your breath. With each exhalation, allow your body to release its weight into the support beneath you. With each inhalation, fill your body with breath, inviting a sense of receptivity and growth. Balance the grounding of the exhalation with the expansion of the inhalation.

Spine: Bring your awareness to your spine. As you inhale, lengthen your spine so the top of your head extends toward the sky. As you exhale, keep this sense of length as you release down into your support.

Stay here for a few breaths, feeling a wavelike release radiating from the center of your body.

2. Mountain Pose

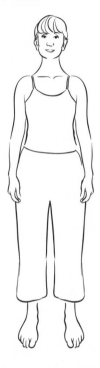

The most basic standing posture, Mountain Pose teaches us, literally, how to stand on our own two feet. Many common aches and pains, including back and neck pain, are often linked to poor posture. Practicing the healthy alignment of Mountain Pose can offer profound relief.

Anytime you're standing, whether waiting in line, cooking dinner, riding an elevator, or chatting at a party, take a minute to come into Mountain Pose:

1. Place your feet hip-width apart and distribute your weight evenly on both legs.

2. Feel the ground under your feet. From that place of rootedness, activate your leg muscles and lengthen upward through your spine.

3. Extend the top of your head (called the crown) up toward the sky. Don't lift your chin; keep it parallel to the ground.

4. Relax your shoulders down away from your ears and release any tension in your face and throat.

5. Stack your joints, so that if someone were looking at you from the side, your ear would be over your shoulder, your shoulder would be over your hip, your hip would be over your knee, and your knee would be over your ankle.

6. Imagine a light shining out from your breastbone (sternum) or heart center and direct it forward, not down at the ground.

7. Take a few full, easy breaths, filling and emptying your lungs, so that the entire circumference of your rib cage expands on each inhalation and relaxes back on the exhalation.

Variation 1: Standing in Mountain Pose, inhale as you extend your arms up, then exhale as you bring them down. Repeat three to five times, synchronizing your movement with your breath.

Variation 2: Standing in Mountain Pose, inhale as you extend your arms up and clasp your hands overhead. If it's comfortable, exhale as you rotate your wrists to turn your palms up toward the sky. If this isn't comfortable, keep your palms facing your head. From here, inhale and lengthen upward, then exhale as you bend to the left side, keeping length in both sides of your waist—avoid crunching to one side. Inhale and return to center, then exhale as you bend to the right side in a similar manner. Repeat three to five times, synchronizing your movement with your breath.

3. Seated Mountain Pose

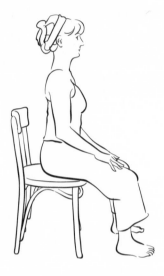

In our sedentary culture, people typically spend most of the day sitting down. Poor postural habits, such as sitting on the sacrum and rounding the spine, can lead to back and neck pain and headaches and can also contribute to respiratory, circulatory, and digestive problems. Take a minute to find good alignment in Seated Mountain Pose:

1.   Find your sit bones, the two hard knobs at the base of your pelvis. (The anatomical term is ischial tuberosities.) You may need to shamelessly reach your hands under your bottom to feel for these knobs, then gently move the flesh of your buttocks aside so you can feel your sit bones

releasing down onto surface on which you're sitting.

2. Rest your hands in your lap or on your thighs.

3. Place the soles of your feet on the floor or, if they don't comfortably reach the floor, on a footstool or folded towel. Take a moment to get grounded: root down through your sit bones and feel the soles of your feet connect with the support underneath them.

4. From this place of grounding, extend the top of your head up toward the sky, creating length in your spine. As with Mountain Pose (Yoga Spark 2), be sure to keep your chin parallel to the floor—avoid tilting it up or tucking it in.

5. Relax your shoulders down away from your ears and release any tension in your face, jaw, and throat.

6. Stack your joints, so that if someone were looking at you from the side they'd see your ear over your shoulder and your shoulder over your hip.

7. Imagine a light shining out from your breastbone (sternum) or heart center and direct it forward, not down at the ground.

8. If your chair doesn't support this good posture, consider placing a support (such as a rolled towel) at your lower back in the area of your lumbar spine.

4. Tree Pose

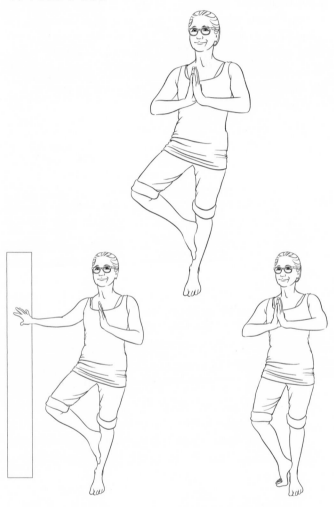

Balance poses teach some of yoga's most important lessons: getting grounded, finding your center, staying focused, maintaining concentration, and steadying the mind. The process of learning to balance, with its inevitable falling and trying again, cultivates patience, persistence, humility, and good humor. These qualities help us do more than stay balanced in the posture; they help us stay balanced in life.

1. Come to Mountain Pose (Yoga Spark 2). Lightly touch a countertop, wall, or chair back for support if you like.

2. Find a fixed spot at eye level to focus your gaze. Anchoring your gaze on a specific focal point, known as a *drishti*, can help stabilize your balance.

3. Send imaginary roots down into the earth from your right foot and pick up your left heel. Bend your left knee and slide the sole of your left foot against your right ankle, keeping the ball of your left foot on the ground. Bring your palms together at your heart center or extend your arms up to the sky, keeping your shoulders relaxed and down.

4. Balance here for a few breaths. Or, to increase the challenge, place the sole of your left foot against the inside of your right leg anywhere but at the knee, then balance for several slow, easy breaths. Feel free to lightly touch your hand to a support if that's useful.

5. Repeat on the other side.

5. Shoulder Shrugs

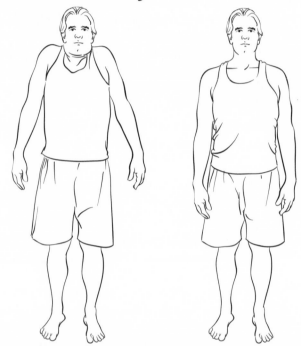

Many of us carry the weight of the world on our shoulders, and this is apparent in tension held in the neck, shoulders, and upper back. If you carry stress in these areas, play with this practice throughout your day:

1. Come into Mountain Pose or Seated Mountain Pose (Yoga Spark 2 or 3) and tune in to your breath.

2. On an inhalation, lift your shoulders up toward your ears.

3. As you exhale, drop them down.

4. Repeat three to five times, synchronizing your movement with your breath. Keep your arms as relaxed as possible so they simply go along for the ride.

Variation 1: On each exhalation, say "haaa," visualizing this action expelling tension from your body and mind.

Variation 2: Circle your shoulders in one direction for a few breaths, then switch directions.

Variation 3: Bicycle your shoulders—one shoulder circling forward and the other shoulder circling back—then switch directions.

6. Gentle Twist

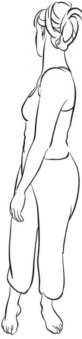

An often-recited yogic teaching says, "You are as young as your spine." This gentle twist will help keep your spine supple. Be sure to lengthen your spine before you twist. Keep the quality of movement smooth and easy—avoid forcing or pushing.

1. Stand tall in Mountain Pose (Yoga Spark 2) and tune in to your breath.

2. Turn your body gently to the right so that, if possible, you can see behind you over your right

shoulder. Breathe comfortably and keep your arms relaxed as you turn, so they hang like empty sleeves or soft noodles.

3. Come back to the starting position, then turn your body gently to the left in the same way.

4. Continue gently turning to each side for six to ten slow, easy breaths.

7. Lips Together, Teeth Apart

Clenching or grinding your teeth, a common habit known as bruxism, can be painful and result in permanent tooth damage. While experts don't agree on the cause, stress is thought to be a contributing factor. As a practice of awareness, yoga can be useful in relieving this problem by bringing attention to this often-unconscious pattern and inviting relaxation in the affected area.

1. Bring your attention to your mouth and notice how you're holding your jaw, teeth, lips, and tongue. Are your teeth clenched? Is your tongue pressed to the roof of your mouth? Are your shoulders up by your ears?

2. Take an easy, full breath and relax your shoulders down away from your ears. Soften the muscles of your face.

3. Lightly close your mouth and let your lower jaw gently relax downward, creating space between your upper and lower teeth.

4. Relax your tongue and soften the inside of your mouth.

5. Close your eyes if you like or leave them open, then take a few easy breaths. On each inhalation, mentally tell yourself, "Lips together," and notice that your lips are together. As you exhale, tell yourself, "Teeth apart," and notice that your teeth are apart.

8. Lion's Face

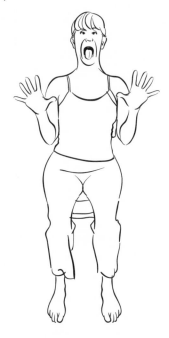

Our facial muscles get quite a workout from smiling, frowning, talking, and going through various other contortions throughout the day. In addition, many of us develop habitual patterns of expression that we may not even be aware of, such as furrowing the eyebrows or pursing the lips when concentrating. Lion's Face helps stretch and release facial muscles. It's also a breathing practice and has the added benefit of strengthening an important abdominal muscle.

1. Take a deep, full breath in through your nose.

2. As you begin to exhale, open your mouth and eyes as wide as you comfortably can, stick your tongue out as far as possible, and spread your fingers widely, palms facing away. Make a "haaa" sound with your exhalation and draw your belly in toward your spine. When you've exhaled completely, relax and take a few easy breaths.

3. Repeat three to five times.

Variation 1: On each exhalation, extend your tongue out in a different direction—up toward your nose, down toward your chin, as far to the right as possible, and as far to the left as possible.

Variation 2: Instead of making a "haaa" sound on exhalation, roar loudly. (Be sure you've notified anyone within hearing range that you're okay before you do this.)

9. Relaxation

This brief adaptation of Savasana, or Corpse Pose, may seem pretty simple since it involves being still and doing nothing. But it's actually among the most difficult poses to master because it requires totally letting go of all physical tension, quieting the mind, and surrendering completely to the earth.

1. Lie down or sit comfortably, with your body completely supported by your bed or the floor if you're lying down or by the chair if you're sitting.

2. Close your eyes and take a full, easy breath, then let it go with a sigh.

3. Bring your awareness to the back of your body—every place that's touching the floor or your chair—and feel the connection with the support holding you up. Recognize that, in this position, there's very little you need to do.

4. As you exhale, allow your body weight to drop into the support beneath you, so that with each exhalation your body becomes heavier and more relaxed.

5. With each inhalation, fill your body with breath, and with each exhalation, relax, release, and let go.

BREATHING SPARKS

10. Relaxed Abdominal Breath

Many people in Western cultures tend to breathe shallowly, using only the middle and upper portions of the lungs, a habit known as chest breathing. Trying to look thin by sucking in the gut and puffing out the chest is sometimes responsible. In addition, stress often contributes, since it causes muscles to tense and respiration rate to increase. This can result in a vicious cycle: We breathe shallowly because we're under stress, which makes the body feel as if it's not getting enough air. This, in turn, can cause more stress, prompting faster, shallower breathing.

In contrast, breathing by relaxing the abdomen – which is more elastic than the bony rib cage – helps you slow and deepen the breath. This, in turn, triggers a cascade of calming changes in the body and mind. That's why relaxed abdominal breathing, sometimes called belly breathing, is one of nature's best antistress medicines.

1. Lie down if possible, or sit tall. If you're lying down, feel free to bend your knees or put a rolled towel under your knees if that's more comfortable.

2. Breathe in and out through your nose and take a moment to notice the sensations of your breath coming into and leaving your body.

3. Place your palms on your lower belly, resting them comfortably below your navel. Relax your abdomen.

4. When you're ready, inhale and notice how your belly rounds and your hands gently rise. Observe how your navel moves away from your spine.

5. As you exhale, notice how your belly releases inward and your hands gently fall. Observe how your navel moves toward your spine.

6. Continue for a few more slow, full breaths, watching this gentle rise and fall. Avoid pushing your belly out or straining. Be patient and relaxed. Your body knows how to do this.

It's fine to breathe through your mouth if you must, but because the nose has little hairs that warm and filter the air, nose breathing is preferable. As yogis often say, "The nose is for breathing; the mouth is for eating."

11. Three-Part Breath

Sometimes called the Complete Yoga Breath or Dirga Pranayama (*dirga* means "slow and deep"), Three-Part Breath involves focusing attention on movement of the diaphragm, rib cage, and upper chest. This practice builds on Relaxed Abdominal Breath (Yoga Spark 10), so please familiarize yourself with that practice first. Start with Relaxed Abdominal Breath for a few cycles of breath, then add these steps:

1. Slide your hands up to your ribs, resting your right palm on the right side of your rib cage and the left palm on the left side of your rib cage. Continue breathing slowly and deeply, so your belly rounds as you inhale, and now feel how your rib cage expands out to the sides—left and right—under your hands as you inhale and relaxes as you exhale. Continue for a few breaths, observing how your rib cage expands like an accordion on inhalation and releases back on exhalation.

2. Move your hands to your upper chest, resting your palms below your collarbones. Continue breathing slowly and deeply, so your belly rounds and your rib cage expands as you inhale. Feel the movement of air in the uppermost portion of your lungs, observing the rise and fall of your upper chest. Continue for a few breaths.

3. Leave one hand on your chest and move the other hand to your belly. Continue this slow, deep

breathing, observing how your belly rounds, your rib cage expands out to the sides, and your upper chest fills and broadens as you inhale. Then notice how everything softens down as you exhale. If you like, at the end of each exhalation gently engage your abdominal muscles so that your belly hugs in toward your spine to help press out old, used air. Then relax your belly completely on the inhalation so that it's soft and receptive as you fill up once again with fresh, new breath.

12. Even Breath

Also called Sama Vritti Pranayama or Equal Breath, Even Breath is a basic breathing practice that helps focus the mind and calm the body.

1. Lie down or sit tall and turn your attention to your breath. Close your eyes if you like to help concentrate your focus.

2. Mentally count the length of your inhalation and the length of your exhalation. For example, you may count "one, two, three, four" on your inhalation and "one, two, three, four" on your exhalation. Or you may count to two, five, or six; the number doesn't matter. Just observe and count the length of your inhalation and exhalation.

3. Without forcing or straining, try to make your inhalation and exhalation equal in length. Pick a length that's comfortable for even inhalation and exhalation. Continue for a few breaths, then let your breath return to its natural rhythm.

13. Extended Exhalation

When your exhalation is longer than your inhalation, it's a signal to your nervous system to relax—that everything is fine. Just as a natural reaction to finally sitting down after working hard is to let out a long sigh (*Ahhh…*), extending your exhalation invites the relaxation response. This practice builds on Even Breath (Yoga Spark 12), so become familiar with that practice first to help you figure out a comfortable length for your inhalation. Then add these steps:

1. Play with making your exhalation longer than your inhalation. For example, if you inhale to the count of four, try exhaling to the count of five or six.

2. Once this is easy, try to make your exhalation up to twice as long as your inhalation: If you're inhaling to the count of three, try to exhale to the count of six. If you're inhaling to the count of four, try to exhale to the count of eight. As with all yoga practice, don't strain. Longer isn't necessarily better. Just play with finding a ratio that's comfortable and relaxing for you.

MEDITATION SPARKS

14. Mindful Awareness of Breath

In our stressful, rushed culture, we're often caught up in planning or worrying about the future or ruminating about the past. As a result, we often miss out on what's going on in the only moment that's actually available to us—the present moment.

Mindfulness is an ancient practice that helps us learn to be present for our lives. As Jeffrey Brantley, MD, my colleague at Duke Integrative Medicine, explains in his excellent guide *Five Good Minutes in Your Body*, "Mindfulness is the name for the awareness that arises from paying attention on purpose, in a gentle and welcoming way, moment by moment" (Brantley and Millstein 2009, 5).

One of the most basic mindfulness practices is observing the breath. Unlike the Breathing Sparks, which involve directing the breath, Mindful Awareness of Breath invites us to simply pay attention, mindfully, to our breath without trying to change, control, or manipulate it.

1. Lie down or sit comfortably, or if necessary, you can practice while standing.

2. Turn your attention to your breath, observing the movement of the air going into and out of your body.

3. Without judging, labeling "good" or "bad," or trying to change your breath in any way, notice

the sensations associated with your breathing. Perhaps you feel the coolness of the air as it enters your nostrils and the warmth as it exits. Maybe you feel your breath more through one nostril than the other. What places and spaces in your body move with your breath? Is your breath deep and slow? Is it short and choppy? Just notice.

4. If your thoughts wander off to the past or future or otherwise drift away from your breath, notice without judgment that your mind is chattering, then bring your focus back to your breath again. You may need to do this over and over again— and that's the practice.

15. Conscious Breathing with a Smile

A central teaching of Zen master Thich Nhat Hanh is awareness of each breath. In his classic guide *Peace Is Every Step* (1991), he explains, "While we practice conscious breathing, our thinking will slow down, and we can give ourselves a real rest" (11).

To help keep the focus on the breath, he suggests mentally reciting a word or phrase with each inhalation and exhalation—even just saying "in" on the inhalation and "out" on the exhalation.

Nhat Hanh also recommends adding a smile, which he calls "mouth yoga," to relax muscles in your face. Indeed, research suggests that moving facial muscles into an expression of joy can produce feelings of happiness. Smiling "affirms our awareness and determination to live in peace and joy" (6), he writes. "Wearing a smile on your face is a sign that you are master of yourself" (10).

To incorporate conscious breathing and a smile, he suggests reciting these phrases as you inhale and exhale: "Breathing in, I calm my body. Breathing out, I smile" (10).

16. Mantra Meditation

Building on the practices Mindful Awareness of Breath and Conscious Breathing with a Smile (Yoga Sparks 14 and 15), in this meditation you add your own meaningful word or phrase, said in conjunction with the inhalation and exhalation. This helps strengthen the mind-body connection. The name for a thought or intention, expressed as a sound and used as a focus of meditation, is "mantra." One of the most well-known mantras is the syllable "om" or "aum," considered by Hindus to be a sacred sound.

Virtually any sound, word, or phrase can be used as a mantra. Consider picking something that's meaningful to you, such as an inspiring word, a line from a poem or song, or a prayer from your religious tradition. Examples might be "Peace," The Lord is my shepherd," or "I am loved."

1. Lie down or sit comfortably, or if necessary, you can practice while standing.

2. Turn your attention to your mantra and begin reciting it either silently or out loud.

3. If you like, link your recitation with your breath— reciting your mantra once on your inhalation and once on your exhalation. Or, for a variation of Extended Exhalation (Yoga Spark 13), recite it once as you inhale and twice as you exhale.

4. If other thoughts arise, notice without judgment that your mind is chattering, then return your focus to your mantra.

17. In and Out Visualization

Visualization can be a useful complement to breath-linked meditation. This practice, taught in *Yoga Journal* by Kate Holcombe, founder and president of the nonprofit Healing Yoga Foundation in San Francisco, involves breathing in an intention and letting go of obstacles as you exhale (2011, 60):

1. Sit comfortably and take a few conscious, relaxed breaths.

2. As you inhale, imagine bringing into your system whatever is most supportive for you—for example, strength or confidence.

3. As you exhale, imagine letting go of what no longer supports you—for example, fear or doubt.

4. Continue for several breaths, being sure to focus on what you're bringing in. As you exhale, imagine releasing whatever feels like an obstacle, doing so gently to avoid giving obstacles too much power.

18. Loving-Kindness

Many people equate self-love with selfishness and tend to be very hard on themselves, often feeling frustration and even self-loathing about their perceived flaws. Loving-kindness meditation, sometimes called *metta* (Pali) or *maitre* (Sanskrit) meditation, "can help you break mental habits of meanness and self-judgment," write Mary Brantley and Tesilya Hanauer in *The Gift of Loving-Kindness* (2008, 4). "Loving-kindness practice helps develop positive feelings and lets us embrace all aspects of ourselves and others unconditionally. [It] shows us how to meet our inner critic with love instead of hate" (2).

Loving-kindness meditation helps us learn the art of "inner friendliness, expressed by being kind toward ourselves and finding good in others" (7). Brantley and Hanauer suggest that you mentally recite the following loving-kindness phrases toward yourself:

May I be happy.

May I be healthy.

May I be peaceful.

May I be safe.

Repeat these phrases several times. For further practice, repeat these phrases aimed at a loved one, then a person you feel neutral about, then a difficult person, and, finally, all living things.

19. Riding the Waves

When confronted with a wave of feeling that seems overwhelming or unmanageable, psychotherapist Stephen Cope recommends this technique as a way to skillfully navigate difficult emotions. A senior Kripalu yoga teacher and author of several books, Cope teaches this five-part practice on his audio CD *Yoga for Emotional Flow* (2003):

1. **Breathe:** Relax your belly and breathe fully and deeply. Place your palms just below your navel and feel the long, slow wave of breath fill your body. Allow it to draw your awareness away from your mind and into your body. Continuing this full yogic breath, close your eyes and notice where the difficult feeling or sensation is located in your body—perhaps in your belly, throat, chest, or head. Visualize your breath moving into the center of this feeling, let the feeling drop into the wave of your breath, and let your whole body be washed by this wave.

2. **Relax:** Notice your posture. Where are you holding some kind of constriction? Adjust your body so the constrictions can be released and your breath can move freely. Scan your body and notice any areas of holding or tightness, perhaps in your face, jaw, shoulders, or belly. Consciously invite these muscles to let go.

3. **Feel:** Bring your awareness toward the feeling and explore it. Does it have a color? Is it dense, or transparent? Feel the raw energy of the feeling,

visualize it as a big wave moving through, and recognize that it would be safe to ride it. There's no need to fight the feeling or push it away; let go of any judgments you may feel about it and visualize yourself diving into the feeling.

4. **Watch:** Shift your attention so you become a witness to your own practice, keeping yourself company as you ride on this wave. Observe yourself without any judgment. If you're experiencing aversion to the feeling, that's okay; just notice that. Let this witness be your friend, coaching you to stay on this wave of feeling—helping you recognize that it's safe to ride with it and surf it.

5. **Allow:** Surrender to the wave of sensation. For a moment, can you risk letting go and not having any control at all? Visualize yourself plunging into a river and just let go, floating on the river. The river is intelligent and has wisdom, so relax your grip and let it take you to just the right place.

20. Preferred Place

Even if your body must be in an uncomfortable situation, that doesn't mean you have to be miserable. Using the power of your mind, you can invite your body to inhabit another, more pleasant environment. This has many benefits. For example, studies show that surgical patients who use mind-body therapies such as relaxation and guided imagery may require less medication, feel less pain, experience faster wound healing, and have shorter hospital stays (Astin et al. 2003).

The heart of this meditation on a preferred place is cultivating a particular mental state through visualization, a practice known as *bhavana* in yogic terms. It can be particularly useful when undergoing medical or dental treatment, but can also offer a mental vacation virtually anytime you find yourself in an unpleasant situation.

1. Close your eyes and turn your attention to your breath.

2. Visualize a special place where you feel peaceful and safe. It can be somewhere real, such as your bedroom at home; someplace imaginary, such as a tropical island; or a place from memory, such as your grandmother's kitchen.

3. Imagine the scene in exquisite sensory detail: see the colors, hear the sounds, smell the aromas, taste the flavors, and feel the tactile sensations.

4. If there is a person or animal with whom you have a loving connection, consider inviting that dear one into the space.

5. Breathe easily and comfortably as you experience this special place.

6. When you're ready, open your eyes, feeling nourished by a sense of peace and support.

PRINCIPLE SPARKS

21. Body Scan

The niyama of self-study (svadhyaya) is at the heart of yoga's teachings, since self-study leads to self-understanding, which is essential for transformation. If, like many people, you tend to live from the neck up, a quick course of self-study through a body scan can get you out of your head and into your body. This allows you to identify any places of tension, tightness, or discomfort and helps you learn to release it.

1. Sit comfortably or lie down, or if necessary, you can practice while standing.

2. With an attitude of detached curiosity, take a journey throughout your interior landscape, looking for any places of tension, tightness, pain, discomfort, or "dis-ease." Pay particular attention to areas where you tend to hold your stress, such as your neck and shoulders, lower back, or stomach.

3. If you find a tense area, try your best to describe the sensation: Is it sharp or dull, achy or sore? Is it knotty, warm, or tingly? If you feel pain, how intense is it on a scale of 1 to 10, with 1 being mild and 10 being severe? Are you experiencing discomfort in more than one place? If so, do all the places feel similar, or are some areas more painful than others? Do these painful areas

appear connected or disconnected? Avoid spiraling into worry over any sensation; just notice each and let it be.

4. Make a mental note of any discoveries. If you like, jot your observations in a notebook, along with any associations, such as where you are, what you've been doing, or what you've been thinking about.

5. Practice a few rounds of Relaxed Abdominal Breath (Yoga Spark 10). Imagine your breath moving through the uncomfortable areas and helping them soften and release.

22. Awareness

From sound waves to brain waves, ocean waves, and heartbeats, "everything in the universe vibrates in wave-like patterns," write Jim and Kimberly Carson, creators of the innovative Yoga of Awareness program. "Yoga is the art of learning how to ride all the varied waves of life skillfully," they note, "finding our balance and keeping our poise amidst the tumult of life's ever-changing challenges" (Carson and Carson 2012).

Central to our ability to surf these waves is developing greater awareness, according to Jim Carson, PhD, a clinical psychologist and former yogic monk, and Kimberly Carson, a health educator and yoga therapist. Their eight-week Yoga of Awareness course is designed to teach people how to become more aware in daily life and use this awareness to deal with a specific challenge, such as cancer or low back pain. In a recent study of Yoga of Awareness for fibromyalgia, more than half of the participants in the weekly, two-hour yoga class experienced 30 percent reductions in symptoms such as pain, fatigue, and stiffness (Carson et al. 2010).

The Carsons recommend the following approach to practicing awareness:

- Watch yourself in daily life with alert interest.

- Notice bodily sensations, thoughts, feelings, and actions.

- Observe all this with the intention to *understand* rather than to judge.

23. Self-Talk

Yoga's first principle, ahimsa, or nonviolence, applies to more than just physical violence; it also relates to the emotional violence of name-calling, insults, and other forms of hateful speech. It's surprisingly common for people to commit this kind of violence against themselves. When we label our body parts as "bad" or "stupid" (for example, "my bad back" or "these stupid thighs"), we're engaged in a form of self-violence that can negatively impact our health. This applies to our inner dialogue—the way we think and feel about our bodies—as well as to how we describe our bodies to others.

If there's a body part you've been fighting with, call a truce and make peace:

1. Sit comfortably, lie down, or stand and take a few easy, full breaths.

2. Turn your attention to the embattled area and set an intention to treat it with kindness. Invite your breath to help you soften and release any physical or emotional tension you feel in that place and throughout your entire being.

3. Vow to stop the name-calling. Instead of labeling this area as somehow "bad," think of it as challenged or special.

4. Throughout your day, if you catch yourself saying unkind things to yourself, apologize and try to be more compassionate. Vow to speak to yourself as you would to a beloved friend.

24. Letting Go

In our "all-you-can-eat" consumer culture, cultivating aparigraha, or greedlessness, can be challenging. This principle, literally translated as "not grasping all around" and often referred to as "nonhoarding," involves not taking more than is necessary and getting rid of things you don't need.

On the yoga mat, this entails letting go of unnecessary tension and distracting thoughts. Off the mat, it's an opportunity to eliminate excess possessions—decluttering our closets, our pantries, and our lives. Avoiding taking more than is necessary also extends to behaviors. For example, piling huge amounts of food on your plate can be a form of greed, as can taking up two parking spaces or being too possessive of someone else's time.

This yogic notion of voluntary simplicity can help free us from being possessed by our possessions. As yoga master T. K. V. Desikachar writes in his classic book *The Heart of Yoga*, "The more we have, the more we need to take care of it. The time and energy spent on acquiring more things, protecting them, and worrying about them cannot be spent on the basic questions of life" (1995, 178).

Adopting the habit of greedlessness—of being willing to let go of possessions, expectations, or even your special spot in a yoga class—offers the opportunity to recognize that true happiness doesn't depend on things. As a bonus, getting rid of excess stuff often provides the added blessing of being able to give to others.

The opportunities for a quick Letting Go practice are endless. Here are a few suggestions:

- When purchasing food to go, take only one napkin, fork, cup, condiment pack, and so on.

- Whenever you add new clothing to your wardrobe, give something old away.

- Watch portion sizes and avoid supersizing.

- Spend sixty seconds putting excess items from a junk drawer into a giveaway bag.

- Purchase mindfully. Ask yourself if the item is something you actually need or just something you want, and if you can really afford it.

25. Acceptance: It Is What It Is

An increasingly common response, often to unpleasant circumstances, is the blunt statement "It is what it is." This phase is at the heart of the principle of acceptance: the seemingly simple, yet often quite difficult, practice of surrendering to the reality of a challenging situation.

When confronted with something unpleasant, whether it's a minor parking ticket or a major health problem, it's common for our minds to spin with resistance: *This is unfair. It must be a mistake. If I do X, Y, or Z, it will go away.* Yet all this effort we put into resistance actually increases our suffering. Instead, we can practice acceptance, surrendering to the reality of what is. However, this doesn't mean giving up. Acceptance is simply being willing to have the experience you're already having.

When we stop wishing that things were different from how they are, we avoid wasting energy on resistance and can instead focus on positive ways to deal with the situation. We can see more clearly and decide on a beneficial course of action.

A key Buddhist teaching is "Pain is inevitable, but suffering is optional." In other words, pain plus resistance equals suffering. Freeing ourselves from suffering involves releasing our resistance and accepting that it is what it is.

Whenever you find yourself resisting the reality of a situation or wishing something were different, try this practice:

1. Pause and observe your thoughts.

2. Practice a few rounds of Relaxed Abdominal Breath (Yoga Spark 10).

3. With each exhalation, release your resistance to the situation.

4. Be willing to have the experience you're already having.

26. Contentment and Gratitude

Cultural messages tend to encourage discontent: our hair isn't shiny enough, our belly isn't flat enough, our car isn't cool enough, even our teeth aren't white enough. This sense of dissatisfaction tends to spill into our everyday lives, where we often fixate on what's "wrong" and frequently look for something better or different.

The yogic principle of santosha—or contentment—invites us to view the world through a different lens, to focus on what's right and be grateful for our many blessings. It's not so much a change in reality as a change in perception. For example, if you fall out of Tree Pose, you might chastise yourself for your poor balance, decide you're not good enough, and give up. However, you could instead applaud yourself for attempting something difficult, be grateful that you have two legs, and joyfully try again.

When you recognize that gratitude is an attitude, you'll find countless opportunities for contentment practice. Here are a few to get you started:

- Mindfully notice your breathing. Take a moment to be grateful for the precious gift of breath.

- Before each meal, practice gratitude for the food you'll be eating.

- Recognize that the best way to have what you want is to want what you have. Practice gratitude for things you may take for granted, including your home and family.

- Say "thank you" whenever possible—for example, to someone who opens a door, bags your groceries, checks you in, or delivers a package.

- If you're feeling anxious or having trouble sleeping, try counting your blessings.

27. Cultivating the Opposite

When disturbing thoughts threaten to tense your body and cloud your mind, consciously substituting positive thoughts can help you find peace and calm. In modern psychology this technique of shifting your mental perspective is called cognitive reframing, and it's a popular stress-reduction practice. It's also an ancient yogic approach known as *prakti paksha bhavana*, described in Yoga Sutra 11.33: "Unwholesome thoughts can be neutralized by cultivating wholesome ones" (Hartranft 2003, 33).

Rooted in the recognition that stress is often related to your *perception* of a situation, prakti paksha bhavana helps you defuse potentially upsetting experiences by adjusting your attitude and changing your point of view. Even though the situation may stay the same, if you think about it differently, you're likely to feel better. For example, if a snowstorm causes your flight to be canceled, you could be furious at the airlines or the weather, or you could choose to enjoy the snow and be grateful that you're safe. Faced with a mountain of dirty dishes, you might feel resentful and overwhelmed, or you could decide that washing dishes is fun and appreciate having plates, utensils, hot running water, and food to eat and share with your loved ones.

Practicing prakti paksha bhavana invites you to pay close attention to your thoughts and feelings and, when a disquieting emotion arises, to cultivate an opposite, positive attitude. In other words, to change your mood, change your mind.

28. Cleanliness 1: Hand-Washing Practice

One of yoga's niyamas, or disciplines of self-control, is saucha, which means "purity." It relates both to the internal practice of keeping our hearts and minds pure and to external habits of good hygiene. The ancient proverb that places cleanliness next to godliness aligns with this yogic teaching that keeping your body, your home, and your world clean is more than just a chore; it's a sacred discipline.

On a practical level, practicing saucha through habits such as hand washing and hygienic food handling can reduce the risk of illness. In fact, the Centers for Disease Control and Prevention (CDC) says hand washing is one of the most effective ways to prevent infection and illness and recommends frequent hand washing, including before, during, and after preparing food; before eating; after using the toilet; after blowing your nose, coughing, or sneezing; after touching an animal, animal feed, or animal waste; and after touching garbage (Centers for Disease Control and Prevention 2012).

Rather than viewing hand washing as a boring task, turn it into an opportunity to cultivate saucha with this practice, adapted from the CDC's recommendations on how to wash your hands most effectively:

1. Stand tall and take an easy breath.

2. Wet your hands with clean running water and apply soap.

3. Rub your hands together to make a lather and scrub them well, including the backs of your hands, between your fingers, and under your nails.

4. Continue rubbing your hands for at least twenty seconds—the time it would take to hum the song "Happy Birthday" twice. Alternatively, you could recite a twenty-second prayer, devotional song, or mantra. Be creative—consider reciting (mentally or out loud) something that makes you smile, such as a verse from a favorite poem.

5. Rinse your hands under running water, then dry them with a clean towel.

29. Set an Intention

Our culture encourages us to set goals—for example, to lose ten pounds by swimsuit season, to achieve a certain grade point average, or to get a promotion at work. While these are noble aims, if we fail to meet our goals we're often filled with disappointment and self-blame.

Yoga offers a different, less result-oriented approach to moving in the direction of our heart's desires. Rather than striving for a specific goal, which may be beyond our control, the yoga tradition encourages us to concentrate on actions that we can commit to doing, such as taking a thirty-minute walk every day or eliminating soft drinks from our diet.

Shifting our focus from the results we want, which may be difficult or impossible to achieve, to behaviors that are within our control, is an empowering and helpful attitude adjustment. Too often, people become discouraged when they fail to meet goals and as a result give up on healthy behaviors entirely. Instead, yoga invites us to let go of the desire for a specific end result and focus our energies on living more skillfully in the present moment.

To sharpen and clarify this focus, yoga practice invites us to set an intention—a process called *sankalpa*. Holding this intention in your heart and mind helps channel your energies to move in a particular direction. Consider ways in which you'd like to move in the direction of health, whether physically, emotionally, or economically, and explore specific actions you can commit to doing that would help you on that path. Here are some examples of specific intentions:

- Stand up and stretch once an hour when you're working at your computer.

- Set aside a percentage of your paycheck to put into savings or give to charity.

- Read to your child every night before bed.

- Listen to your spouse without interrupting.

- Laugh heartily at least once a day.

Be sure to set an intention that's realistic, meaningful, and achievable. Pick a healthy behavior you can and will do and that can become a permanent part of your life. Avoid the common mistake of promising to do too much. Even small changes can have profound benefits.

· 2 ·

AROUND THE HOUSE PRACTICES

More than just a residence, your home is also a refuge. It's where you let down your hair, put up your feet, and find shelter from life's storms. In the privacy, comfort, and security of your home, your yoga practice can blossom.

This chapter is geared toward helping you bring the teachings of yoga home, literally—right into your bedroom, kitchen, living room, and even bathroom. It includes practices designed to turn housework into a moving meditation and to make brushing your teeth an opportunity to find balance. These Yoga Sparks invite simple acts, such as getting up from a chair or picking up a laundry basket, to become opportunities to strengthen your legs and back. There are breathing practices to calm your nervous system and help you sleep, and meditations that can transform everyday activities into sacred rituals. Some of the practices are designed to help you organize and declutter your surroundings so your home can better support your physical, emotional, and energetic health. Play with these practices—and perhaps be inspired to create some of your own.

POSTURE SPARKS

30. Rise and Shine

The way you start your day sets the tone for the rest of your waking hours. The common practice of jumping out of bed and rushing around is not only hard on your nervous system, it also establishes a frantic, hurried tone that adds stress to your life. Just getting out of bed can be stressful enough—particularly if it's Monday morning, the time when heart attacks are most likely to occur (Watson 2009).

Start your day right by setting your alarm to go off at least five minutes before you need to rise so you can make the important transition from horizontal to vertical in a mindful, gradual manner. If possible, choose a pleasant sound for your alarm—a favorite song or an appealing tone. If you have a "snooze" feature, use the second ring to let you know that you really must get out of bed.

When you wake—either from the alarm or on your own—invite your first conscious thought to be an expression of gratitude for the blessing of waking to a new day. Then, when you're ready, lie on your back, knees bent if you like or with your legs straight, and try this practice:

1. Rest your palms on your belly below your navel and tune in to your breath. With eyes closed, mindfully breathe fully and deeply so that your hands rise as you inhale and fall as you exhale.

2. Consider saying a prayer or setting an intention for your day, making a choice about how you

want to move through the next twelve hours. (For more on this topic, see Set an Intention, Yoga Spark 29.)

3. Open your eyes and take a few more mindful breaths as you extend your arms overhead and stretch whatever body parts need attention.

4. Roll onto your side, then use the strength of your arms to lift your torso as you lower your feet to the floor and come to a sitting position on the edge of your bed. Take a few easy breaths, then rise and greet your day with a smile.

31. Knee-to-Chest Pose

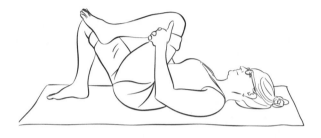

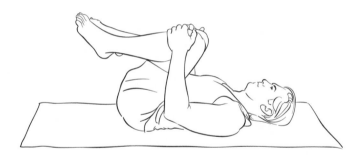

Waking up with an aching back is common in our culture, where back pain affects eight out of ten people at some point in life (National Institutes of Health 2012). Arguably the single best back stretch is this knee-hugging posture.

Try it first thing in the morning, before you get out of bed, or anytime you need to ease out your back.

1. Lie on your back with knees bent and feet about hip-width apart.

2. Take a full, easy breath in. As you exhale, hug your right knee to your chest, holding your leg behind your right thigh. (If this strains your shoulders, use a yoga strap, old necktie, or bathrobe belt to catch your leg.) Stay here for a few breaths, drawing your right thigh toward your body each time you exhale. Relax your shoulders, arms, and face, inviting your breath to help soften any tension you might feel.

3. Release and repeat with the left leg.

Variation 1: While hugging your knee to your chest, draw circles with the toes of the same foot to "wake up" your ankle.

Variation 2: Hug both knees at the same time and rock gently from side to side.

32. Apanasana: Wind-Relieving Pose

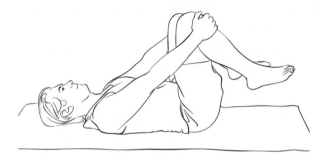

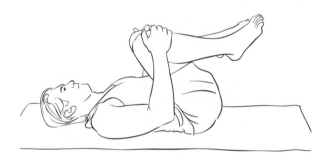

This simple posture can be profoundly helpful in both stretching out your back and relieving constipation, bloating, and other symptoms of digestive distress. In yogic teachings, *apana*, for which this posture is named, is the energy of elimination that governs expulsion of wastes.

This pose is designed to enhance the flow of apana—so don't get embarrassed if it lives up to its name in "wind relief"! (If you're pregnant, skip this pose.)

1. Lie on the floor or in bed with your knees bent and take a few easy breaths.

2. Bring your thighs in toward your torso, with your hands resting on your knees. If this is uncomfortable, hold your legs behind your thighs or use a yoga strap to catch your legs.

3. As you take a full, easy inhalation, straighten your arms and let your thighs move away from your body while continuing to lightly hold your knees.

4. As you exhale, bend your elbows and draw your thighs back toward your body, bringing them as close as comfortably possible.

5. Continue for five to ten breaths, synchronizing your movement with your breath to create a gentle pumping action.

6. If you have a round body, feel free to open your thighs wider to make the pose more comfortable.

33. Standing Salutation

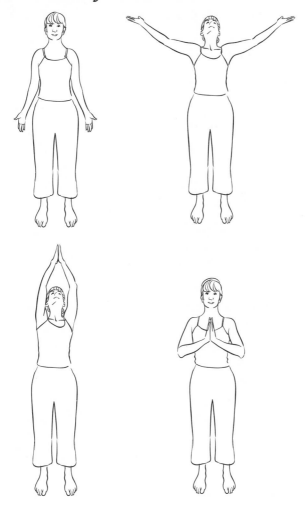

This practice is a small piece of the classic yoga sequence called the Sun Salutation, or Surya Namaskar, which moves the major muscles and joints of the body through a full range of motion. Here, the focus is on energizing the arms, shoulders, and upper body. This practice is a lovely way to start the day or to take a break if you've been sitting still.

1. Stand tall in Mountain Pose and turn your attention to your breath.

2. On an inhalation, rotate your arms from the shoulders so your palms turn out and your shoulder blades move toward each other, simultaneously extending your arms out to the sides and up overhead until your palms touch, lifting your heart toward the sky and gazing up at your thumbs. Keep your neck long; don't drop your head back.

3. As you exhale, keep your palms together and bring your hands down past your forehead and throat, resting them at your heart center—a position called Anjali Mudra.

4. Repeat five times, synchronizing your movement with your breath. On each inhalation, visualize yourself gathering in positive energy. On each exhalation, bring this energy into your heart.

34. Chair Pose

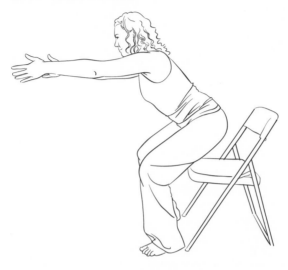

Most of us get up and down from sitting many times throughout the day. Chair Pose can turn each of these moments into an opportunity to build strength in the quadriceps, the muscles in front of the thigh. Strong quads are a key determinant for an older adult's ability to live independently, which is why they are sometimes called the "muscles of independence." In fact, the chair stand test for older adults counts how many times someone can come to standing in thirty seconds as a way to determine lower body strength and fall risk (Rikli and Jones 2001). Practicing Chair Pose can enhance strength and balance.

1. Sit toward the front of a chair with both feet planted firmly on the floor.

2. Take an easy, full breath in, then exhale as you hinge forward from your hips, keeping length in your spine (*not* rounding your back). At the same time, press your feet into the floor and use the strength of your legs to come to a standing position.

3. Standing in front of the chair, inhale as you extend your arms forward to shoulder height, bend your knees, and hinge forward from your hips—not your waist. At the same time, stick your bottom out and, keeping length in your spine (not rounding your back), lower yourself slowly and mindfully into the chair.

4. Repeat five to ten times, coming to a standing position, then slowly lowering yourself back to a sitting position. Be sure to keep the breath flowing; don't hold your breath.

Variation: For more challenge, as you return to the seated position from standing, hover with your bottom a few inches from the seat for several breaths before sitting.

35. Hip Hinge: Lift and Carry

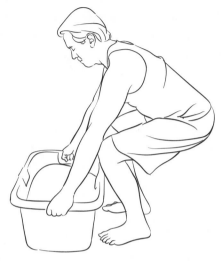

When people hurt their backs, it's often from doing something relatively minor, such as picking up the newspaper from the floor. Poor body mechanics can increase the risk of injuring your back and can also increase the risk of a vertebral fracture in those with osteoporosis. Bending forward can be a particularly problematic movement, which is why the National Osteoporosis Foundation recommends that people with impaired bone strength avoid bending forward from the waist (National Osteoporosis Foundation 2011).

Instead, hinge forward from your hips and bend your knees when you need to reach down for something low or on the floor. Remember, yoga is a practice of awareness, so whenever you're preparing to bend over and pick something up, mindfully use these healthy body mechanics:

1. Turn your body so your feet face the object. This keeps you from having to twist your spine.

2. Bend your knees and hinge forward from your hips—not your waist—sticking your bottom out and keeping length in your spine (avoid rounding your back).

3. Pick up the item and bring it in toward your body.

4. Use the strength of your legs to stand back up.

36. Puppy Pose

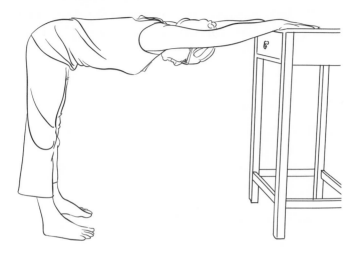

Many yoga postures are named for animals, who have a great deal to teach us about living well in our bodies—including the important lesson of stretching whenever we get up from a fixed position. This pose is a variation of the classic yoga posture Downward-Facing Dog, inspired by the canine's paws-down, tail-up stretch. Puppy Pose offers a similar stretch without requiring you to put your hands on the floor:

1. Rest your palms on a wall, countertop, or shelf, shoulder-width apart.

2. Walk your feet back and hinge forward from your hips until your arms are fully extended, your

torso is parallel to the floor, and your hips are directly over your ankles.

3. Inhale deeply, then exhale as you press your palms into the wall and draw your hips back, keeping your neck in line with your spine. Stay here for a few breaths.

Variation: To add more stretch in the lower legs, step your right foot forward and left foot back while still drawing your hips back evenly. For more intensity, lift the toes and ball of the front foot, keeping the heel on the floor. Stay here for a few breaths, then switch legs.

37. Nondominant Hand Practice

If you check the soles of an old, favorite pair of shoes, they're likely to be worn down in a way that reflects your habitual patterns of movement. Our bodies can also reflect wear patterns. After years of using your muscles in a specific way—often related to using your dominant hand—you may become asymmetrical or lopsided, which can be a setup for injury and pain. Yoga can remedy this situation, as it's designed to help balance your body so that all areas—right and left, front and back, top and bottom—have equal or appropriate strength and flexibility.

This practice is designed to help you cultivate strength and coordination on your nondominant side while also offering relief from any repetitive tension you may experience on your dominant side. Being mindful to keep good postural alignment in Mountain Pose or Seated Mountain Pose (Yoga Spark 2 or 3), use your nondominant hand to perform various tasks:

- Brushing your teeth or combing your hair

- Performing kitchen chores, such as stirring, mashing potatoes, or washing dishes

- Answering the phone or using the TV remote

- When using both hands for activities such as sweeping or raking, switch the hand that's on top.

38. Tightrope Walking

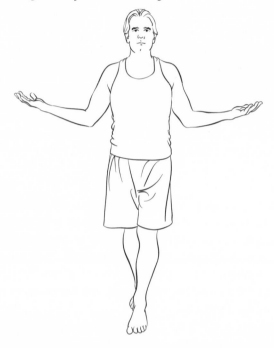

In yoga we place our bodies in challenging positions and learn how to relax and breathe through the difficult pose. Then, when life places us in challenging positions, we can draw upon this experience to relax and breathe through the difficult situation. Tightrope walking is a prime example of this principle—and also a wonderful metaphor for life—since it's about learning to keep our balance in challenging circumstances.

You might recall the astonishing high-wire performance of tightrope artist Philippe Petit, who walked between New York's Twin Towers in 1974, as you play with this pose:

1. Stand tall in Mountain Pose (Yoga Spark 2), then bring your left heel directly in front of the toes of your right foot. If this feels unsteady, widen up your stance a bit—more like walking a plank than a tightrope.

2. Gaze at a spot at eye level. Extend your arms out to your sides, bend your elbows, and turn your palms up. Alternatively, you can lightly touch a wall or countertop for support if you like.

3. Feel your weight evenly distributed on both legs, then shift your weight to your front foot and pick up your back heel. Keeping your breath flowing, take a step forward, placing your right heel in front of the toes of your left foot and redistributing your weight evenly on both legs.

4. Continue slowly and mindfully walking forward in this way for a few steps.

Variation: For more challenge, try walking backward. Stand with your weight evenly distributed on both legs, then shift your weight to your back foot and pick up the ball of your front foot. Keeping your breath flowing, take a step backward and redistribute your weight evenly on both legs. Continue slowly and mindfully walking backward in this way for a few steps.

39. Palm Tree

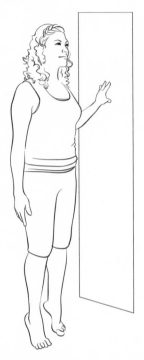

Sometimes called heel raises by physical therapists, this posture helps strengthen your ankles and calves and improve your balance. Try it in the kitchen, perhaps while waiting for water to boil, in the bathroom while brushing your teeth, or anywhere in your house while on the phone:

1. Stand tall, lightly touching a chair back, counter-top, or wall for support if you like.

2. Focus your gaze on a spot at eye level.

3. On an inhalation, slowly lift your heels up as high as they'll go.

4. On an exhalation, bring your heels back to the ground.

5. Continue for several breaths, synchronizing your movement with your breath.

6. When you're ready, stay in the heels-up position, keeping your breath flowing.

Variation: For more challenge, take one or both hands away from the support and balance on the balls of your feet.

40. Crane Pose

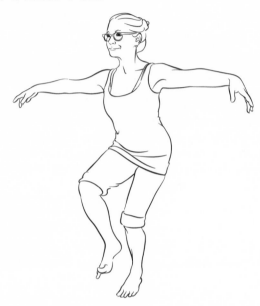

Named for the long-necked bird that mates for life and is considered a symbol of good luck and fidelity, this posture helps strengthen the legs and abdominals while enhancing balance.

1. Stand tall in Mountain Pose (Yoga Spark 2) with your palms together in front of your chest.

2. Soften your knees and engage your abdominal muscles, drawing your belly in toward your spine.

3. Inhale and lift your right knee up, slightly bending your left knee and extending your arms out to your sides.

4. Exhale and place your foot back down, returning to Mountain Pose with your palms together at your chest.

5. Repeat with the other leg.

6. Continue, alternating legs six to ten times, synchronizing your movement with your breath.

Variation: For extra challenge, stay in the balance position for several breaths.

41. Legs up the Wall or on a Chair

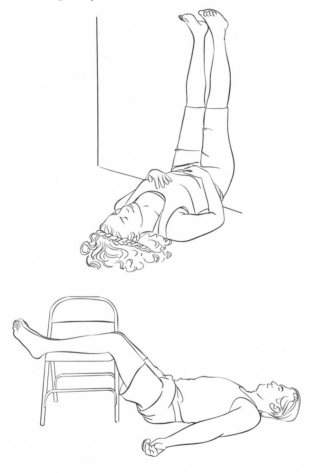

Inverted postures literally turn our world upside down, reversing the effects of gravity on our muscles, bones, and bodily fluids. Unfortunately, some well-known inverted poses, such as Headstand and Shoulder Stand, are often inadvisable for people who are overweight or have health challenges such as osteoporosis. However, this simple practice of elevating the legs on a wall or chair can provide many of the welcome "antigravity" effects without the risks for most people. (If you have a serious health condition or are unsure whether this is safe for you, please check with your health care provider.)

A variation of the posture Viparita Karani, a name that translates as "reversed doing," Legs up the Wall helps calm the nervous system and relieve fatigue of body and mind. It's particularly useful if you've been on your feet for hours—for example, working in the kitchen or the yard. Ideally, it's nice to rest in this restorative pose for ten, twenty, or even thirty minutes. But even if you have just sixty seconds, it's worth taking a load off and elevating your legs.

To practice at a wall: Sit on the floor about one hand's width away from the wall with your legs parallel to the wall. Swing your legs up on the wall as you ease your back onto the floor. Adjust the distance between your bottom and the wall so that you feel comfortable. Some people like to have their sit bones almost pressed to the wall, while others like their bottom to be six to twelve inches away.

To practice with a chair: Lie on the floor and rest your lower legs on a chair. It's fine to cushion your calves with a blanket or towel if that's more comfortable.

In either variation, adjust your arm position for comfort, relaxing them out at your sides or placing your palms on your belly or chest. If you like, place an eye pillow over your eyes. Set a timer so that you can relax completely. Turn your attention to your breath, inviting it to slow and deepen. As best you can, release any distracting thoughts and invite yourself to surrender completely into the support of the floor and wall or chair.

BREATHING SPARKS

42. Shower Om

The most basic mantra in the yoga tradition is "om," a syllable that's said to represent the sound made at creation and considered to be the fundamental sound of the universe. (For more about mantras, see Mantra Meditation, Yoga Spark 16.) Hindus revere "om" as a sacred syllable, and other religious traditions embrace similar sounds, such as the Jewish "shalom," the Islamic "salaam," and the Christian "amen." Feel free to substitute any of those in the following practice; you can even use the word "home" if you like.

Reciting these sounds creates a vibration throughout the body that can loosen tension from the inside out. This resonance is enhanced when you practice in an enclosed space, such as a shower stall. As those who love singing in the shower have discovered, the acoustics created in that small boxlike space amplify the resonance and reverb of certain tones, producing a deeper, fuller sound. Tile and glass tend to reflect the sound back and forth, boosting the intensity.

Try this practice in the privacy of your home shower, possibly with the water streaming onto your back or chest:

1. Stand tall in Mountain Pose (Yoga Spark 2), with your hands at your sides or your palms together in front of your breastbone, and take a few easy breaths.

2. Inhale deeply.

3. Begin your exhalation by making a long "oh" sound. As you continue exhaling, close your lips to hum an "mmm" sound. As you continue humming the "mmm" sound, feel the vibration in your head and neck and invite it to travel down to the base of your spine.

4. Inhale when you need to, and when you exhale again, continue playing with the sound, observing the vibrational quality throughout your body.

5. When this feels complete, stand quietly and notice the echoes of this practice.

43. Bee's Breath

Sometimes called the Humming Breath, or Bhramari in Sanskrit, this practice creates a vibration in the skull that can help release tension in the face, neck, and shoulders. It can be particularly useful during allergy season or anytime the sinuses feel blocked, and for relief from tension headaches.

1. Stand or sit tall and take a few easy breaths.

2. Inhale through your nose, then, with your mouth lightly closed, exhale and make a humming sound, letting your lips vibrate.

3. Make your exhaling hum as long as comfortably possible and focus on the sensation of vibration.

Variation: To enhance the sensation, practice with your eyes closed and your fingers gently closing your ears.

44. Alternate Nostril Breathing

According to yogic tradition, two of the body's most important energy channels, or *nadis*, are connected to the nostrils. At the right nostril is the *pingala nadi*, or sun channel, which corresponds to the energy of warming and masculinity. At the left nostril is the *ida nadi*, or moon channel, which corresponds to the energy of cooling and femininity. They are said to wind around the central channel, called the *sushumna*, in a manner similar to a caduceus, the medical symbol with two snakes coiled around a central staff.

The practice of Alternate Nostril Breathing, called Nadi Shodhana, which means "channel cleaning," helps balance the body and mind, restoring equilibrium between our right and left sides, including the right and left hemispheres of the brain. A calming and soothing technique, Nadi Shodhana is often recommended to ease anxiety and insomnia.

When you begin, use your index fingers to gently close each nostril. Once you're comfortable with the practice, try closing the nostrils with one hand. Traditionally, the right hand is held in Mrigi Mudra (Deer Face Mudra), with the index and middle fingers folded into the palm; the right thumb is used to close the right nostril, and the right pinkie and ring finger are used to close the left nostril.

1. Sit comfortably in Seated Mountain Pose (Yoga Spark 3) and take a few easy breaths.

2. Gently close your right nostril and inhale through your left nostril.

3. Gently close your left nostril, open your right nostril, and exhale through your right nostril.

4. Inhale through your right nostril.

5. Gently close your right nostril, open your left nostril, and exhale through your left nostril.

6. Continue alternating in this manner for several rounds of breath, finishing with an exhalation through your left nostril.

45. Chanting or Singing Breath

When I teach yoga breathing, the people who catch on easily are often singers or musicians who play wind instruments. Typically, they've learned how to completely fill and empty their lungs because it's essential to their craft, enabling them to achieve rich, full tones and get through long phrases or hold long notes.

Singing, chanting, or even whistling can be a wonderful form of breathing practice, since all three require taking full, deep breaths and often involve extending the exhalation for as long as possible, which can invite relaxation (see Extended Exhalation, Yoga Spark 13). If you add in the mood-brightening effect music often has (think of the song "I Whistle a Happy Tune," from *The King and I*), it's clear that singing or chanting can be a truly uplifting yogic practice. Here are a few suggestions on how you can create your own mood music:

- Whistle while you work.

- Sing a child or pet to sleep.

- Sing or chant while you do housework.

- Conclude your yoga practice with a song or chant.

MEDITATION SPARKS

46. Housework or Yard Work Meditation

The practice of mindfulness—of paying attention, on purpose, in a gentle and welcoming way—can transform virtually any activity into a meditation. (See Mindful Awareness of Breath, Yoga Spark 14.) Mindfulness invites us to be fully present in the moment, with heart and mind absorbed in the activity at hand. This can be a very different experience than the common practice of going through the motions while thinking about something else, the mind busy planning, worrying, scheduling, judging, and so on. Perhaps you've had the common experience of pulling your car into a parking space at your destination and then realizing you don't recall the details of the drive. This is just one example of how, all too often, we tend to space out in our lives.

To turn a routine chore into a meditation, set your intention on keeping your mind focused on whatever you're doing and enjoying all the sensations associated with the task. This can be applied to any activity, from cooking and cleaning to raking and weeding. To practice a mindful dishwashing meditation, for example, focus on enjoying the task of washing dishes, noticing the sensations involved: the roughness of the scouring pad, the sound and heat of the water, the fragrance of the suds. If anxieties about the past or worries about the future intrude, gently let them go and return your attention to washing the dishes. If you find yourself hurrying to get to your next activity, slow your pace and truly be present, enjoying the here and now.

Consider adding some awareness of your posture. If you're rounding your back over the sink, with your head forward, adjust your alignment so you're standing tall in Mountain Pose (Yoga Spark 2), with your head balanced over your shoulder girdle. If you must lean forward, bend your knees, hinge forward from your hips, and keep your spine long. Consider switching the sponge to your non-dominant hand.

The heart of the practice is staying present in the moment. Anytime your mind wanders off to the future or the past, notice without judgment that your mind is chattering. Release those distracting thoughts and bring your attention back into the present moment. Remind yourself that there's no place to be but right here, right now.

47. Mindful Eating

In our fast-food culture, many of us eat quickly, and often while doing something else, such as watching TV, working, or driving. Emerging research suggests that this kind of mindless, hurried eating may be associated with a host of negative health implications, ranging from weight gain to digestive distress (Vangsness 2012).

According to yoga's sister science, ayurveda (sometimes called traditional Indian medicine), poorly digested food is a major contributor to disease. For this reason, ayurvedic medicine recommends that you pay attention not just to *what* you eat but also to *how* you eat it. For example, it's recommended that meals be eaten with a relaxed, calm mind, preferably in silence, after a prayer of gratitude has been said over the food, and that all food be chewed well (Tirtha 1998, 128).

Teaching people how to eat slowly and mindfully has become a key component of many weight-loss programs in recent years, as our nation struggles with an epidemic of obesity. Mindful eating involves sitting at a table (not standing or driving a car); eating without TV, radio, reading materials, or other distractions; and eating slowly, paying attention to all the sensations—not just flavor, but also aroma, mouthfeel, chewing, and swallowing. In the popular mindfulness-based stress reduction program created by Jon Kabat-Zinn, PhD, participants are introduced to this practice by mindfully eating one single raisin.

For a taste of this practice, try the following mindful eating meditation:

1. Choose a small piece of food as the focus for this meditation—for example, a grape, a bite-size piece of chocolate, or one piece of popcorn.

2. Look at the food, examining its texture, color, and shape.

3. Feel the food with your fingers, noting its squishiness or firmness, ridges and smooth areas, and so on.

4. Smell the food, noticing details of its fragrance.

5. Finally, eat the food—slowly, with exquisite attention to every detail of the act, from salivating to chewing and swallowing.

6. Take a moment to reflect on this experience.

48. Sacred Space

We tend to take time in our lives and make space in our homes for things that are important to us. Clearly TV is of great importance, forming the centerpiece of many American living spaces. The same is often true of computers, game systems, and other electronic devices.

Consider setting aside some time to create a sacred space in your home that will provide an inviting ambiance for yoga practice. If possible, devote a room or part of a room to your practice and decorate the area with inspirational pictures or pleasing artwork to enhance the meditative quality of the space. Keep your yoga mat and any props, such as blocks or straps, nearby. You might have a cushion, stool, or chair available for seated meditation and breathing practice. Consider having appropriate music available if it helps set the mood.

Ideally, you'll spend at least fifteen minutes a day practicing postures, breathing, and meditation. But even on days when you truly don't have time for more than a minute of practice, sit or lie down quietly in your sacred space. Set a timer for sixty seconds and turn your attention inward, observing your breath and any sensations that arise.

49. Three Good Things

Humans have evolved to spend more time thinking about things that have gone wrong than appreciating what has gone right, notes renowned psychologist Martin Seligman (2002), who has done extensive research on depression and happiness. Pondering past problems and how to fix them may have given us an evolutionary advantage, Seligman notes. But this "bad news" focus has an unfortunate side effect: it minimizes life satisfaction and maximizes anxiety and depression.

To correct our negative bias, Seligman created the Three Good Things exercise, which redirects thoughts toward positive events. His research into the practice suggests that becoming more conscious of good events increases happiness and decreases depression. Noticing and being grateful for our many blessings aligns with the yogic principle of santosha, or contentment, which invites us to cultivate the habit of gratitude for what's right in our lives (see Contentment and Gratitude, Yoga Spark 26).

Seligman's exercise, which is also known as Three Blessings, is designed to be done at night, before you go to sleep. Here's how to practice:

1. Think of three good things that happened over the course of your day. These can be anything that seems positive, from something small, like eating an especially great bowl of oatmeal at breakfast, to something major, like your child saying his or her first word.

2. Write down these three positive things.

3. Reflect on why they happened. Maybe the oatmeal was good because your partner made it for you just the way you like it, with nuts and berries. Come up with reasons for each event that make sense to you.

PRINCIPLE SPARKS

50. Cleanliness 2: Tidy Home Practice

Chances are, you're already cultivating saucha, the yogic self-discipline of cleanliness, with good personal hygiene habits such as brushing and flossing your teeth, showering, and hand washing (see Cleanliness 1: Hand-Washing Practice, Yoga Spark 28). Keeping your environment clean can also reduce the risk of illness and have a profound impact on your energy and emotions. For example, consider how it feels to come home to a messy house compared to walking into a clean one. Taking time to tidy up our mess—whether the clutter is dishes, toys, or negative thoughts—offers the opportunity to move forward with a clean slate, or at least a clean countertop.

Recognize that your cleanliness habits contribute to your physical and emotional well-being and embrace opportunities to practice saucha around the house. Here are a few examples:

- Use your comb to clean hair from your brush. Clean both with a dab of shampoo, then let them dry on a towel.

- Clear away clutter from kitchen countertops. Wash kitchen sponges and dishrags at least once a week in hot water in the washing machine.

- Carefully clean your TV remote control with a cotton swab dipped in alcohol and your telephone receiver with a clean cloth and an all-purpose cleanser.

51. Unplug: Restraint of the Senses

Our senses help us navigate the outer world, stimulating our mind and body with information essential for our survival. Yet this sensory input can be a distraction on the inward journey of connection with our deepest self. The yogic principle of *pratyahara*, or sensory inhibition, sometimes likened to a turtle retracting into its shell, involves making a conscious choice to withdraw from the outside world and focus inward. By detaching ourselves from the pull of worldly distractions, we are freed from being controlled by whatever is going on around us.

In today's world our senses are amplified electronically (by computers, phones, TV, and radio), allowing us to see and hear events, both imaginary and real, from around the globe—from natural disasters and wars to talent contests, sports events, and virtually anything you can imagine. Research suggests that the stimulation from watching a screen can contribute to sleep disturbance, which is why many sleep experts recommend avoiding TV and computer use right before bed (Dotinga 2011).

Unplugging can be difficult, but it's a rewarding practice that helps break habits of overstimulation. For some people, technology addiction has become a powerful compulsion that consumes many waking hours and distracts them from being involved in whatever is happening in the present moment.

One of my favorite ways to practice unplugging is to not check email on the Sabbath. It's interesting to feel myself reflexively reach for the mail icon on my smartphone, then consciously not touch it. This practice has helped me recognize my often compulsive impulse to check email and develop a more balanced relationship with this service. Here are some other ways to practice unplugging:

- Consider establishing "cell phone free" areas in your home, where any cell phone use—including texting, calls, and game playing—is off limits.

- Limit broadcast news to no more than thirty minutes a day.

- Turn off the TV when you're finished watching a show.

- Go off-line for a specific period of time, from one minute a day to one day a week or more. During this time, don't use or respond to electronics. Free yourself from the habitual pull of computers, phones, and other distracting devices and notice your reactions. Welcome whatever arises without judgment and with the intention of seeking to understand yourself better.

- As Google executive Eric Schmidt urged graduates at Boston University in his commencement speech, "Take one hour a day and turn that thing off... Take your eyes off that screen and look into the eyes of the person you love. Have a conversation, a real conversation" (Moscaritolo 2012).

52. Clutter-Busting Practice

The cleanliness and orderliness of our homes can both reflect and influence our state of mind. An extreme example is the disorder of compulsive hoarding, a pathological behavior characterized by excessively accumulating possessions—often items without value or usefulness. But acquisition doesn't have to reach this irrational level to become problematic in our lives.

"Americans have been on an acquisition binge for decades," Pulitzer Prize–winning journalist Anna Quindlen notes in a *Newsweek* column headlined "Stuff Is Not Salvation" (2008). An important question we should ask ourselves, she writes, is "Why in the world did we buy all this junk in the first place?"

The yogic principle of aparigraha (greedlessness or nonhoarding) can help free us from the tyranny of being smothered by too much stuff (see Letting Go, Yoga Spark 24). It's useful to periodically do a thorough spring-cleaning and get rid of anything you don't need. Unfortunately, this prospect is often so overwhelming that we do nothing. Instead, take a minute to do quick clutter-busting practices as often as you can. Here are a few examples:

- Find one or two items of clothing, pairs of shoes, or accessories in your closet that you haven't worn in a while and set them aside to donate.

- Check the items on one shelf of your pantry and get rid of anything that's expired or that you won't use.

- Examine one shelf where you store books, DVDs, CDs, games, and so on, and find at least one item to give away or discard.

- Take a trash bag out to your car and get rid of anything you don't need.

53. Self-Study: Journaling

At its heart, yoga is a practice of connecting with your innermost self. One of the best ways to do this is by writing down your deepest thoughts and feelings in a journal. Journaling is more than just listing the events in your day; it involves examining your thoughts and feelings about important and often stressful situations in a manner similar to how you might talk about them with a therapist.

One of the oldest forms of self-inquiry and self-expression, journaling has many benefits. It can help you let off steam and relieve stress. It also serves as an effective tool for problem solving and helps you gain insight into your behaviors and feelings. In fact, research suggests that journaling may improve physical and mental health (Purcell 2012).

From a yogic perspective, journaling is an excellent way to practice the principle of svadhyaya, or self-study, which has the goal of self-understanding and, ultimately, transformation. To practice, keep a journal handy and spend a minute writing in it daily or anytime you find yourself stewing about something. You can buy blank books marketed for this purpose, but my favorite journals are inexpensive composition books, sold with school supplies and at office supply stores.

54. Discipline

Discipline often gets a bad rap because it's frequently associated with punishment. But the word "discipline" has other meanings, including "a branch of knowledge" and "training that develops strength, self-control, and character." This notion is embodied in the yogic principle of *tapas*, a Sanskrit word often translated as "disciplined effort" but that literally means "heat." It's frequently described as a burning effort to pursue goals.

Since yoga is about balance, this notion of disciplined effort offers an ideal counterbalance to the equally important yogic notion of letting go. Yoga teaches us to balance opposites: effort and surrender, courage and caution, doing and undoing. To describe this exquisite balance, many teachers use the analogy of tuning a stringed instrument: to make the ideal sound, the string must be wound neither too loose nor too tight.

To cultivate positive self-discipline in your life, it's helpful to take a moment to identify what's important to you; for example, perhaps you value good health, an orderly home, or strong relationships. To create relevant Yoga Sparks, consider adopting some simple, quick self-discipline practices that will help you reach these goals, as in these examples:

- **Good health:** Substitute water for sugary drinks. Take the stairs instead of the elevator when going up or down a few flights.

- **An orderly home:** Put your dishes and utensils in the dishwasher immediately after you eat. Hang up your clothing rather than tossing it on the floor or bed.

- **Strong relationships:** Phone, text, or e-mail a loved one to check in. Offer to take in your neighbors' mail or newspapers when they're out of town.

· 3 ·

AT WORK PRACTICES

W hether you're staring at a computer screen, standing in front of a classroom, seeing patients, helping customers, building a home, or conducting a symphony, your work is likely to be a major part of your life. It probably takes up much of your time and energy, and it may be a major part of your identity.

Although work is fulfilling and exciting for some and stressful and boring for others, for most people it's a mixed bag of delight and discontent. Even if you're fortunate enough to love your work, it can still be physically, emotionally, and mentally taxing.

This chapter offers stretching and strengthening practices to help you deal with the physical challenges of work, whether that means excessive standing or sitting, long hours of repetitive motions, or having to contort your body into awkward positions. You'll find breathing practices to help energize you when you're tired and calm you when you're stressed, as well as meditations and principle-based practices to help you enhance job performance, improve concentration, get centered, and relax.

POSTURE SPARKS

55. Mini Mountain Pose

Our work often places difficult demands on our bodies, whether it's sitting at a computer for hours, standing up all day, or performing a repetitive motion, such as chopping vegetables, painting walls, or scanning groceries. Maintaining good posture as you work can be extremely helpful in relieving and preventing the musculoskeletal pain that can result from workplace demands. However, many people are completely unaware of their own poor alignment habits and how to make healthy changes.

Awareness is the first step, so from time to time during your workday, take a moment to briefly stop and notice your posture (see Freeze, Ground, Breath, Spine, Yoga Spark 1). You might even set your watch or cell phone to chime every hour as a reminder to do this posture check.

This Mini Mountain Pose brings you into healthy alignment by focusing on three points:

1. **Root down.** Find your roots. Get grounded through whatever part of your body is supporting you. This should be your sit bones if you're sitting or your feet if you're standing.

2. **Lift up.** Extend up from the top of your head. Imagine that the crown of your head is magnetic and is being drawn up toward a powerful magnet in the sky. Avoid the common pitfall of tipping your chin up. As you lift from the top of your

head, be sure to keep your chin level and your shoulders relaxed, down away from your ears.

3. **Shine forward.** Visualize a light shining out from the center of your chest at your breastbone. Shine your light forward, not down toward the ground.

Relax any parts of your body that don't need to be engaged. Depending on what you're doing, this is likely to include your shoulders and jaw. Notice where you habitually hold tension, then let it go.

56. Side Stretch

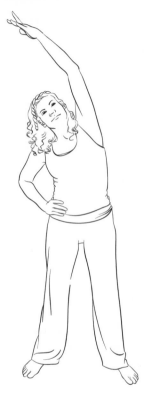

Few activities in daily life stretch out the side of the body, an often-neglected region that can become compressed by excessive sitting and poor posture. Side-bending postures help open the rib cage and the side of the waist, bringing breath into these areas and energizing the entire torso. This basic side stretch can be done seated or standing. If you stand all day, take a break and try it seated. If you sit all day, stand up for your side stretch.

Standing Version

1. Take a wide stance, with your feet a little more than shoulder-width apart and your toes angled out.

2. Bring your hands to your hips (not your waist— feel the bony prominence at the top and front of your pelvis under your fingers). From your hands down, send grounding energy into the earth. From your hands up, lift and lengthen.

3. Inhale and extend the crown of your head up toward the sky.

4. Exhale and bend to the right side, keeping both sides of your waist long—avoid crunching over on the right side.

5. Extend your left arm up and overhead, palm facing in toward your body. Feel a long line of energy up the left side of your body, all the way from your foot to your fingers.

6. Stay in this position for several breaths, then come back to center.

7. Repeat on the other side.

Seated Version

1. Sit tall in a chair and spread your legs out wide, with your feet planted on the floor and your toes angled out.

2. Follow steps 2 through 7 of the standing version, being sure to root down through your left sit bone and buttock when you're stretching to the right and your right sit bone and buttock when you're stretching to the left.

57. Computer Asana

One of the toughest physical challenges the human body can face is sitting all day. Standing is our natural posture. Sitting increases pressure on the lower back, and poor alignment—shoulders rounded, head craned forward, spine slouched—further increases this pressure. This is one reason why so many people in our sedentary society suffer from chronic back and neck pain. Recent research also links excessive sitting to reduced life expectancy (Katzmarzyk and Lee 2012).

If your work requires you to sit for hours in front of a computer, recognize the challenge this poses to your body and sit with good alignment (see Seated Mountain Pose, Yoga Spark 3). Here are some additional tips for maintaining good alignment:

- Enhance the ergonomics of your workstation with a chair that fits your body and has lumbar support to maintain the natural curves of your back. If your chair doesn't have good lumbar support, place a rolled towel or small pillow between your lower back and the chair.

- If you use a laptop, consider using an external monitor and keyboard to avoid crunching your body forward to see the screen. The National Institutes of Health's Office of Research Services (2012) offers an excellent poster showing proper ergonomics for computer workstations through their Division of Occupational Health and Safety. (See *references* for the url).

- If your feet don't rest flat on the floor, use a footrest.

- Be sure your head is balanced over your shoulder girdle, so that if someone were looking at you from the side, your ear would be directly over your shoulder. It's common for the head to drop forward when people have trouble seeing or get tired. If you find yourself straining to see the screen, consider investing in a pair of computer glasses. If you're slumping due to fatigue, get up and stretch if possible. If that isn't possible, do some of the seated stretches in this section.

- Take brief walking breaks as often as you can, or at least stand up and stretch frequently, preferably for a few minutes every hour. When you're talking on the phone, use a headset and stand up. An easy way to add extra walking is to use the bathroom farthest from your work area, preferably climbing stairs to get there.

- Consider investing in a standing desk or adjustable-height workstation that allows you to stand or sit.

58. Seated Back Bend

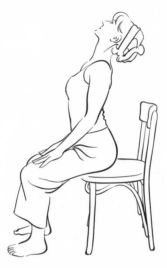

When we're intensely focused on something in front of us, we often lean forward—a tendency that's exacerbated if we're straining to see or hear. Add deadline pressure, tension, or fatigue, and this lean often collapses into a slump. Doing a gentle back bend counters this poor posture by reversing the curve in the upper back, replacing the slumping forward with an arching back. It also stretches out the chest and shoulders, which can become compressed by poor seated posture.

1. Sit tall in Seated Mountain Pose (Yoga Spark 3).

2. Place your palms on your thighs and tuck your elbows in close to your sides. Press your sit bones into the chair and your feet into the floor.

3. On an inhalation, press down with your palms and lift your chest, arching your upper back. Keep your shoulders down and your neck long (don't drop your head back) and gaze up.

4. Exhale and return to sitting tall.

5. Repeat several times, moving with your breath.

6. If you like, stay in the back bend position for a few breaths. Be sure to keep your breath flowing; don't hold your breath.

Variation: Rest your forearms on your desk, elbows shoulder-width apart and hands clasped. Press down with your forearms as you lengthen your spine and arch your upper back.

59. Angel Wings

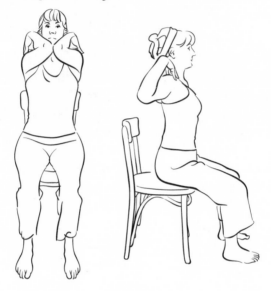

We rarely see our own backs except in a dressing room, where the view is often less than flattering. The Angel Wings practice focuses on this unseen area, the upper back and shoulders, which often become stiff and rigid from extended sitting. As you practice, try to get as much movement as possible in your shoulder blades, the two triangular bones on either side of your spine.

1. Begin by standing or sitting tall in Mountain Pose or Seated Mountain Pose (Yoga Spark 2 or 3).

2. Extend your arms forward, then bend your elbows and place your fingertips on your shoulders.

3. On an inhalation, open your elbows out to the sides and draw your shoulder blades together in the back of your body, as if you had a nut on your spine and your shoulder blades were moving together like a nutcracker to squeeze it.

4. As you exhale, bring your elbows forward and together (or as close as they'll comfortably come) in front of you. Feel your shoulder blades sliding to either side, away from each other.

5. Continue for several breaths, synchronizing your movement with your breath.

Variation: With your fingers resting on your shoulders, draw large circles in the air with your elbows.

60. Wrist, Arms, and Hands Stretch

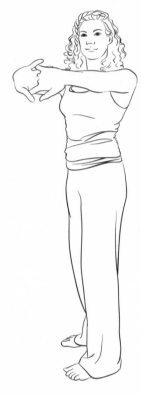

If you've been using your hands in a repetitive motion, such as operating machinery, working at a computer, or playing an instrument, this practice offers a refreshing "counterpose," stretching out your wrists, arms, and hands.

1. Stand or sit tall and bring your palms together in front of your chest. Take a few easy breaths.

2. Clasp your hands and, on an inhalation, extend your arms forward and turn your palms away, keeping your fingers interlaced. (If this is uncomfortable, keep your palms facing in.)

3. Exhale and gently turn to the right. If you're sitting, press your left sit bone into your chair. If you're standing, press your left foot into the floor.

4. Inhale and return to center.

5. Exhale and gently turn to the left. If you're sitting, press your right sit bone into your chair. If you're standing, press your right foot into the floor.

6. Inhale and return to center.

7. Exhale and bring your palms together as you bend your elbows and place your clasped hands in front of your chest. Notice which set of fingers you have on top—which thumb, index finger, and so on. Then switch so the other set of fingers is on top and repeat the stretch.

61. Forearm Stretch

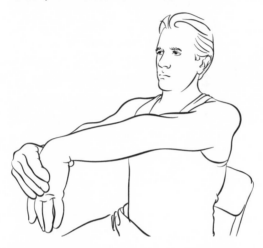

Relieve tension in your forearm muscles with this stretch, which can be particularly helpful for people who work long hours at a computer:

1. Stand or sit tall and extend your right arm forward at shoulder height.

2. Bend your wrist so your fingers point down.

3. Place your left hand over your right hand with the fingers of the left hand pointing toward the right and your left thumb on the inside of your right wrist. Keeping your right arm straight and your fingers pointed down, use your left hand to gently press your right hand down and in toward your body, stretching the top of your right wrist and forearm.

4. Repeat on the other side, gently stretching your left wrist and forearm.

62. Hand Jive

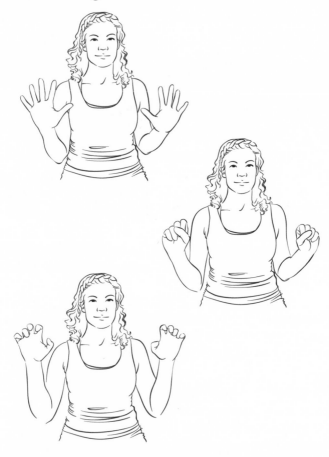

Take a break from a hand-intensive activity, such as key-boarding, and stretch out your hands and fingers with this practice:

1. Sit or stand tall, extend your arms comfortably in front of you, palms facing away, and turn your attention to your breath.

2. Inhale and spread your fingers as wide apart as you can.

3. Exhale and bring your hands into a light fist. If your knuckles are white or there's tension in your arms and shoulders, your fists are too tight. Soften your grip so your fingers remain curled but the tension is released—as if you were holding a baby bird.

4. Continue for five more breaths, inhaling and spreading your fingers, then exhaling and curling them.

5. Rest your hands in your lap or by your sides, relax them completely, and notice any echoes of the movement.

Variation 1: Inhale and spread your fingers wide, then exhale and bend just the top two joints of each finger, making a shape like a bear claw. Continue for several breaths.

Variation 2: Play with moving through all three positions—fingers wide, bear claw, and light fist—being sure to keep your breath flowing.

Variation 3: Turn your palms toward you and move through the three hand positions, then turn your palms so they're facing in, toward each other, and move through the three hand positions again.

63. Modified Cow's Face

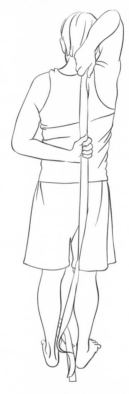

This practice involves the upper body portion of Gomukhasana, or Cow's Face Pose. It's one of the best ways to stretch the front of the shoulders, an area that's often tight in people who sit all day. Most people need to use a strap to do this practice; an old necktie or bathrobe belt works well.

1. Holding the strap in your right hand, sit or stand tall and extend the crown of your head up toward the sky.

2. Raise your right arm and bend your elbow as if you were going to pat yourself on the back. Let the strap rest along your back.

3. Reach your left arm behind you, palm facing out, and lightly grasp the strap.

4. Walk your hands toward each other along the strap. (Clasp your hands together only if you're able to do so without contorting your spine.) Invite your right elbow to point up and your left elbow to point down. Be sure to keep your head balanced over your shoulder girdle (don't duck your head forward) and continue to lift the crown of your head upward.

5. Take a few easy breaths, inviting any tight areas to soften and release.

6. Relax and repeat on the other side.

64. Spread Your Wings

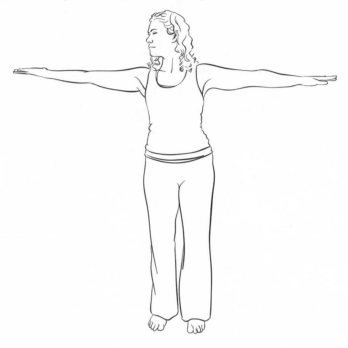

Take a break from sitting in a fixed position with this posture, which will stretch out your upper back, chest, arms, and shoulders:

1. Sit or stand tall and tune in to your breath.

2. Inhale and extend your arms out to the sides at shoulder height, palms down.

3. Exhale and relax your shoulders down away from your ears, continuing to reach your arms out and extending the fingers of your right hand to the right and the fingers of your left hand to the left.

4. Stay here for a few breaths as you spread your wings, extending your "wingspan" as wide as you can.

5. On an inhalation, rotate your right palm up and turn your head to the right, gazing out over your palm.

6. On an exhalation, rotate your right palm down and turn your head back to center.

7. Repeat on the other side, gazing to the left over your palm, then returning to center.

8. Continue for six to ten breaths, then relax your arms to your sides and notice the effects of the practice.

65. Eye Play 1: Clock Eyes

Our work often demands a great deal of our eyes, requiring that we spend hours staring at a computer screen, reading documents, focusing on traffic, and so on. This practice and the next two can relieve eyestrain or even prevent it.

For this practice, which can be done standing, sitting, or lying down, keep your nose pointed forward and only move your eyes, as the focus of this posture is on stretching and strengthening the muscles supporting your eyeballs.

1. Gaze straight up, past your forehead to an imaginary twelve o'clock.

2. Gaze straight down, past your chin to an imaginary six o'clock.

3. Gaze as far to the right as you can, to an imaginary three o'clock.

4. Gaze as far to the left as you can, to an imaginary nine o'clock.

5. *Slowly* let your gaze make a complete circle around this imaginary clock face several times, starting at twelve o'clock and moving clockwise for a few circles. Keep your breath flowing smoothly and evenly; don't hold your breath.

6. Reverse the direction and circle counterclockwise several times.

66. Eye Play 2: Fingertip Push-Ups

Help boost your ability to focus with this practice:

1. Extend your right arm with the index finger pointing forward and the other fingers clasped.

2. Gaze at the fingernail on your right index finger as you *very* slowly bend your right elbow and touch your finger to your nose.

3. Keep gazing at your fingernail as you extend your arm back to the starting position.

4. Repeat with your left hand.

67. Eye Play 3: Palming

Soothe tired eyes with this practice, which uses your hands to create a nourishing environment of darkness and warmth. It's especially effective after doing Eye Play 1: Clock Eyes (Yoga Spark 65), Eye Play 2: Fingertip Push-Ups (Yoga Spark 66), or both of those practices. If you wear glasses, set them aside for a moment while you do this practice.

1. Sit or stand tall and tune in to your breath.

2. Rub your palms together as you take three slow, easy breaths.

3. Cup your hands and place them gently over your eyes. Don't press into your eyes; rather, invite the warmth and darkness created by your palms to help your eyes relax and rest. If you like, support your elbows on a tabletop. Be sure to keep your breath smooth and easy. Send some gratitude to your eyes for all the important work they do for you.

68. Neck Side Stretch

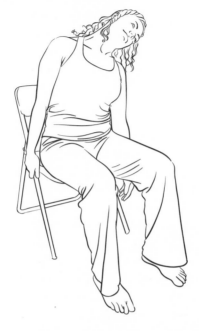

Neck pain is common in our culture, where many people are sedentary and spend countless hours in front of a computer. This often puts stress on muscles and ligaments of the upper body, frequently due to poor postural habits such as jutting the head forward so that it protrudes in front of the shoulders and the upper back rounds. (For a comprehensive guide to preventing and relieving neck pain, please see my book *Healing Yoga for Neck and Shoulder Pain*.)

This practice helps stretch muscles on the sides of the neck, which are often tight and stiff in people who have neck pain. You'll need to sit on a stool or in a chair without arms to do this practice.

1. Sit tall in Seated Mountain Pose (Yoga Spark 3) with your hands on your thighs.

2. Inhale and extend the crown of your head up toward the sky.

3. Exhale and release your right ear down toward your right shoulder, keeping your neck long. (Be sure to drop the right ear toward the right shoulder—avoid lifting the shoulder up toward the ear.)

4. Keeping your breath flowing, press your left shoulder down and breathe into the left side of your neck. Let your left arm dangle down at your side and gently swing it like a pendulum, inviting your left arm and shoulder and the left side of your neck to relax and release.

5. Lightly hold the bottom of the chair with your left hand. Shift your weight into your right buttock and lean to the right. Let the weight of your head help bend your body over to the right side, extending only to the point where you feel a nice, comfortable stretch up the left side of your arm and neck.

6. Inhale and return to center.

7. Repeat on the other side.

69. Restorative Forward Bend

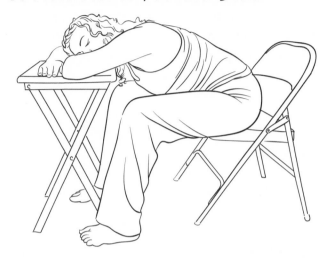

Remember how nice it felt to put your head down on your desk back in grade school? Even now, this posture can provide a mini relaxation break during a busy workday.

1. Sit toward the front of your chair with your feet on the floor and your hands resting on your desk.

2. Hinge forward from your hips and slide your forearms onto your desk, arranging your arms and hands to comfortably cushion your head.

3. Ease your forehead onto your hands or arms; if necessary, slide your chair back so you can rest comfortably with your head and arms supported by your desk.

4. Close your eyes and turn your attention to your breath. As you exhale, allow your body weight to drop into the desk and chair so that with each exhalation your body becomes more relaxed and feels heavier.

5. With each inhalation, invite your breath into your back, feeling the expansion in the back of your rib cage.

6. With each exhalation, relax, release, and let go.

Variation: Turn your head so one cheek rests on your hands. Stay here for a few breaths, then turn your head and rest the other cheek on your hands.

BREATHING SPARKS

70. Breath Surfing

There are four parts to the breath: inhalation, exhalation, and two pauses in between—one as the inhalation makes the transition to exhalation; the other as the exhalation makes the transition to inhalation.

Many teachers liken this breath cycle to the movement of ocean waves lapping onto and then away from the shore. A wave rolls onto the beach, then there's a slight suspension as it prepares to recede. The wave rolls out, then there's a slight suspension as the next wave gets ready to roll onto the shore.

Visualize your breath as a wave during this practice and imagine yourself riding the waves of breath. Like riding on ocean waves, riding your breath can be both relaxing and energizing.

1. Sit or stand tall and turn your attention to your breath. Observe the four parts of your breath cycle: inhalation, pause, exhalation, pause.

2. Focus on the transitional pauses and see if you can lengthen the sense of suspension—*without holding your breath.*

3. Continue breathing in this manner, inviting your breath to be easy, full, and comfortable as it takes you for an enjoyable ride.

71. Sun Channel Breathing

While many breathing practices can help you relax and calm down, such as Relaxed Abdominal Breath (Yoga Spark 10) and Extended Exhalation (Yoga Spark 13), Sun Channel Breathing, or Surya Bhedana Pranayama, can help you become alert, energized, and warm.

The practice involves breathing through the right nostril, which is said to stimulate the pingala nadi, or sun channel, one of the body's three main energy channels. (For more on nadis, or energy channels, see Alternate Nostril Breathing, Yoga Spark 44.) Translated as "tawny current," the pingala nadi corresponds to the sympathetic nervous system, the part of the body's autonomic nervous system that mobilizes the fight-or-flight response, revving us up in response to a perceived threat. The sun channel, which is similar to the yang element of traditional Chinese medicine, is associated with masculine attributes and warming, solar energy.

Try this practice as an alternative to caffeine if you need a midday pick-me-up:

1. Sit tall and bring your attention to your breath.

2. Exhale normally, then use your left index or middle finger to gently close your left nostril.

3. Inhale through your right nostril.

4. Use your right index or middle finger to close your right nostril, release your finger from your left nostril, and exhale through your left nostril.

5. Close your left nostril, open your right nostril, and inhale through your right nostril.

6. Continue for several rounds of breath, finishing with an exhalation.

Once you're comfortable with the practice, try closing the nostrils with one hand. Traditionally, the right hand is held in Mrigi Mudra (Deer Face Mudra), with the index and middle fingers folded into the palm; the right thumb is used to close the right nostril, and the right pinkie and ring finger are used to close the left nostril.

72. Moon Channel Breathing

The opposite, or balancing, practice to Sun Channel Breathing (Yoga Spark 71) is Moon Channel Breathing, or Chandra Bhedana Pranayama. This cooling and quieting practice involves breathing through the left nostril, which is said to stimulate the ida nadi, or moon channel, one of the body's three main energy channels. (For more on nadis, or energy channels, see Alternate Nostril Breathing, Yoga Spark 44.) Translated as "channel of comfort," the ida nadi corresponds to the parasympathetic nervous system, the part of the body's autonomic nervous system that is responsible for "rest-and-digest" activities, such as slowing the heart rate, lowering blood pressure, and promoting digestion. The moon channel, which is similar to the yin element of traditional Chinese medicine, is associated with feminine attributes and cooling, lunar energy.

Try this practice to calm down if you're feeling wired or stressed:

1. Sit tall and bring your attention to your breath.

2. Exhale normally, then use your right index or middle finger to gently close your right nostril.

3. Inhale through your left nostril.

4. Use your left index or middle finger to close your left nostril, release your finger from your right nostril, and exhale through your right nostril.

5. Close your right nostril, open your left nostril, and inhale through your left nostril.

6. Continue for several rounds of breath, finishing with an exhalation.

Once you're comfortable with the practice, try closing the nostrils with one hand. Traditionally the right hand is held in Mrigi Mudra (Deer Face Mudra), with the index and middle fingers folded into the palm; the right thumb is used to close the right nostril, and the right pinkie and ring finger are used to close the left nostril.

73. Victorious Breath

The distinctive, rhythmic sound of this breathing technique has given it imaginative nicknames including "ocean breath," "Darth Vader breath," and "snoring breath." However, the actual translation of the Sanskrit name of this practice, Ujjayi Pranayama, is Victorious Breath. It's cited in ancient yogic texts for its ability to strengthen the respiratory and digestive systems. Often used during flowing asana practices, including ashtanga yoga and some forms of power yoga, Victorious Breath creates an audible anchor for harnessing attention to the breath, which enhances the meditative quality of the practice.

Although calming and balancing, Victorious Breath is a bit tricky to learn, so just play with it—don't work too hard. Over time, it becomes easier. To create the sound that accompanies the breath, open your mouth and exhale a soft "haaa" as if you were trying to fog a mirror or clean a pair of glasses. Now close your mouth and make the same sound; it's a bit like sighing with your mouth closed. Making this distinctive sound involves contracting your glottis, which is comprised of the vocal cords and the space between them. Yogic texts describe the action of inhalation during Ujjayi Pranayama as "drawing up the breath from the heart and the throat" (Feuerstein 1997, 313). As always, avoid forcing, straining, or holding your breath.

Once you have a feel for the sound, you're ready to try the practice:

1. Inhale through your nose with your mouth closed, slightly constricting your throat so you hear a soft "ocean" sound.

2. Exhale through your nose with your mouth closed, again slightly constricting your throat so you hear a soft "ocean" sound.

3. Continue for several breaths, then rest.

MEDITATION SPARKS

74. Boot Up, Download, or On Hold Meditation

Our workdays often contain small islands of downtime. Perhaps we're waiting for a computer to boot up, a file to download, or the arrival of students or a teacher, or maybe we're on hold on the phone. Turn downtime into meditation time with this centering practice, adapted from the teachings of Sarah Powers, who blends yoga and Buddhism in her approach, called Insight Yoga (Powers 2011).

Place your palms on your belly about two inches below your navel. This area, called the *hara* in Japanese and the *dan tien* in Chinese, is considered the body's energy center and repository for life force, prana, or, in traditional Chinese medicine, chi. It is also our center of gravity and a focal point for relaxed abdominal breathing.

Sit or stand tall and turn your attention to your breath. As you inhale, feel your belly gently swell and your hands rise. As you exhale, feel your belly relax back. If your mind wanders, notice this without self-condemnation and return your focus to your breath, mentally reciting, "Breathing in, I'm here now. Breathing out, I'm letting go of distracting thoughts." Continue for several breaths, surrendering to this body-based experience.

75. Telephone Meditation

While the telephone is convenient, "we can be tyrannized by it," notes Zen master Thich Nhat Hanh in his classic guide to mindfulness, *Peace Is Every Step* (1991, 29). "We may find its ring disturbing or feel interrupted by too many calls." The ring can "create in us a kind of vibration, and maybe some anxiety: 'Who is calling? Is it good news or bad news?'"

Rather than be victimized by the phone, he suggests turning its ring into an opportunity to practice telephone meditation:

1. When the phone rings, don't rush to answer.

2. Stay where you are, breathe in and out consciously, and smile.

3. Continue breathing and smiling as you walk to the phone slowly and with dignity. Recognize that if the caller has something important to say, he or she will wait for at least three rings. Answer calmly and joyfully, without anger or irritation. This will benefit not only you, but your caller as well.

76. Rehearse Success Visualization

If you've ever awakened from a scary dream with your heart pounding or imagined biting into a juicy peach and felt your mouth water, you've experienced how your thoughts can affect your physiology. As the Buddha famously said, "We are what we think. All that we are arises with our thoughts. With our thoughts we make the world" (Byrom 1993, xv).

Top athletes use this principle in a form of mental training called visualization or imagery, and many consider this practice essential to success. Golf legend Jack Nicklaus described his use of imagery in his book, *Golf My Way* (2005, 79): "I never hit a shot, even in practice, without having a very sharp, in-focus picture of it in my head. It's like a color movie. First I 'see' the ball where I want it to finish, nice and white and sitting up high on the bright green grass. Then the scene quickly changes and I 'see' the ball going there: its path, trajectory, and shape, even its behavior on landing. Then there's a sort of fade-out, and the next scene shows me making the kind of swing that will turn the previous images into reality."

Worry is also a form of visualization—but not one that supports success. So to enhance your performance at work, don't fret; instead, harness your imagination's positive power with this meditation that focuses your intention on the best possible outcome. You can apply this visualization to anything from giving a great presentation or performing a complicated procedure to handling a difficult customer or requesting something from your supervisor.

1. Close your eyes and bring your attention to your breath.

2. Take a relaxed, centering breath, then continue breathing comfortably as you imagine yourself at the scene where you'll be doing this work, incorporating as many sensory details as you can. Picture the colors, the aromas, any background noises, the feel of anything you're touching, and so on.

3. Imagine yourself moving flawlessly through the situation. As if you were watching a home movie, see yourself mastering each element of the task and doing a great job.

4. When you're ready, open your eyes, continue breathing comfortably, and savor the image of your competence and strength.

77. Walking Meditation

Despite the popular image that meditation must be practiced sitting cross-legged in Lotus Pose, you can meditate in virtually any position, or even while moving. More important than the position of the body is the disposition of the mind.

Walking meditation takes the practice of mindfulness off the cushion and onto any path, from hallway to sidewalk to hiking trail. (For more on mindfulness, see Mindful Awareness of Breath, Yoga Spark 14.) At work, turn a trip to the restroom or any short walk into an opportunity to practice mindfulness, paying careful attention to the movement of your body in the present moment in a compassionate and nonjudgmental way.

1. Stand tall and feel your feet on the ground and your head extending up toward the sky. Relax your shoulders and let your arms hang comfortably at your sides. Soften your face.

2. Move slowly and deliberately: Lift one foot, swing it forward, and place it in front of you. Then do the same with the other foot, lifting it, swinging it forward, and placing it in front of you. Notice the subtle shifts in your balance and any sensations you feel in the heel, arch, ball, and toes of each foot.

3. Walk simply to enjoy the process of walking. Keep your focus on the present moment, noticing the sensations in your body and the environment around you. If your mind starts spinning off to

thoughts of the past or the future or begins chattering with planning, organizing, or judging, release those thoughts and come back to the present moment.

PRINCIPLE SPARKS

78. Sympathetic Joy

In our competitive culture, it's not uncommon to feel envy or jealousy at a coworker's success. In fact, there's even a German word—*schadenfreude*—to describe feeling pleasure at someone else's bad fortune. Some work environments play on this cutthroat sense of competition, pitting individuals or work teams against each other in performance contests.

However, these selfish, negative attitudes separate us from others and impair our ability to open our hearts, love, and feel compassion. The antidote to destructive attitudes of envy, bitterness, resentment, jealousy, and spite is the practice of sympathetic joy. In the Buddhist tradition, learning to feel joy for others, known as *mudita* in Sanskrit, is considered one of the four *brahmaviharas*, or heavenly abodes, along with compassion, loving-kindness, and equanimity. The Yoga Sutras also encourage an attitude of being "joyful with those doing praiseworthy things" (Desikachar 1995, 159).

Rejoicing in the happiness and accomplishments of others can be challenging in our dog-eat-dog world, where there's often a tendency to view someone else's success as our own failure. "Judgment and envy, comparisons and insecurity: these narrow our world and make sympathetic and altruistic joy difficult to experience," notes Roshi Joan Halifax, founder of the Upaya Institute and Zen Center, a Buddhist monastery in Santa Fe, New Mexico

(Halifax 2011). "We can learn and practice offering joy to others, even though there might be a touch of pretending there at the beginning," she notes. "From recent research in neuroscience we have learned that these areas of the brain can be intentionally cultivated. Like a violinist whose talent for playing increases with practice, we can also increase our joy with practice."

Rather than begrudge the success of others, take delight in their well-being, success, good fortune, and accomplishment. To do so, Roshi Joan suggests mentally reciting phrases such as these:

- I am happy that you are happy.

- I wish you all the best.

- May your success continue.

79. Concentration

Although we often pride ourselves on our ability to multitask—for example, texting while talking on the phone while checking email—we're actually not doing several things at once. Instead, the brain is ping-ponging attention among activities. Research involving MRI scans of the brain shows that we can't focus on more than one thing at a time and instead switch rapidly between tasks (Hamilton 2008). So it's not surprising that eating lunch at our desk while working on one project and talking on the phone about another can leave us feeling tense, exhausted, and unbalanced.

The yogic principle of *dharana*, or concentration, invites us to "monotask"—to do only one thing at a time and to train our full attention on that task. This is the sixth limb of the ancient sage Patanjali's Eightfold Path of yoga. *Dharana* comes from the Sanskrit root *dhri*, meaning "to hold or retain," and the practice involves holding attention on one point. It's an essential skill for meditation, or *dhyana*, which is the seventh limb, and for ecstasy, or *samadhi*, which is the final limb and ultimate goal of the path.

"A one-pointed mind can be cultivated throughout the day by giving your complete attention to whatever you are doing," writes spiritual teacher Eknath Easwaran in *Take Your Time* (1994, 78). He points to the Buddha's teaching: "The Buddha said, 'When you are walking, walk. When you are sitting, sit. Don't wobble.'... We need this advice today because we spend most of our time wobbling," he says. "We find it all but impossible to do just one thing at a time" (76).

Learning to stay focused is essential to success, notes Easwaran, who says "no skill in life is greater than the capacity to direct your attention at will… If you have trained your mind to give complete attention to one thing at a time, you can achieve your goal in any walk of life. Whether it is science or the arts or sports or a profession, concentration is a basic requirement in every field. And complete concentration is genius" (66).

Training your attention is like training a puppy, he says. "When something distracts your attention, you say, 'Come back' and bring it back again." As with puppy training, he notes, it's important to be kind and avoid yelling. "With a lot of training, you can teach your mind to come running back to you when you call, just like a friendly pup" (87).

So the next time you're tempted to multitask, pick one of the jobs and devote yourself to it fully. When you've completed that task, move on to the next.

80. Integrity

While integrity is important in all aspects of life, it's particularly essential in the workplace, where dishonesty, deception, and misconduct can severely damage, if not destroy, your career. In the yogic tradition, the concept of *arjava*—which is variously translated as "integrity," "straightforwardness," "honesty," and "rectitude"—is considered a central moral principle.

Integrity clearly involves obeying laws, paying taxes, and dealing fairly with others. Many professions also have a code of ethics outlining standards specific to a particular occupation.

The yogic principle of arjava encompasses avoiding even small acts of dishonesty, such as using the office copier to duplicate personal materials, embellishing your resume with a white lie, borrowing supplies from a coworker and not returning them, or taking credit for someone else's idea.

Creating the habit of acting with integrity in our professional and personal lives keeps us grounded in the truth and is essential to good relationships with others, from bosses to coworkers, clients, students, and customers. It's also central to a good relationship with oneself.

• 4 •

ON THE GO PRACTICES

Even when you're on the go—driving to work, flying across the globe, hanging onto a subway strap, or speeding along on a train—you can practice yoga. In our mobile society, yoga practices can help you feel at home no matter where you are, allowing you to find strength and stability, peace and equanimity, anytime, anywhere, in any situation.

Although travel can be fun and exciting, it can also be exhausting, boring, and scary. This chapter offers practices to help you counter the stress of travel, from sitting in a cramped seat for hours to waiting in long lines and from navigating unclean environments to sleeping in a strange bed. Some of the practices are designed to help you cool down in a hot situation, others can help you slow down in a rushed situation, and all will help you find balance and ease.

POSTURE SPARKS

81. Driving Asana

Sitting in a fixed position for an extended period of time is hard on your body in any situation, and it can be particularly challenging if you're behind the wheel. Research suggests that those who spend more than twenty hours a week driving are at increased risk of back pain and other musculoskeletal disorders (Porter and Gyi 2002). And even short periods of driving—especially in bumper-to-bumper traffic—can trigger a cascade of physical and emotional tension.

Yoga invites you to bring the same awareness to your driving posture as you do to poses on the mat. As best you can, arrange the ergonomics of your driver's seat to allow you to sit on your sit bones and keep length in your spine, just like in Seated Mountain Pose (Yoga Spark 3). Adjust your seat so your legs can move freely to reach the pedals while your back remains snug against the seat. If there's not a good lumbar support for your low back, use a lumbar roll designed for this purpose or place a small pillow or rolled towel between the small of your back and the seat. Adjust your mirrors so you don't have to round forward to use them. Adjust your head restraint so the top of it is even with the top of your head; if it won't reach that height, lift it as high as it will go. The distance from the back of your head to the restraint should be as small as possible, preferably less than four inches, according to the Insurance Institute for Highway Safety (2012).

Here are some other tips on proper driving posture:

- Sit tall, extending up from the crown of your head, especially when you need to turn your head, as when changing lanes.

- Hold the wheel with your hands on opposite sides. Many experts now advise that you place your hands at three and nine o'clock, rather than at two and ten o'clock, as was formerly recommended. This newer, parallel position will protect your hands if your airbag were to deploy and makes for safer driving in general (Johnson 2012).

- Avoid having a death grip on the wheel. If your knuckles are white and your shoulders are up by your ears, relax your arms, hands, shoulders, neck, and face. Use only as much effort as is necessary for good control of the car, and remember to balance this effort with relaxation.

- Keep your breath easy and flowing. Use red lights and stop signs as opportunities to take a Relaxed Abdominal Breath (Yoga Spark 10).

82. Seat Stretches

Travelers on long trips have a small but very real risk of developing a potentially life-threatening condition called deep vein thrombosis, where blood clots form in a vein deep in the body, generally in the lower leg or thigh. If a clot breaks off and travels through the bloodstream, it can lodge in an artery in the lungs and block blood flow, a serious condition called a pulmonary embolism.

The risk is higher on trips longer than four hours or if you have other risk factors, such as being obese, pregnant, or over age fifty. To decrease the likelihood of developing deep vein thrombosis, the US Surgeon General recommends that travelers frequently walk up and down the aisle of a bus, train, or airplane or stop the car every hour and walk around (US Surgeon General 2012).

Since this behavior is often discouraged on airplanes, moving your legs often while seated can also reduce your risk. Try these seated stretches, being sure to keep your breath flowing. Each one could take about a minute, so consider doing one at a time over the course of a long trip or, if you have time, do several in a row:

- Place both feet on the floor, with your shoes off if possible. Raise your right leg. As you inhale, flex your foot so your toe points up and back, toward your nose. As you exhale, point your foot so your toe points away. Repeat three to five times, synchronizing your movement with your breath, then switch legs.

- With both feet on the floor, inhale and lift your heels up as high as possible. As you exhale, bring your heels down. Repeat five to ten times, synchronizing your movement with your breath.

- With both feet on the floor, inhale and lift your toes up as high as possible while keeping your heels on the floor. As you exhale, bring your toes down. Repeat five to ten times, synchronizing your movement with your breath.

- Raise your right leg and extend your right hand, then slowly rotate your right ankle and wrist for a few breaths, first clockwise, then counterclockwise. Repeat on the other side.

Variation: For extra challenge, continue rotating your wrist clockwise and switch the direction of your ankle, rotating it counterclockwise. Circle in opposite directions for a few breaths, then switch directions of both wrist and ankle. Repeat on the other side.

83. At Ease

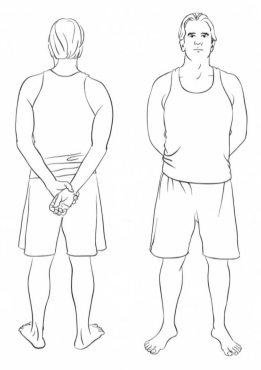

If you find yourself standing for any length of time, moving into this adaptation of the military "at ease" stance can help you maintain good posture. Relaxed yet disciplined, this pose helps keep your shoulders from rounding forward and distributes your weight evenly on both legs.

1. Bring your feet to a comfortably wide stance, a little wider than hip-width apart, with your toes angled out and your knees soft.

2. Lengthen up through the crown of your head and relax your shoulders down away from your ears. Relax your jaw and soften the inside of your mouth.

3. Bring your hands behind you. If you're right-handed, rest the back of your right hand in your left palm and lightly clasp your right hand. If you're left-handed, rest the back of your left hand in your right palm and lightly clasp your left hand.

84. Core Strengthener

Our culture seems obsessed with flat abs, yet the common practice of doing sit-ups primarily targets just one of our four abdominal muscle groups—the most visible and superficial abdominal muscle: the rectus abdominis. Better known as the "six-pack" muscle, it runs vertically from the pubic bone to the breastbone and flexes the spine, bending the body forward.

However, the other three abdominal muscle groups are equally important, if not more important, for good health and appearance. These are the internal and external obliques, on the sides of the torso, and the transversus abdominis (TA), which is deepest, running horizontally underneath the rectus and obliques. Sometimes called the "corset" muscle, the TA is arguably the most important muscle to strengthen because it helps support the lower back and flatten the belly. A strong TA helps you stand with good posture, which can make you look and feel better.

To locate your TA, stand or sit tall and place one palm just below your belly button. Cough gently and feel this muscle contract beneath your hand. Alternatively, imagine that you're trying to zip up "skinny jeans" to experience the drawing-in action of the TA. Yoga teachers often cue students to hug the belly in toward the spine, which activates the TA.

My favorite place to practice the Core Strengthener is while driving, when waiting at a red light, but you can do this isometric contraction virtually anywhere without anyone knowing that you're giving your abs a workout.

1. Stand or sit tall in Mountain Pose or Seated Mountain Pose (Yoga Spark 2 or 3).

2. As you inhale, relax your abdominal muscles, filling your lungs completely so your diaphragm descends and your belly swells.

3. As you exhale, engage your TA muscle and press your belly in toward your spine, completely expelling all of the air.

4. Repeat five to ten times, then rest.

85. Pelvic Floor Strengthener

Sometimes likened to a hammock positioned at the bottom of a bowl, the pelvic floor muscles support the organs in the lower abdomen and provide a foundation for the body's core. Several common conditions contribute to weakness in this area, including excess weight, age, and, for women, pregnancy and childbirth. Weak pelvic floor muscles are linked with numerous health problems, such as organ prolapse and urinary incontinence. Pelvic floor exercises can help alleviate these problems, and, for men, they have been shown to alleviate erectile dysfunction (Dorey et al. 2005).

In the yoga tradition, the pelvic floor is the location of the first of seven main energy centers, or chakras, that are situated along the spine from base to crown. Each chakra corresponds to a particular physical, mental, and energetic aspect of our being. The lowest chakra, also known as the root center or *muladhara chakra*, is located in the subtle body at an area corresponding to the perineum and is related to material security and safety. Cultivating strength and balance in the pelvic floor is considered important for feeling grounded and secure.

This practice is best learned while lying down on your back. Then, once you've become familiar with the movements and breath, you can do it virtually anywhere— sitting, standing, or lying down—without anyone knowing.

1. Lie on your back with your knees bent or straight and bring your attention to your pelvic floor. If you're not sure where this is, imagine a diamond

formed by four points—your two sit bones, your pubic bone, and your tailbone. The area inside this diamond is your pelvic floor.

2. Tune in to your breath, allowing it to come into an easy, natural rhythm.

3. When you're ready, inhale and invite the muscles in your pelvic floor to soften, lengthen, and relax.

4. As you exhale, gently draw these muscles up and in.

5. Continue for five to ten breaths, synchronizing your movement with your breath. Inhale as you relax and soften, and exhale as you gently squeeze up and in. You might visualize your pelvic floor moving down with each inhalation and moving up with each exhalation.

6. Don't strain. If other muscles, such as the buttocks or shoulders, get involved, you're probably working too hard. Relax and try to isolate just the pelvic floor muscles.

86. Self-Massage of the Head and Neck

The face, head, neck, and shoulders tend to hold a great deal of tension, particularly on days when we're interacting with others, talking, smiling, frowning, and making other expressive faces. This self-massage can help relax physical and emotional tension in the head and neck. You can do it in the privacy of your hotel room or while traveling by plane, bus, or car. (If you're driving, please pull over or save this for a long red light or traffic jam, when you're not moving.)

1. Sit or lie down with your back supported and comfortable. Bring the tips of your middle fingers (the index fingers can be too strong) to the "third eye" space between your eyebrows and gently stroke your eyebrows in an outward direction, toward your ears. Do this a few times, smoothing out any worry lines between your eyebrows.

2. Move to your temples and gently massage in a circular pattern.

3. Slide your fingers down to your temporomandibular joint (TMJ); to find it, open and close your mouth a few times and feel for an area that protrudes out when your mouth opens. Give this area a gentle rub.

4. Let your mouth go slack and massage the strong jaw muscle, the masseter, noticing if one side feels tighter than the other. (To find the masseter,

place your fingers on your cheek where the upper and lower jaw meet and slide them slightly toward your mouth.)

5. Ease your fingers back behind your skull and massage the occipital ridge area, where the skull and neck meet. Rub in the hollows and any sore spaces and turn your head from side to side to find any particularly tight spots that need attention.

6. Slide your fingers down your neck, massaging any tense places.

7. Gently pull on your ears, rubbing and massaging any stiff areas.

8. If you like, finish with Eye Play 3: Palming (Yoga Spark 67).

87. Shake Hands with Your Feet

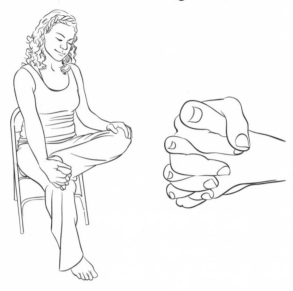

Yoga's sister science of ayurveda, sometimes called traditional Indian medicine, recommends massaging the feet at bedtime to calm the nervous system and enhance sleep. This practice can be particularly welcome for travelers after a long day of sight-seeing, standing in line, or walking on challenging surfaces, such a cobblestones.

1. Soak or wash your feet if possible, then sit comfortably and place your right foot on your left thigh.

2. Massage oil or lotion into your foot, being sure to attend to the top, soles, heels, and lower leg.

3. Use your thumbs and fingers to smooth out any sore spots you find.

4. Weave the fingers of your left hand between the toes of your right foot, with each finger between two toes, and gently stretch and spread your toes.

5. Repeat with the other foot.

6. You may want to wear cotton socks to bed to keep the oil from rubbing off onto the sheets.

BREATHING SPARKS

88. "Ha" Breath

One of the best ways to expel pent-up energy or emotions is through a forceful breathing technique with a vocalization. Martial artists use this kind of breath-supported sound, known as kiai, to add power to a punch or kick, and ancient masters were said to be able to drop a bird from the sky with their kiai alone. The grunts released by tennis players and weight lifters are another common example of this principle.

Making the "haaa" sound while exhaling is part of Lion's Face (Yoga Spark 8), but it can also be a stand-alone breathing practice.

1. Sit or stand tall and inhale fully through your nose.

2. Exhale through your mouth, making a "haaa" sound for as long as you comfortably can, simultaneously drawing your belly in toward your spine.

3. Relax your abdominal muscles and allow your belly to round as you inhale, then repeat.

In her book *Yoga and You*, my mentor Esther Myers wrote, "Said loudly, [this practice] discharges emotional stress; said more quietly it has a quality of relief and unwinding" (1997, 68). If you're shy about vocalizing, she suggests practicing in the shower, in the car with the windows closed, or with the vacuum cleaner on.

89. Cooling Breath

Animals that can't sweat cool off by sticking out their tongues and panting. This principle underlies the breathing practice of Sitali Pranayama, or Cooling Breath, which is one of the few yogic breathing techniques that involve inhaling through the mouth. In addition to helping cool the body, this practice also is recommended for people who are hotheaded or agitated, as well as those experiencing hot flashes and fevers.

1. Sit tall and take a few easy breaths.

2. Exhale normally.

3. To inhale, stick out your tongue and, if possible, curl in the sides so that you suck the air in over your tongue as if it you were drinking from a straw. It's fine to make a hissing sound; in fact, this practice is sometimes called hissing breath. (The ability to curl the tongue is genetic, so if you can't curl yours, leave it flat as you inhale.)

4. Relax your tongue, close your mouth, and exhale through your nose. If possible, make your exhalation longer than your inhalation.

5. Repeat for several rounds, being sure not to strain.

90. Timing the Breath

When you're feeling emotional or mental turmoil, steadying your breath can help steady your mind. Practices that use the breath to ease the mind and body generally involve bringing inhalations and exhalations into a particular rhythm. For example, in Even Breath (Yoga Spark 12), the inhalation and exhalation are equal in length, while in Extended Exhalation (Yoga Spark 13), the exhalation is up to twice as long as the inhalation.

While mentally counting the breath is often the easiest way to practice, it can be challenging to keep a steady mental count without veering into fluctuating speeds and rhythms. You can use your pulse to time your breath, but that may also fluctuate. For these reasons, a clock or metronome can be particularly helpful, especially if you're feeling distracted or emotionally charged. (You need not own or purchase a metronome; online and app versions are available.)

1. Sit tall and turn your attention to your breath, taking a few easy breaths to establish a natural rhythm.

2. Watch the second hand of a clock or count the beats of a metronome to determine your normal breathing pace. How many seconds or beats does a typical inhalation last? How many seconds or beats does a typical exhalation last?

3. Continue breathing naturally for one minute, counting how many breaths you take during this time.

4. This knowledge of your baseline breathing rate can inform your breathing practice. Try timing your breath at different times of the day or in different states of mind and notice any variations that may occur.

Over time, as you continue to play with the Breathing Sparks, you may find that your ability to slow and deepen your breath increases, and your baseline breathing rate may even change. However, don't struggle or strain to manipulate your breath, and recognize that longer isn't necessarily better. Instead, focus on finding patterns and rhythms that enhance your sense of well-being.

91. Square Breath

The stabilizing and grounding practice of Square Breath involves making all four parts of the breath equal in length, which is why it is sometimes called Sama Vritti Pranayama, or equal breath. Before you try this, practice Breath Surfing (Yoga Spark 70) to get comfortable with the four components of the breath: inhalation, pause, exhalation, pause. Then play with making all four parts of the breath equal in length with this practice:

1. Sit tall and take a few breaths to establish a natural rhythm.

2. When you're ready, begin to pause briefly after each inhalation and exhalation.

3. Gradually lengthen the pauses until all four parts of the breath are equal in length.

Don't hold your breath in the pauses; rather, allow them to be a gentle suspension of the breath without tension. This is particularly important if you have high blood pressure, heart disease, or glaucoma. For most people, it's advisable to practice Square Breath with short breaths, perhaps two or three seconds for each part of the breath. For example, inhale for two seconds, pause for two seconds, exhale for two seconds, and pause for two seconds.

MEDITATION SPARKS

92. Waiting Meditation

While it's lovely to have a daily meditation practice, many people say it's hard to find the time. Yet life typically offers us chunks of downtime throughout the day in the form of waiting: in line at the store, for a restaurant table, while baggage is unloading, in the doctor's office, sitting in traffic, and so on.

Embrace these moments as opportunities to practice meditation. Mindful Awareness of Breath (Yoga Spark 14) and Mantra Meditation (Yoga Spark 16) are particularly portable. Or try this waiting meditation:

1. Stand or sit tall and turn your attention to your breath.

2. Observe the sensations of your breath as it moves into and out of your body.

3. Notice any sounds around you—the hum of an air conditioner, music, ringing phones, and so on—without making any judgments or creating stories about their meaning. Just notice the sounds. Then bring your attention back to your breath.

4. Notice any activity around you—birds flying, people moving, lights blinking—without making any judgments or creating stories about their meaning. Just notice the activity. Then bring your attention back to your breath.

5. Use this waiting time to enjoy simply being present in the moment, allowing life around you to unfold.

93. Sacred Objects

Sacred objects can help you stay connected to your highest values and deepest beliefs. They can be especially useful when you're out in the world, away from home. Jewelry often serves this purpose, reminding us of that which we hold most dear—from a wedding ring or family heirloom to a bracelet of prayer beads for meditation or a necklace with a religious symbol, such as a cross or a Star of David.

Consider bringing one or more small sacred objects with you when you travel. Virtually anything that helps you find peace, comfort, and joy can be helpful, whether a picture of a loved one, a stone from your favorite place, a shell from a beloved beach, or a special note from your child.

Having an object available in your pocket or around your neck can be useful for a quick meditation anytime you'd like a calming moment—for example, if you're in a plane that encounters turbulence or if you get lost in a foreign city. You can also create a small altar or sacred space in your hotel room by arranging one or more special objects there, turning a sterile environment into a familiar sanctuary. You might light some incense or a candle. If you're in a nonsmoking room, use a small LED candle or aromatic oil.

Amid the often-hectic pace of travel, allow your sacred objects to help you connect with your true self. Take a moment to sit quietly and turn your attention inward, observing your breath and any sensations, emotions, or thoughts that arise. If you like, offer a prayer or set an intention for how you'd like to move through the world.

94. Pause: Inner Listening

Yoga is a practice of inner listening, according to renowned California yoga teacher Erich Schiffmann, who outlines his approach in *Yoga: The Spirit and Practice of Moving into Stillness* (Schiffmann 1996). Posture practice is the training ground for learning this skill, which you then apply throughout your day.

"Physical yoga…is essentially an awareness process wherein you attend to subtle shifts in sensation and feeling," he notes (Schiffmann 1995). "In so doing you exercise your sensitivity and cultivate the ability to 'listen' inwardly."

To practice inner listening, pause and ask for guidance frequently, advises Schiffmann, who suggests doing this whenever you have a decision to make, even something as minor as whether to wear a red or blue shirt. Another option is to set a timer to sound every half hour and, when it goes off, pause and ask for guidance about whatever you're facing in that moment.

Schiffmann offers these instructions for inner listening: "Stop moving physically. Relax your body, breathe gently, and be aware of the feeling-tone of your body… Listen inwardly as though you were waiting to hear a message. The inner feeling will give you a subtle, internal prompting about what to do or not do. All you need to do is pay attention and listen" (1996, 343).

PRINCIPLE SPARKS

95. Slow Down

Many years ago, my husband and I arrived in the Bahamas after a long and stressful trip. We boarded a small bus filled with grumpy, rumpled travelers who, like us, were agitated and anxious to get to our hotel. Our smiling young Bahamian driver calmed us all with this cheerful pronouncement, which has become one of my favorite travel mantras: "We have three speeds here in the Bahamas: we have slow, we have stop, and we have reverse. So relax! You're on vacation."

This wise recognition that life is lived in this moment, and isn't about getting somewhere else but about being where you are right now, fully and completely, is central to yoga practice. In her classic book *Awakening the Spine*, legendary yoga master Vanda Scaravelli describes the appropriate yogic attitude as one of "infinite time and no ambition" (1991, 34).

Put simply, yoga is not in a hurry.

Yet for many people in our rushed, striving culture, making this critical downshift from a hurried, full-speed-ahead mentality into a relaxed, moment-by-moment awareness is a tremendous challenge. Rushing has become second nature for many people, and they are often oblivious to their "need for speed" attitude.

As with many addictions, the first step in breaking free of habitual rushing is simply to become aware of your pace. When you find yourself hurried and stressed, ask yourself, *Where's the fire?* Is it really necessary to rush, or is this just a bad habit you should break? In other words, are you rushing because you're stressed, or are you stressed because you're rushing?

If you're habitually hurried, try these practices for slowing down:

- When doing yoga postures, notice the speed at which you tend to move. For example, if you're making ankle circles, do you tend to make rapid circles? If so, try slowing down to half the speed, then to one-quarter the speed.

- Anytime you find yourself rushing, pause and turn your attention to your breath—at first without trying to change or control it in any way. Just allow your breath to tell you the story of what's going on in your body. Chances are, your breath will be shallow and your muscles will be tense. Take a moment to come into Mountain Pose or Seated Mountain Pose (Yoga Spark 2 or 3), then practice a few rounds of Relaxed Abdominal Breath (Yoga Spark 10). Savor the way this feels.

- Counter the tendency to hurry by mentally downshifting. If you're in overdrive, imagine yourself downshifting to fourth gear, then third, then second, and finally neutral.

- Aim to do things at an appropriate pace. Rather than always rushing, consciously move at a suitable speed—sometimes fast, sometimes slow, sometimes in between.

- Give yourself more time to get where you're going. Use any extra time to breathe deeply and smile.

- Do less and enjoy more. Avoid the tendency to overschedule so you won't be continually concerned about being late for your next activity.

- Remember that life isn't a race. As Mahatma Gandhi is reputed to have said, "There is more to life than increasing its speed."

96. Cultivate Patience

Have you ever pushed a lighted elevator button in a futile attempt to speed it up? Or perhaps you've fumed at having to wait in line, be put on hold, or drive behind a slow car. If so, you've experienced some symptoms of the modern malady known as time urgency/impatience, sometimes called "hurry sickness." Chronic impatience is not only hard on those around you, it can also increase your risk of hypertension and heart disease (Yan et al. 2003).

Becoming impatient with people or circumstances is frowned upon in the yoga tradition, which encourages cultivation of the quality of *kshama*—a Sanskrit term meaning "patience" or "forbearance." Considered among the noblest of virtues, this practice is defined as having equanimity in all circumstances—pleasant and unpleasant—and remaining kind, calm, and serene even when facing hardship.

Bumps in the road are inevitable in life, and delays are common, especially when you're traveling. When faced with a traffic jam, long line, or delayed flight, you can wait impatiently and be miserable, or you can wait patiently and be happy; the choice is yours.

"Without patience, we can't truly learn from the lessons life throws at us; we're unable to mature," notes M. J. Ryan in *The Power of Patience* (2003, 6). "We remain at the stage of irritable babies, unable to delay gratification more than momentarily."

A synonym for "patience" is "self-possession," Ryan writes. "I love that word; it helps me remember that, with patience, we are in charge of our selves. We can choose how to respond to a given event, rather than being hijacked by our emotions" (12).

Ryan offers these patience practices:

- Ask yourself, *What's the worst possible thing that could happen?* In other words, what's the worst-case scenario if you're late, the plumber doesn't show up, and so on? Chances are it won't be as harmful as the aggravation of getting worked up about a delay.

- If you're working on a big project, choose to notice what you've done rather than what you've got left to do. This increases patience by tapping into a sense of positivism.

- In heated situations, count to ten before speaking. If you still feel upset after counting to ten, count to twenty.

- Put a pebble in your pocket. When you start to feel irritation rise, break the anger cycle by moving the pebble from one pocket to another.

- Thank others for being patient when you've been fumbling for change and holding them up.

97. After You

One of the loveliest features of living in a small college town is the courtesy of drivers. They're typically willing to let you merge, make a turn, or even take a parking space. This behavior was a pleasant surprise for us when we moved to Chapel Hill, North Carolina, from Washington, DC, back in 1988, and I soon learned that both accepting the courtesy and extending it to others made driving much more pleasant and safe. As our town has grown in recent years, we've seen an increase in rudeness on the road, but I still treasure the practice of letting someone else go ahead of me. Dropping the "me first" mentality in favor of an "after you" attitude brings a smile to the other person's face and warms my heart.

From a yogic perspective, this involves both the principle of aparigraha, or greedlessness (see Letting Go, Yoga Spark 24), and the principle of kshama, or patience (see Cultivate Patience, Yoga Spark 96). Aparigraha entails recognizing that there is plenty for all. There's no need to hog the road or take more than one parking space; instead, we can share the highway, yield the right of way, and so on. Kshama asks us to be patient and kind. Rather than honk our horn or cut in front of another car, we can wait patiently while another driver takes his or her turn.

Adopting an "after you" attitude can ease your own stress and also make life more pleasant for others, on or off the road. You can practice in many situations, such as in lines at the bank or in shops or passing food at the table. Here are some ways to practice:

- Release the need to be first. Make it a habit to be courteous and safe on the road.

- Pay attention to those who might need assistance, such as an elderly person or a mother with young children, and allow them to go ahead of you.

- If you find yourself racing someone else for something, from a parking space to the last brownie on the plate, stop, smile, and let the other person have it.

98. Cleanliness 3: Sanitizing Practice

The principle of saucha, or purity, is particularly important when traveling, since public areas can put you at increased risk of exposure to disease-causing pathogens. This is particularly true of certain travel environments such as airplanes, where the air is very dry and contains recirculated particles and germs, and air-conditioned cruise ships that may have high levels of mold in the cabins (American Academy of Otolaryngology 2012).

Frequent hand washing is one of the best ways to reduce your risk of illness (see Cleanliness 1: Hand-Washing Practice, Yoga Spark 28). But for those times when soap and clean water aren't available, carry an alcohol-based hand sanitizer with you, preferably one with the FDA-recommended concentration of 60 to 95 percent ethanol or isopropanol (Reynolds, Levy, and Walker 2006). In addition, consider these cleanliness practices to reduce your exposure to germs while traveling:

- Carry alcohol-based sanitizing wipes to clean hard surfaces near your seat on an airplane, including the tray table, seat belt, and seat arms.

- In public restrooms, use a paper towel to open the stall door and flush the toilet, then throw the towel away as you leave.

- Breathe through your nose. The yogic practice of breathing through the nose rather than the mouth can help reduce risk of illness, since the nose filters, warms, and humidifies the air you breathe.

·5·

PRACTICES WITH OTHERS

The fruits of yoga practice go far beyond chiseled abs and better balance, extending to the deeper gifts of a peaceful mind and a joyful heart. Relationships are key here, as they are central to our health, tranquility, and happiness.

Yoga Sutra 1.33 offers timeless wisdom on relating to other people in one comprehensive sentence: "The mind becomes quiet when it cultivates friendliness in the presence of happiness, active compassion in the presence of unhappiness, joy in the presence of virtue, and indifference toward error" (Bouanchaud 1997, 49).

At the heart of this teaching is the recognition of our common humanity with all people, which helps remove the barriers posed by selfishness and egoism. The benefits of these attitudes extend beyond helping another person; they also serve to open our own hearts and calm our own minds, freeing us from the tight grip of anger, hatred, and resentment. In addition, learning to treat others with kindness enhances our ability to be kind to ourselves.

This chapter offers practices to help strengthen your relationships with others, from family, friends, pets, and people you love to colleagues, acquaintances, strangers, and people you dislike. There are postures and breathing practices designed to encourage intimacy, meditations to foster closeness, and principles for cultivating compassion and love.

POSTURE SPARKS

99. Smiling Eyes

Americans spent nearly ten billion dollars on cosmetic procedures in 2011, according to the American Society for Aesthetic Plastic Surgery (2011). Yet one of the easiest ways to boost appearance is free.

A genuine smile—not just from the mouth, but from the heart—lights the eyes, softens the face, and releases tension from the brow and jaw. This simple form of "mouth yoga" benefits much more than just how we look; it's also a powerful way to brighten the lives of others and to feel better ourselves. (See Conscious Breathing with a Smile, Yoga Spark 15.)

Mother Teresa noted that "joy shows from the eyes," and said that "when people find in your eyes that habitual happiness, they will understand that they are the beloved children of God" (Stern 2009, 125). When she accepted the 1979 Nobel Peace Prize, Mother Teresa advised, "Let us always meet each other with a smile, for a smile is the beginning of love."

Cultivate the habit of wearing a gentle smile during your yoga posture practice by paying attention to the expression on your face. It's not uncommon for students struggling with a difficult pose to reflect this tension with scowls and grimaces, clenching the jaw or furrowing the brow. I often crack silly jokes when I'm teaching yoga to encourage smiles. Learning how to find ease amid challenge and to stay connected with a sense of joy is central to yoga, and our facial expressions can signal how adept we are at this practice.

Off the mat, having a cheerful countenance can be a powerful way to make yourself feel better, and it can also bring smiles to the faces of those around you. Universally recognized across all cultures, a smile can be infectious and spread joy to everyone in your path. To practice, first make eye contact and really see the other person. Then offer a genuine smile. It doesn't have to be a huge Cheshire cat grin to be effective. In fact, a gentle smile—slightly turning up the corners of your mouth or just smiling with your eyes—may be more welcome.

100. Namaste

Yoga classes typically end with a gesture of respect and connection performed by bringing the palms together in front of the chest and bowing—student to teacher, teacher to student, and students to one another. Unlike the Western practice of shaking hands, this salutation is a noncontact form of greeting that can be appropriate between people of different genders, ages, and social standing.

This practice, which is common in India and throughout Asia, is called *namaste*, which translates, in short form, to "I bow to you" or "I honor you." When this is done at the end of a yoga class, people often say "namaste" to one another, although the gesture itself signifies this meaning.

A more complete translation of the meaning of "namaste" is offered in this anonymous explanation:

I honor the place in you that is the same in me.

I honor the place in you where the whole universe resides.

I honor the place in you of love, light, truth, and peace.

When you are in that place in you, and I am in that place in me,

We are one.

To practice, bring your palms together—slightly cupped, with fingers pointed up—in front of your heart chakra, at the center of your chest. This hand position is called Anjali Mudra (*anjali* means "offering," and *mudra* means "seal" or "sign"). Allow this sacred gesture to help you connect with your deepest self. Then bow gently toward the other person and offer your heartfelt respect.

As an especially deep form of honoring an esteemed person, such as a teacher or spiritual leader, make the Anjali Mudra gesture first in front of the "third eye" space on your forehead between your eyebrows, then move it down to your heart.

101. Pet Poses

Meaningful relationships need not be exclusively with humans. Animals can offer companionship and comfort, which help relieve stress, brighten mood, and enhance health. A growing body of evidence supports the therapeutic value of the human-animal bond. For example, studies show that petting your dog can lower your blood pressure, and that interacting with animals can increase your level of oxytocin, sometimes called the "love hormone" (Rovner 2012).

Animals help bring us closer to nature, ground us in the present moment, and offer a sympathetic ear and trusting gaze—without judgment or criticism. Compassion, known as *daya* in Sanskrit and considered one of the foundational moral behaviors, is a quality that many animals, including dogs, cats, and horses, can both give and receive. In fact, animals can be master teachers of many healthful habits, including stretching when you get up from sitting or lying in a fixed position, lapping up plenty of water, and taking time to smell the roses—or the rabbit holes.

Here are some ways to bring your relationship with animals into your yoga practice:

- **Pet your pet.** Assume a mutually comfortable position and mindfully stroke your companion animal. Be present to the sensations: soft fur, easy breath, warmth or coolness, purring or sighing. Let your hands give and receive loving energy.

- **Emulate an animal.** Watch something appealing an animal does and copy it. For example, our beagle, Sheba, is a master of the yoga stretch Downward-Facing Dog, or Adho Mukha Svanasana, modeled on the canine paws-forward, tail-up pose. I've learned a great deal about this posture from watching her. You might also try sniffing your food before you eat it, standing perfectly still and listening deeply, or taking a nap in the sun.

BREATHING SPARKS

102. Laughter Yoga

Laughter is often likened to "inner jogging." This connection between humor and health gained national attention in the 1970s when the late journalist Norman Cousins described how he healed himself from a life-threatening disease with a diet of positive emotions and laughter. Stimulated by funny movies and TV shows, including Marx Brothers comedies and episodes of *Candid Camera*, Cousins discovered that "ten minutes of genuine belly laughter had an anesthetic effect and would give me at least two hours of pain-free sleep" (Cousins 1979, 43).

Today, a growing body of scientific evidence confirms the notion that laughter is good medicine, offering a wide range of health benefits including improving respiration, stimulating circulation, decreasing stress hormones, boosting the immune response, elevating the pain threshold, relieving anxiety, elevating mood, and enhancing mental functioning (Mora-Ripoll 2011).

Supported by this scientific research, physician Madan Kataria of Mumbai, India, created Laughter Yoga International in 1995 to promote health, joy, and world peace through laughter, according to the group's website (www.laughteryoga.org). This well-being workout involves doing exercises that simulate laughter, which then turns into real and contagious laughter. It's practiced in more than six thousand Laughter Yoga Clubs in about sixty countries, run by volunteers trained as laughter yoga teachers. Emerging research suggests the practice may boost mood and life satisfaction in elderly depressed women (Shahidi et al. 2011) and improve heart rate variability in patients awaiting organ transplantation (Dolgoff-Kaspar et al. 2012).

Here are a few laughter yoga practices you might try:

- Speak in gibberish and encourage childlike playfulness, in keeping with the slogan "Fake it until you make it," since the body can't differentiate between real and pretend emotions.

- Fake laughter by making different laughing sounds, such as "ha-ha" and "hee-hee," which typically prompts genuine laughter.

- For a wonderfully silly way to encourage laughter among friends, try a "ha-ha line," which is particularly fun with a large group of people. The first person lies on the ground, the second person lies with his or her head on the first person's belly, then the third person lies with his or her head on the second person's belly, and so on. The first person says "ha," the second person says "ha ha," the third person says "ha ha ha," and so on, until the entire group erupts in laughter.

103. Mindful Listening

Communication involves far more than just taking turns talking. To truly understand another person, listening is key. Yet all too often we listen halfheartedly, while engaged in another task, lost in our own thoughts, or planning what we're going to say next. In an age of social networking, many people are willing to express themselves—whether by talking, tweeting, blogging, or posting—yet those willing to really *listen* are rare.

Mindful listening brings the principles of mindfulness—paying attention to the present moment, kindly and without judgment—to the act of listening. This allows you to focus completely on understanding what someone is telling you. Taking the time and expending the energy to sincerely listen to others—hearing their story and honoring their truth—is one of the greatest gifts we can give.

You can practice mindful listening with anyone, from a loved one to a stranger. It can be a particularly meaningful tool for enhancing relationships with family members, friends, or coworkers. Here are the basics for this practice:

1. Pay full attention to what the other person is saying. As best you can, let go of any other thoughts, such as how you'll respond or your own experiences that are similar to what the person is

telling you. Give your undivided attention and don't interrupt.

2. Listen to the emotions and meanings being expressed. Recognize that words are only part of what's being communicated.

3. Be open and kind. Let your body language express your intention to avoid being judgmental.

4. Don't talk. Just listen.

Mindful listening often requires more time than the sixty seconds allotted for a Yoga Spark. When this is the case, tell the person you only have a minute right now, and set a time in the near future where you can give him or her your full attention for longer. At that time, follow the steps above, and also remove any barriers to listening. Turn off the TV or radio, and sit close if possible. You can also listen on the phone or computer, although it's helpful to be able to see the person's body language and other forms of nonverbal communication.

When the other person is completely finished, consider speaking only if he or she asks for your reaction. You might restate what you heard the person say to make sure you understand. Recognize that you don't have to—and may not be able to—solve specific problems or fix anything. What you *can* do is be there and let the person know you care.

104. Honor a Difficult Person

When I was a young reporter at the *Washington Post*, I sometimes felt intimidated by the prospect of interviewing celebrities and politicians. Then one of my editors suggested that I visualize the person sleeping peacefully in polka-dot pajamas. The vulnerability and humanity created by this image helped me relate to powerful people more comfortably and with greater ease.

Along similar lines, Nischala Joy Devi, one of my yoga teachers and a good friend, suggests a practice to improve your relationship with a difficult person by visualizing him or her as a personal deity. In her book *The Secret Power of Yoga*, Devi recalls being in charge of a large department and having difficulty interacting with a grumpy person who resented taking orders from a woman. "I designed a spiritual practice in which he was the principal deity," she writes. "Each day as he entered my office, I would imagine placing a garland of flowers over his head and touching his feet. As he turned to walk away, murmuring under his breath, my hands joined together...to wish him well" (2007, 172).

One week into the practice, she says, she felt many positive effects, including no longer having to stifle a visceral reaction to run when she saw him. Eventually, he approached her and confessed that, although he didn't like her very much, he was starting to look forward to seeing her. "I cannot say we became best friends," she writes, "but we were both able to say, 'We like each other'" (173).

Here are some practices that can help you improve your relationship with a difficult person:

- Imagine the person as a young child, innocent and vulnerable, or as a revered elder.

- Notice something you like about the person, even if it's as simple as the color of his or her eyes.

- Offer compassion toward the person and resist the urge to judge.

- Breathe in a positive quality, such as peace or joy. As you breathe out, direct a kind wish toward the person.

105. Extend Compassion

Compassion benefits both the receiver and the giver, according to His Holiness the Dalai Llama, who advises, "If you want others to be happy practice compassion; and if you want yourself to be happy practice compassion" (2009, x).

Recent studies involving brain imaging support this notion, suggesting that meditation practices geared toward enhancing compassion may decrease stress-induced distress and have a positive impact on health (Hofmann, Grossman, and Hinton 2011). Emerging research also suggests that compassion meditation changes the brain, making people more empathetic to others, and may help those suffering from various psychological disorders, including depression (Land 2008).

In his book *The Power of Compassion* (1981), the Dalai Lama writes that compassion is based "on a clear acceptance or recognition that others, like oneself, want happiness and have the right to overcome suffering. On that basis one develops some kind of concern about the welfare of others" (62–63). He says that, despite fundamental differences between different religious ideas, compassion, love, and forgiveness are the common ground for all religions.

The Sanskrit word for compassion, *daya*, embraces the concept that someone else's suffering causes us to suffer too, and involves the wish to relieve another's suffering. This notion is supported by a University of Wisconsin study, which found that cultivating compassion and kindness through meditation has effects in the brain that can make a person more empathetic to other people's mental states (Lutz et al. 2008). You can practice extending compassion with this variation on a traditional loving-kindness meditation:

1. Think about someone you care about, such as a parent, sibling, or other loved one.

2. Allow your mind to be filled with wishes of well-being and freedom from suffering for this person.

3. Turn your attention toward all beings, without thinking about any specific person or creature.

4. Allow your mind to be filled with wishes of well-being and freedom from suffering for all beings.

PRINCIPLE SPARKS

106. Nonharming

The first, and arguably most important, of the yamas (yogic principles of respect toward others) is ahimsa. Translated as "nonharming" or "nonviolence," *ahimsa* encompasses much more than just avoiding acts of physical violence. It also includes abstaining from emotional violence—for example, verbal assaults, such as shouting or yelling, and hurtful behaviors, such as bullying or ignoring. In fact, the true spirit of ahimsa extends beyond abstaining from harmful actions and speech to cultivating respect and love for all, even those we view as enemies. For many people, this is the most challenging aspect of the practice.

Mahatma Gandhi famously embraced ahimsa as a political practice, using nonviolence without hatred to liberate India from British rule. Yogic texts say that when we act, speak, and think with respect and kindness, it can calm aggression in others. In particular, Yoga Sutra 2.35 notes, "Around one who is solidly established in nonviolence, hostility disappears" (Bouanchaud 1997, 119).

While many people are accustomed to avoiding physical violence, practicing ahimsa also invites us to abstain from other forms of violence that may be less obvious yet all too common in daily life, such as starting or listening to gossip, aggressive driving, killing harmless insects, making mean-spirited jokes, name-calling, or being sarcastic at others' expense.

107. Nonstealing

If you've ever waited for someone who is habitually late, felt drained after listening to a chronic complainer, or heard that someone else took credit for your work, you know that it's possible to steal more than material goods. The principle of *asteya*, translated as "honesty" or "nonstealing," asks us to not take anything that isn't freely given. This includes time, energy, and praise.

Practicing asteya is rooted in deep respect and consideration for other people's possessions and needs. Here are some examples of how you might practice:

- **Pay debts promptly.** Avoid making people who provide goods or services wait for payment.

- **Be on time.** Gandhi was known for being punctual and "considered it a mark not only of courtesy but of mastery to be on time wherever he went" (Easwaran 1994, 19).

- **Honor copyright.** Duplicating copyrighted music, games, photographs, print materials, and so on is a form of stealing.

- **Be honest.** If a cashier gives you too much change or forgets to charge you for an item, let him or her know.

- **Pay attention.** If you're speaking with someone, give that person your undivided attention.

- **Be generous.** A principle related to asteya is *dana*, or generosity, which involves giving without thought of reward. Consider giving generously of your money, time, or talents. Research suggests that generosity may have numerous health benefits, including enhancing immune function and boosting mood, creating what psychologist Robert Ornstein and physician David Sobel (1989) call a "helper's high."

108. Right Speech

Strong relationships are built on trust, and at the heart of trust is truthfulness. *Satya*, which translates as "truth" or "truthfulness," is the second of the five yamas—principles of respect toward others—outlined in Patanjali's Yoga Sutras. Yogic texts consider truth the highest virtue and advise that "all actions should be rooted in truthfulness" (Feuerstein 1997, 264). Yoga practice is designed to help you stay calm and peaceful, and lying can disturb this sense of ease by activating physiologic symptoms of arousal. (This is the basis of the lie detector, or polygraph, test.) Telling a falsehood often requires vigilance, and sometimes more lying, to keep your story straight.

But while it's important to stay grounded in truth—avoiding even white lies and distortions—it's equally important to be sensitive in the communication of truth, balancing satya with ahimsa, or nonharming (see Nonharming, Yoga Spark 106). When the truth could cause harm, the yama of nonharming has priority. This concept is illustrated in a saying from the ancient Sanskrit epic the Mahabharata: "It is better to tell the sick person what he or she can bear with gentleness, and as agreeably as possible" (Bouanchaud 1997, 112).

The practice of speaking with honesty and kindness is called "right speech," says author and meditation teacher Sally Kempton, who notes that "the Buddha made Right Speech one of the pillars of his Eight-fold Noble Path" (Kempton 2006). Practicing right speech "is essentially to approach speaking as a form of yoga," Kempton says. "You can change the world, or at least your experience of it, by becoming conscious of the words coming out of your mouth." To practice right speech, she suggests the following approaches:

- Eavesdrop on yourself. Become conscious of what actually comes out of your mouth—without activating your inner critic. Try to notice not just what you say, but also the tone with which you say it.

- Try to sense the emotional residue your words create. How do you feel after making certain remarks? How do others react?

- Ask yourself, *What makes me say what I say?* Is a buried emotion, such as anger or sadness, masking what you really want to say?

- Ask yourself these three questions before you speak: *Is it true? Is it kind? Is it necessary?*

EPILOGUE

In our ever-more-complex world, going to the gym or out for a run is easily sidelined. Going to church or even finding meaningful time with friends is a challenging accomplishment. But everyone, everywhere, can find a minute. And as every practice in this book illustrates, in taking a minute to find yourself, you can find yourself literally and spiritually in the moment—a practice and a process that can transform even the most maddening and mundane corners of life itself.

The masters of virtually every mystical tradition teach the transformational power of spiritual realization in the moment. This realization is achieved through practices that connect us to the deepest of spiritual resources. Such practices are not intended to separate us from life, but to imbue life with purpose, meaning, beauty, and joy.

The corollary to this timeless wisdom is that transformational practices do not actually change the human being. Rather, they uncover within us a spiritual Light that is already present within the human condition—a Light that is always shining, and thus always ready to be uncovered in the present.

Perhaps the most illuminating theme of this book is that this connection can be made, this Light can be uncovered, not through twenty-five years spent alone on a mountaintop but by opening the heart in a single minute. Perhaps the most reassuring theme of this book is that there is not one way, but a wide variety of avenues and lenses through which a single minute can spiritually transform the moment.

The diversity of practices in this book also reminds us that devoting a minute to concentrate the spirit—to touch peace of mind, to heal, to energize—fits well into all of life's moments: in quiet times or in stressful times, during activity or during rest, in the face of horror or in the face of beauty, to give thanks, to surrender. We are reminded that, for many reasons and through many portals, we can connect to our spiritual Source in any minute of any hour of any day.

As variable as is the human condition, so are there many avenues of practice in this book. As universal as is the human condition, so in every practice is the power of finding and taking a minute to reconnect ourselves to the Source of meaning, beauty, and peace of mind. Through a minute's practice in the moment is the path to living within the reality of impermanence by uncovering the eternal Light that shines within it. In that one minute, we can recover both joy in life and the ability to repeatedly restore our connection to the Source of that joy.

I see this book as a collection of flowers from many beautiful gardens—flowers that are gifts of God and nature. And within their diversity, they share a singular truth: it takes about sixty seconds to grow these blossoms.

—Mitchell W. Krucoff, MD, FACC, FAHA
Professor, Medicine/Cardiology
Duke University Medical Center

REFERENCES

American Academy of Otolaryngology—Head and Neck Surgery. 2012. "Fact Sheet: Your Nose, the Guardian of Your Lungs." www. entnet.org/HealthInformation/lungGuardian.cfm (accessed October 8, 2012).

American Society for Aesthetic Plastic Surgery. 2011. "Fifteenth Annual Cosmetic Surgery National Data Bank Statistics." www. surgery.org/sites/default/files/ASAPS-2011-Stats.pdf (accessed October 8, 2012).

Astin, J., S. L. Shapiro, D. M. Eisenberg, and K. L. Forys. 2003. "Mind-Body Medicine: State of the Science, Implications for Practice." *Journal of the American Board of Family Medicine* 16(2):131–147.

Bouanchaud, B. 1997. *The Essence of Yoga: Reflections on the Yoga Sutras of Patanjali.* Portland, OR: Rudra Press.

Brantley, J., and W. Millstine. 2009. *Five Good Minutes in Your Body: 100 Mindful Practices to Help You Accept Yourself and Feel at Home in Your Body.* Oakland, CA: New Harbinger.

Brantley, M., and T. Hanauer. 2008. *The Gift of Loving-Kindness: 100 Meditations on Compassion, Generosity, and Forgiveness.* Oakland, CA: New Harbinger.

Byrom, T. 1993. *Dhammapada: The Sayings of the Buddha.* Boston: Shambhala Pocket Classics.

Carson, J. W., and K. M. Carson. 2012. "The Practice of Riding the Waves." www.yogaofawareness.org/program/overview (accessed October 7, 2012).

Carson, J. W, K. M. Carson, K. D. Jones, R. M. Bennett, C. L. Wright, and S. D. Mist. 2010. "A Pilot Randomized Controlled Trial of the Yoga of Awareness Program in the Management of Fibromyalgia." *Pain* 151(2):530–539.

Centers for Disease Control and Prevention. 2012. "Wash Your Hands." www.cdc.gov/features/handwashing (accessed October 7, 2012).

Cope, S. 2003. *Yoga for Emotional Flow: Free Your Emotions through Yoga Breathing, Body Awareness, and Energetic Release.* Audio CD. Louisville, CO: Sounds True.

Cousins, N. 1979. *Anatomy of an Illness as Perceived by the Patient.* New York: W. W. Norton.

Dalai Lama. 1981. *The Power of Compassion: A Collection of Lectures by His Holiness the Dalai Lama.* San Francisco: Thorsons.

Dalai Lama. 2009. *The Art of Happiness, Tenth Anniversary Edition: A Handbook for Living.* New York: Riverhead Books.

Desikachar, T. K. V. 1995. *The Heart of Yoga: Developing a Personal Practice.* Rochester, VT: Inner Traditions International.

Devi, N. J. 2007. *The Secret Power of Yoga: A Woman's Guide to the Heart and Spirit of the Yoga Sutras.* New York: Three Rivers Press.

Dolgoff-Kaspar, R., A. Baldwin, M. S. Johnson, N. Edling, and G. K. Sethi. 2012. "Effect of Laughter Yoga on Mood and Heart Rate Variability in Patients Awaiting Organ Transplantation: A Pilot Study." *Alternative Therapies in Health and Medicine* 18(5):61–66.

Dorey, G., M. J. Speakman, R. C. Feneley, A. Swinkels, and C. D. Dunn. 2005. "Pelvic Floor Exercises for Erectile Dysfunction." *British Journal of Urology International* 96(4):595–597.

Dotinga, R. 2011. "Using Electronics before Bed May Hamper Sleep." HealthDay, *US News & World Report*, March 7. http://health.usnews.com/health-news/family-health/sleep/articles/2011/03/07/using-electronics-before-bed-may-hamper-sleep (accessed October 7, 2012).

Easwaran, E. 1994. *Take Your Time: Finding Balance in a Hurried World*. Tomales, CA: Nilgiri Press.

Feuerstein, G. 1997. *The Shambhala Encyclopedia of Yoga*. Boston: Shambhala.

Halifax, J. 2011. "Sympathetic Joy: The Third Abode." Upaya Institute and Zen Center website, December 17. www.upaya.org/news/2011/12/17/sympathetic-joy-the-third-abode-by-roshi-joan-halifax (accessed October 13, 2012).

Hartranft, C. (translator). 2003. *The Yoga-Sutra of Patanjali: A New Translation with Commentary*. Boston: Shambhala.

Hamilton, J. 2008. "Think You're Multitasking? Think Again." NPR, October 2. www.npr.org/templates/story/story.php?storyId=95256794 (accessed October 7, 2012).

Hofmann, S. G., P. Grossman, and D. E. Hinton. 2011. "Loving-Kindness and Compassion Meditation: Potential for Psychological Interventions." *Clinical Psychology Review* 31(7):1126–1132.

Holcombe, K. 2011. "Making Space: Clear the Pathway to Achieving Your Goals with the Practice of Detachment." *Yoga Journal*, November, 60.

Insurance Institute for Highway Safety. 2012. "Q&A: Neck Injury." www.iihs.org/research/qanda/neck_injury.aspx (accessed October 7, 2012).

Iyengar, B. K. S. 1979. *Light on Yoga: Yoga Dipika*. New York: Schocken Books.

Johnson, M. A. 2012. "Get with the Times: You're Driving All Wrong." http://www.nbcnews.com/business/get-times-youre-driving-all-wrong-518710 (accessed March 16, 2013).

Joyce, J. 2006. *Dubliners*. Clayton, DE: Prestwick House.

Katzmarzyk, P. T., and I. M. Lee. 2012. "Sedentary Behaviour and Life Expectancy in the USA: A Cause-Deleted Life Table Analysis." *BMJ Open*, July 9. doi:10.1136/bmjopen-2012-000828 (accessed October 7, 2012).

Kempton, S. 2006. "Me Talk Pretty." *Yoga Journal*, May, 57–62. Available at http.sallykempton.com/resources/articles/me-talk-pretty (accessed October 13, 2012).

Krucoff, C. 2007. "Positively Healing: Everything That Happens in Your Mind Is Reflected in Your Body, Says T. K. V. Desikachar." *Yoga Journal*, March, 111–115.

Land, D. 2008. "Study Shows Compassion Meditation Changes the Brain." *University of Wisconsin–Madison News*, March 25. www.news.wisc.edu/14944 (accessed October 9, 2012).

Luo, Y., L. C. Hawkley, L. J. Waite, and J. T. Cacioppo. 2012. "Loneliness, Health, and Mortality in Old Age: A National Longitudinal Study." *Social Science and Medicine* 74(6):907–914.

Lutz, A., J. Brefczynski-Lewis, T. Johnstone, and R. J. Davidson. 2008. "Regulation of the Neural Circuitry of Emotion by Compassion Meditation: Effects of Meditative Expertise." *PLoS One* 3(3):e1897. doi:10.1371/journal.pone.0001897 (accessed October 9, 2012).

Macy, D. 2008. "Yoga in America Study." Press release, February 26. www.yogajournal.com/press/yoga_in_america (accessed October 4, 2012).

Mayo Clinic Staff. 2011. "Meditation: A Simple, Fast Way to Reduce Stress." www.mayoclinic.com/health/meditation/HQ01070 (accessed October 7, 2012).

Mora-Ripoll, R. 2011. "Potential Health Benefits of Simulated Laughter: A Narrative Review of the Literature and Recommendations for Future Research." *Complementary Therapies in Medicine* 19(3):170–177.

Moscaritolo, A. 2012. "Google's Schmidt Urges Graduates to Unplug 'One Hour a Day.'" www.pcmag.com/article2/0,2817,2404682,00.asp (accessed October 7, 2012).

Mother Teresa. 1979. "Mother Teresa Nobel Lecture." www.nobelprize.org/nobel_prizes/peace/laureates/1979/teresa-lecture.html (accessed October 8, 2012).

Myers, E. 1997. *Yoga and You: Energizing and Relaxing Yoga for New and Experienced Students.* Boston: Shambhala.

National Institutes of Health. 2012. "Back Pain." www.nlm.nih.gov/medlineplus/backpain.html (accessed October 7, 2012).

National Institutes of Health, Office of Research Services. 2012. "Ergonomics Program: The Computer Workstation." www.ors.od.nih.gov/sr/dohs/Documents/ORS_Ergonomics_Poster_Rd5.pdf (accessed December 16, 2012).

National Osteoporosis Foundation. 2011. "Live with Osteoporosis: Moving Safely." www.nof.org/aboutosteoporosis/movingsafely/moving (accessed October 7, 2012).

Nhat Hanh, T. 1991. *Peace Is Every Step: The Path of Mindfulness in Everyday Life.* New York: Bantam Books.

Nicklaus, J., with K. Bowden. 2005. *Golf My Way: The Instructional Classic, Revised and Updated.* New York: Simon and Schuster.

Ornstein, R., and D. Sobel. 1989. *Healthy Pleasures.* New York: Perseus Books.

Porter, J. M., and D. E. Gyi. 2002. "The Prevalence of Musculoskeletal Troubles among Car Drivers." *Occupational Medicine* 52(1):4–12.

Powers, S. 2011. *Insight Yoga Earth: Balancing Yin Energy.* DVD. San Francisco: Pranamaya.

Purcell, M. 2012. "The Health Benefits of Journaling." http://psych central.com/lib/2006/the-health-benefits-of-journaling (accessed October 7, 2012).

Quindlen, A. 2008. "Stuff Is Not Salvation." *Newsweek/The Daily Beast,* December 12. http.thedailybeast.com/news-week/2008/12/12/stuff-is-not-salvation.html (accessed October 7, 2012).

Reynolds, S. A., F. Levy, and E. S. Walker. 2006. "Hand Sanitizer Alert" [letter]. *Emerging Infectious Diseases* 12(3):527–529. http://dx.doi.org/10.3201/eid1203.050955 (accessed on October 8, 2012).

Rikli, R. E., and C. J. Jones. 2001. *Senior Fitness Test Manual.* Champaign, IL: Human Kinetics.

Rovner, J. 2012. "Pet Therapy: How Animals and Humans Heal Each Other." NPR, March 5. www.npr.org/blogs/health/2012/03/09/146583986/pet-therapy-how-animals-and-humans-heal-each-other (accessed October 8, 2012).

Ryan, M. J. 2003. *The Power of Patience: How to Slow the Rush and Enjoy More Happiness, Success, and Peace of Mind Every Day.* New York: Broadway Books.

Scaravelli, V. 1991. *Awakening the Spine: The Stress-Free New Yoga That Works with the Body to Restore Health, Vitality, and Energy.* New York: Harper Collins.

Schiffmann, E. 1995. "An Interview with Erich" (interviewed by J. Dreaver). http://freedomstyleyoga.com/articles/an-interview-with-erich-3 (accessed October 8, 2012).

Schiffmann, E. 1996. *Yoga: The Spirit and Practice of Moving into Stillness.* New York: Pocket Books.

Seligman, M. E. P. 2002. *Authentic Happiness: Using the New Positive Psychology to Realize Your Potential for Lasting Fulfillment.* New York: Simon & Schuster.

Shahidi, M., A. Mojtahed, A. Modabbernia, M. Mojtahed, A. Shafiabady, A. Delavar, and H. Honari. 2011. "Laughter Yoga versus Group Exercise Program in Elderly Depressed Women: A Randomized Controlled Trial." *International Journal of Geriatric Psychiatry* 26(3):322–327.

Stern, A. 2009. *Everything Starts from Prayer: Mother Teresa's Meditations on Spiritual Life for People of All Faiths.* Ashland, OR: White Cloud Press.

Tirtha, S. S. 1998. *The Ayurveda Encyclopedia: Natural Secrets to Healing, Prevention, and Longevity.* Bayville, NY: Ayurveda Holistic Center Press.

US Surgeon General. 2012. "Fact Sheet: Deep Vein Thrombosis and Pulmonary Embolism." US Department of Health & Human Services, www.surgeongeneral.gov/library/calls/deepvein/factsheetdvt_pe.html (accessed October 8, 2012).

Vangsness, S. 2012. "Mastering the Mindful Meal." www.brighamand womens.org/Patients_Visitors/pcs/nutrition/services/healthe-weightforwomen/special_topics/intelihealth0405.aspx (accessed October 7, 2012).

Wang, D. 2009. "The Use of Yoga for Physical and Mental Health among Older Adults: A Review of the Literature." *International Journal of Yoga Therapy* 19:91–96.

Watson, S. 2009. "Amazing Facts about Heart Health and Heart Disease." www.webmd.com/heart/features/amazing-facts-about-heart-health-and-heart-disease_ (accessed October 7, 2012).

Yan, L. L., K. Liu, K. A. Matthews, M. L. Daviglus, T. F. Ferguson, and C. I. Kiefe. 2003. "Psychosocial Factors and Risk of Hypertension: The Coronary Artery Risk Development in Young Adults (CARDIA) Study." *Journal of the American Medical Association* 290(16):2138–2148.

Carol Krucoff, ERYT, is a yoga therapist, fitness expert, and award-winning journalist. She creates individualized yoga programs for people with health challenges at Duke Integrative Medicine in Durham, NC, where she also co-directs the Therapeutic Yoga for Seniors teacher training. A frequent contributor to Yoga Journal, Krucoff served as founding editor of the health section of the Washington Post, where her syndicated column, Bodyworks, appeared for twelve years. She has written for numerous national publications, including the *New York Times* and *Reader's Digest*, and is author of the book *Healing Yoga for Neck and Shoulder Pain*. Krucoff is creator of the home practice CD *Healing Moves Yoga* and cocreator of the DVD *Relax into Yoga for Seniors*. Certified as a personal trainer by the American Council on Exercise, she also has earned a second-degree black belt in karate and sits on the peer review board for the *International Journal of Yoga Therapy*. Krucoff has practiced yoga for more than thirty-five years. Visit her online at www.healingmoves.com.

Foreword writer **Kelly McGonigal, PhD**, is an award-winning instructor at Stanford University, where she teaches yoga, psychology, and healthy back classes. She is a leader in mind-body science and practice, and provides teacher trainings and continuing education for yoga, fitness, and health care professionals. McGonigal is editor-in-chief of the *International Journal of Yoga Therapy* and a frequent writer for publications such as *Yoga Journal* and *IDEA Fitness Journal*. Visit her online at www.kellymcgonigal.com.

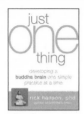
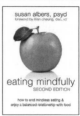
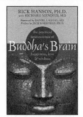
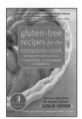
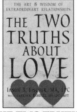
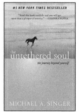

"This is a wonderful collection of micro-practices designed to elicit the meaning of the teachings [of yoga]. Who would want more? Pause, feel the truth, be glad. Keep it simple, short, and frequent."

—**Erich Schiffmann**, author of YOGA: *The Spirit and Practice of Moving into Stillness*

"With a lighthearted understanding and compassion, we are offered 108 easy practices to 'spark' our remembering, connecting us to our spiritual source, each and every moment."

—**Nischala Joy Devi**, international teacher and author of *The Healing Path of Yoga* and *The Secret Power of Yoga*

"Krucoff's *Yoga Sparks* is a simple, powerful tool for you to move from 'doing' yoga to 'being' yoga. For too long in the West we've separated yoga as something we do, when by practicing Sparks you will discover that yoga is in fact what you are, moment to moment. My sense is you will soon be creating your own Sparks as you delight in your realization that 108 is really only just a good start! Let your fire burn brighter with *Yoga Sparks*!"

—**Matthew J. Taylor, PT, PhD, ERYT**, former president of the International Association of Yoga Therapists, and the 'mindbody' rehab guy bridging traditional rehab with yoga

"*Yoga Sparks* is the perfect book for anyone interested in a practical way to incorporate yoga into his or her daily busy life. Krucoff goes beyond the poses and really provides a guide to experiencing all of the benefits that yoga has to offer for improving health and wellbeing."

—**Adam Perlman**, associate vice president for health and wellness for the Duke University Health System and executive director at Duke Integrative Medicine

"Yoga is popularly described as a practice for on and off the mat, but how many people actually integrate and transfer their insights from yoga to ordinary moments? Our reactivity easily eclipses our ease and calm when triggered by the unexpected, or worse, the unwanted details of life. If yoga is to become more than merely exercise, we need to inhabit mini moments with awareness and find ways to reconnect ourselves in body and mind. In *Yoga Sparks*, Krucoff offers profound wisdom in sparkling bites that can easily be applied while moving through our day, enhancing our capacity for mindful living. She teaches us that our busy life is not in the way of our yoga practice, and in fact the way to live yogically is through the everyday moments of our life."

> —**Sarah Powers**, author of *Insight Yoga*

"It is so easy to go from zero to sixty and stay in high gear until you break down. *Yoga Sparks* generously offers a way for you to make a Uturn: quickies that translate into quick ease of posture, concentration, joy, and presence. Krucoff's sensitive sparks jump off the page and inject moments of repose into your days, nights, and life."

> —**Jill Miller, ERYT**, creator of Yoga Tune Up® and the Therapy Ball System™

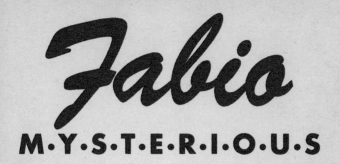

Fabio

M·Y·S·T·E·R·I·O·U·S

in collaboration with

Wendy Corsi Staub

Pinnacle Books
Kensington Publishing Corp.

http://www.pinnaclebooks.com

Chapter One

The sun had been shining when she left Manhattan three hours ago, with temperatures expected to hit sixty-five by noon.

Sixty-five and sunny, in November.

Jorey Maddock sighed and impatiently reached to adjust the Range Rover's windshield wipers. She realized that they were already at top speed, sweeping rapidly back and forth across the glass in a futile attempt to clear the snowflakes.

Snowflakes . . .

Ha!

Snowflakes was too benign, too pleasant, a word for what was happening out there.

Blizzard was more like it.

A blizzard, in November.

Hardly unusual way up here along the Adirondack Northway, Jorey supposed. She should have expected it. She should have checked The Weather Channel or the news this morning before she left the city.

But then, Jorey certainly had never been the look before you leap type.

If she were, she most definitely wouldn't have broken things off with Kurt Govan.

After five months of dating a world-famous, gorgeous, action movie star who was, quite possibly, even wealthier than she was, she probably could—and should—have given some thought to what a break up would mean.

For one thing, it meant she was spending this particular Saturday morning driving through a blinding, white snowstorm instead of basking on the dazzling, white sands of a Caribbean beach.

She wondered if Kurt had gone, anyway, then wondered why she bothered to wonder.

Of course he had gone.

He'd just wrapped an exhausting five month shoot in New York, and he only had two weeks off before he started filming his next two movies back-to-back, one in South America and the other in Ireland. He desperately needed this vacation, and he'd rented a private beachfront villa with two pools, a spa, tennis courts, and a riding stable.

So, Jorey thought, slowing the Rover as the road curved ahead, he was there right now. That was for certain.

And the weather in St. Thomas was a helluva lot better than it was here, in northern New York State. That, too, was for certain.

Was he alone?

She snorted and shook her head.

"No way," she said.

No way was Mr. Movie Star alone.

They had broken up—let's see . . . Wednesday. That gave him almost two full days to have replaced her.

She was only mildly surprised to find that the thought of Kurt sharing his tropical paradise with another woman didn't necessarily bother her. It wasn't even that their relationship had been so horrible, or anything like that.

In the beginning, in fact, it had been exhilarating. Falling in love was *always* exhilarating.

In the middle, it had been good. *Being* in love was always good. Sometimes even great.

But then, over the past six weeks or so, little things about him had started bothering her. Not big things, like the strange hours he kept as an actor filming a movie, or the way flashbulbs were always exploding in their faces when they were in public.

No, little things.

Things she had found adorable in the beginning.

Like his habit of calling her "love" and the bathroom the "loo"—courtesy of the British accent he had developed for his current film.

And his penchant for pistachios, not the white, civilized kind, but the red ones that stained his fingertips.

And the way his dark hair spiked straight up in the morning.

And his citrus-scented cologne.

And his laugh.

And . . .

Okay, so he was really getting on your nerves, Jorey told herself, shaking her head. *And the thought of spending two solid weeks alone with him, even in paradise, made you feel positively queasy.*

She was beginning to wonder if she would ever want to spend two weeks alone with *anybody*.

In her twenty-six years, she had gone through more men than pairs of shoes. And that was really saying something, considering that she happened to be the granddaughter of the late Mayville Maddock, founder of one of Manhattan's most famous upscale department stores.

The thought of dear Papa May unexpectedly brought tears to her eyes, and Jorey took one hand off the steering wheel to swipe them away. Why was she crying about him *now*? It had been nearly a decade since she'd watched him clutch his chest and drop dead on that sultry August afternoon.

But the memory suddenly felt fresh, and Jorey realized it was because of *where* she was.

Here, on the Northway. Heading for Blizzard Bay.

Before Papa May died she had spent every summer of her life in the tiny, lakeside village in the Adirondacks, where her grandparents had owned an estate. How carefree those summers had been.

So different from her life in Manhattan.

For one thing, city life meant constant moving around—her parents had transported the family from one home to another, from one neighborhood to another, never seeming satisfied with what they had. Something better was always waiting—that was their philosophy.

So the Maddocks had gone from the Chelsea brownstone where Jorey, the youngest of their three daughters, was born, to the Upper-East-Side high-rise to the renovated carriage house in the Village to the SoHo loft to the penthouse on Central Park South. At one point, they'd lived in the Dakota; at another, in a Sutton Place duplex that had once belonged to a former president of the United States—Jorey could never remember which one.

And after the divorce, which had happened the year she graduated from high school—the year her whole life changed—there had been even more homes that Jorey couldn't call home. She bounced from her mother's place to her father's place, to the various estates each of them rented every summer and the ski chalets each of them rented every winter.

Then there were the various private schools Jorey had attended over the years. She had left some because she insisted, and others because the administration insisted.

Of course, being expelled was all very civilized when you were a Maddock. It wasn't as if they opened the door and kicked you out into the street. There were meetings with your parents, during which the headmaster and various teachers delicately discussed your various "behavioral difficulties." Then everyone involved would agree that things simply weren't working out, that young Ms. Maddock would be better suited to a more "creative and flexible" environment.

The trouble was, Jorey realized in retrospect, that no school was creative and flexible enough for a free spirit like her.

Nor was any career.

Nor any relationship.

At least, none that she'd tried so far.

So, here she was. Jobless. Romantically eligible once again. And heading back to rediscover the one and only constant in her life.

Blizzard Bay.

Not that she would be staying in the sprawling, old fieldstone house that had held so many happy memories for her. No, she didn't even have that. Grandmother had sold it within a month of Papa May's death.

It would be enough for Jorey to spend some time in the Adirondack village that was more a hometown to her than New York City could ever be.

At least, she hoped it would be enough.

She hoped that a week or two in Blizzard Bay would bring her . . .

What?

What was it that she was searching for?

She had no idea. She only knew that she was restless, more restless than she had ever been.

And that something, some inexplicable yearning, was drawing her back to this place where she had spent so many happy days.

Sawyer Howland brushed the snow off the back window of his car, noticing that at least six inches had fallen already. The meteorologist on The Weather Channel had predicted over two feet before the storm was over.

That was a helluva a lot of snow.

At least the car's engine had started. The temperature was in the single digits, and this ancient Chevy had been known to stall in frigid weather.

But now it idled reassuringly, exhaust from the tailpipe blackening the drifted snow at Sawyer's feet. Feet that were already numb, despite two pairs of woolen socks and the sturdy L.L. Bean boots he was wearing.

He turned his head slightly and the wind whipped his shoulder-length hair against his face, and he could feel ice crystals stinging his cheeks.

He frowned and glanced back up at the big, fieldstone house, thinking that he could be up in his cozy, third floor apartment, sipping hot chocolate in front of a blazing fire.

No real reason to venture out into a blizzard.

Except that he had no choice.

He *had* to answer the cryptic yet compelling need that had been building inside him ever since he bolted up in bed at dawn, heart pounding and mind racing.

He had at first tried to block it out, to ignore it.

That hadn't worked.

And anyway, he had learned the hard way to listen to his instincts.

So here he was, outside in the gale, shivering in the icy wind despite being dressed in so many layers he'd be lucky if he could fit behind the wheel. Setting out for . . .

Where?

He wouldn't know until he began driving.

He went around to the front of the car, stomping his feet against the cold, opened the door, and tossed the brush onto the floor of the backseat. Then he bent his six-foot-four frame stiffly and got behind the wheel, slamming the door behind him. He'd been running the heater while the car was warming up, but it didn't seem to have done much. He could still see his breath as he shifted into gear and stepped on the gas.

The car skidded several times as he steered along the long, winding, unplowed driveway that led out to the road.

Hard to believe this enormous property had once been a private summer estate, owned by some rich businessman from New York City. The grounds, which were still considerable, had once consisted of acres and acres of meadows and woods and streams. The three-story, gray stone mansion had turrets and gables and a wraparound porch, and was set so far back that you couldn't see it from the road.

It was a shame, in a way, that the once grand place had been chopped up into half a dozen apartments. Then again, Sawyer had felt incredibly fortunate to find it when he first came to Blizzard Bay several months ago.

Not that off-season rentals were scarce up here. There were plenty of cottages and cabins available during the winter months. Once the summer and foliage seasons were over, few tourists ventured to this rugged part of the country.

But Sawyer didn't know how long he'd need to stay in the area, and the last thing he wanted was to be left homeless when summer arrived. He knew he needed a year-round rental, and this was perfect.

Being several miles outside the village, tucked away on a country road, offered a certain degree of privacy, privacy that would undoubtedly be hard to come by in a place the size of Blizzard Bay.

And privacy was what he needed in order to go about his business undisturbed.

Besides, there was something about the big old house that had seemed to beckon him from the moment he laid eyes on it. He had sensed, somehow, that this was where he was meant to live.

He had finally reached the twin stone pillars that marked the end of the long driveway. Beyond, Field-stone Road was freshly plowed but snow-covered, and snow was still coming down so hard the windshield wipers could barely keep up with it.

You're a fool, Sawyer told himself as he headed the Chevy out onto the two lane country road. *You're risking your life, and for what?*

He had no idea.

He just knew that he had to go.

He had to *hurry,* before it was too late. . . .

"Damn, damn, damn," Jorey muttered, staring at the Range Rover upside down in the ditch.

She shouldn't have tried to change the CD. If she'd been content to listen to Soul Asylum, she wouldn't be in this predicament. But Soul Asylum reminded her of Kurt. And Kurt was over.

So she had decided to play the Grateful Dead. Good, classic driving music to take her mind off the poor visibility and treacherous roads.

But the moment she leaned forward to eject the built-in CD player, she had lost control of the car.

She hadn't realized she was on a curve—that was part of the problem. She couldn't see two feet beyond the windshield.

So of course she'd missed the curve.

And of course she'd gone off the road, down the steep embankment, and flipped over.

Thank God she hadn't been hurt, she thought now, tucking her bare hands beneath her armpits and staring at the wreck.

But why couldn't this have happened a few miles back, when she was still on the Northway? At least there was traffic there. Someone would probably have stopped to help her, maybe even a state trooper.

She thought of the officer who had stopped her just before Saratoga Springs. He hadn't given her a ticket, just a warning.

She was hardly speeding. That was what she'd told

him when he leaned in her window and narrowed his eyes at her.

"You're driving too fast for these conditions, young lady," was what he said.

Young lady?

As if she were a naughty twelve-year-old.

Young lady!

At five-foot-one, Jorey was used to strangers not realizing she was a grown woman. But this officer had seen her driver's license and knew how old she was—and called her "young lady" anyway. His condescending attitude made her blood boil.

She opened her mouth to offer an indignant reply when he asked, "Where are you headed?"

"Blizzard Bay."

"Still got about ten miles to go," he'd said dubiously, brushing the snow from his graying hair. "Might be best if you get right off the road now. There are plenty of hotels here in Saratoga."

"Well, I can't do that," she'd told him.

He raised an eyebrow at her. "Any good reason why not?"

"Because. Someone's expecting me in Blizzard Bay. They'll be worried if I don't show up until tomorrow."

"Seems to me like they'll be more worried if you don't show up, *ever*," he said. "The farther north you go, the worse the roads are going to get."

She shrugged. "I'll be fine. I've got four-wheel drive."

It was his turn to shrug. "Look, the state hasn't shut the road down. I can't stop you. But a woman driving alone in weather like this—it's dangerous."

At least he hadn't called her "young lady" again.

Still, his attitude infuriated her. Just because she was a

woman, and alone, didn't mean she was any less capable than anyone else.

Now, as she surveyed the car she'd managed to run off the road, she told herself it could have happened to anyone. Yes, it could have happened to a man.

Unfortunately, it had happened to her.

Now she was stranded on this deserted, snow-covered road, a good three miles outside of town.

Too far to walk, especially without boots and gloves and a decent winter coat. All she had with her was a black leather jacket she hadn't dared put on before climbing out of the Range Rover. Snow like this would definitely ruin the leather.

She wondered how far she was from the Northway exit, whether it would be worth heading back in that direction. Hard to tell. She'd gotten off quite a while ago, but she hadn't been able to cover much road.

"Don't they even plow up here?" she grumbled, turning to look at the snow-drifted, two lane highway behind her.

Hers were the only tire tracks that were visible.

It might be hours before someone else came along. Even days.

If her cell phone battery weren't dead she could call for help, she thought wistfully. But she'd forgotten to recharge it before she left home this morning. And she didn't have one of those thingies used to hook it up to a car's cigarette lighter.

You should definitely get one, she told herself a little belatedly.

She simply hadn't thought of it until now. After all, it wasn't as if she did much driving in Manhattan. In fact, she hardly ever drove. It was too much of a hassle to go all the way down to the parking garage beneath her building, and then deal with the traffic congestion on the city streets.

Cabs and limos made much more sense.

She just kept the Range Rover for emergency situations. Like road trips.

This was the first one she'd taken, and look where she'd landed.

As soon as she got back to New York, she'd sell the stupid car. If she ever wanted to come up here again, she'd just fly into Albany and hire a driver. She should have thought of that in the first place.

It was just that there was something appealing about the idea of setting out on her own in a car, on a solo adventure.

Well, this certainly was shaping up to be an adventure, she thought, shivering.

What if she didn't make it out alive?

What if no one came along to save her?

Blizzard Bay was pretty deserted at this time of year. Not that she'd ever been here off-season. But she knew what it was like, because she had plenty of friends who lived in the area year-round. They complained about it turning into a ghost town the moment the last autumn leaf hit the ground.

No wonder, Jorey thought, glancing around.

Nothing but snow, snow, and more snow. Swirling in the air, drifting on the ground, coating everything, including her, in white.

This is the tundra. And I'm going to freeze to death out here.

She supposed she could go back down to the car. At least that would provide shelter from the weather.

But it was upside down—how comfortable would *that* be?

Besides, no one would even be able to see it down there if they were driving along the road. Already, the snow had nearly filled in the skid marks her tires had made. In no time, there wouldn't be a single sign that there'd been an accident there.

No, she couldn't go back down to the car.

She had to stay up here, on the road.

But you can't just stand here, she decided, hugging herself to keep warm. *You've got to keep moving.*

Moving where?

She supposed she could start walking to town.

Maybe she'd pass a house along the way, and she could stop for help.

The only trouble was, she'd opted to take the back road into town instead of staying on the Northway until the next exit, which was a more widely travelled route. There wasn't much traffic on this particular road, even in the summer. It was a dirt road, too winding, too narrow, lined with dense woods on both sides.

But maybe, tucked away in those dense woods, someone had built a summer house. With any luck she would stumble across it, even if it was boarded up and deserted. Maybe it would even have a phone. *Or at the very least, a couple of blankets,* she thought, her teeth chattering.

That decided it. She had to start walking toward town. But first, she should probably go grab her jacket from the Range Rover. So what if the leather got ruined? She could buy another one.

Though not up here in Blizzard Bay.

The fringed leather jacket was a one of a kind couture piece given to her by the designer himself, a close friend of her mother.

Lord knew she'd never be able to find designer clothing, let alone a decent coat, up here in the boonies.

There *were* some decent boutiques in Saratoga, she remembered. But most of them were probably closed down for the winter.

Well, she reminded herself, the search for fashionable clothing was hardly her most pressing problem at the moment.

Basically, her most pressing problem was *survival.*

She turned abruptly and started down the embankment to the car to get her jacket. She could check her luggage, too, for a sweater or something to put on over the cashmere turtleneck she was wearing. Maybe she could even wrap her head in one of her silk scarves, and put a pair of socks on her hands to keep warm. She should definitely switch her Italian leather pumps for a pair of boots. She'd brought two pairs. She'd have to wear the black suede ones; the heels on her brown leather boots were simply too high for a long walk.

Not that the heels of the black boots were all *that* much lower. Jorey rarely wore flats, relying on heels to make up for what she lacked in the height department.

She tried not to think about what the snow would do to the black suede and what she'd look like, trudging along with socks on her hands and a designer scarf wrapped around her head like a babushka.

Lovely. Just—

Jorey froze, hearing a sound in the distance.

An *engine.*

Was someone coming?

Someone *was* coming!

She turned and scrambled back up the slope, arriving on the road just in time to see headlights come around the bend.

She ran into the middle of the road, waving her arms over her head and shouting, "Help! Help! Stop!"

Then she stepped back as the pickup truck slowed to a stop and the door opened.

"Thank God," she blurted as a man leaned out. "You saved my life."

The stranger was still a few yards away, and at first she couldn't make out his face through the blowing snow. He took a couple of steps toward her, and she toward him, and then she froze.

This was no stranger.

"Hob Nixon," she murmured, staring in disbelief.

Of all the people who could happen along this deserted, middle-of-nowhere road, how could it be Hob Nixon?

He looked exactly the same as he had a decade ago—pockmarked, sunken face, teeth missing, and black, greasy hair falling across his forehead.

He smelled the same, too. Even from there, she inhaled the stench of BO and stale cigarettes.

"You know me?" he asked incredulously, peering at her through the storm.

"I . . . yeah."

"Who are you?"

She hesitated before saying, "Jorey Maddock."

He stared at her, then nodded slowly. The expression in his black eyes and the way he looked her over from head to toe gave her the creeps.

Hob Nixon had always made her uncomfortable—her, and everyone else in Blizzard Bay. He was just a few years older than she. Even as a kid he'd been strange. Starting fires in the woods, torturing animals, that sort of thing. He'd lived in a rundown trailer on the outskirts of town with his alcoholic father, who'd died at one point, leaving him alone.

Jorey remembered how she and her friends used to

take the long way into town on their bikes, just so they wouldn't have to ride by Hob Nixon's trailer. The property the trailer sat on bordered her grandparents' estate, and Hob always seemed to be lurking nearby.

Now, after all these years, Jorey couldn't remember just what it was that they'd feared he'd do to them. She just knew that nobody ever wanted to risk being caught alone with the creepy misfit.

Now, here she was, alone with Hob Nixon after all these years.

"What happened to ya?" he asked.

Wordlessly, she motioned behind her and saw him take a few steps to the edge of the road.

"Looks like ya wrecked yer car," he informed her.

No shit, Sherlock.

She bit back the sarcastic remark and nodded. The last thing she wanted to do was antagonize him.

He tilted his head toward his rusted pickup. "Need a lift into town?"

She paused.

Of course she needed a lift.

If she stayed out here, alone, she could die.

But . . .

How dangerous was accepting a ride from someone like Hob Nixon?

For all she knew, he'd blossomed into his full potential as a psychotic killer or serial rapist. Getting into that pickup truck would just be asking for trouble.

Then again, almost ten years had passed since she'd known him. Maybe her teenage paranoia had been unfounded. Maybe he was just a nice, normal guy.

She looked up at him, found him watching her intently, and saw his lips curl into a grin.

A menacing grin that was missing a few teeth.

A grin that made Jorey want to turn and run in the opposite direction.

But that wasn't even an option.

Calm down, she told herself. *You're getting all worked up for no reason. He's probably harmless.*

Besides, she had no choice.

She had to go with him. . . .

She lifted her head suddenly, her ears picking up a sound other than the howling wind and sifting snow.

Yes.

It was unmistakable.

The sound of an approaching car.

Jorey's heart leapt and she fought to keep from sighing in relief.

She was saved *again.*

This time, for real.

Unless the newcomer was an escaped convict or on the FBI's Ten Most Wanted list.

The car came into view, and her heart sank when she realized it was headed in the opposite direction—coming *out* of Blizzard Bay—which meant the driver wouldn't be very eager to give her a lift back to the town he had just left.

She hesitated, wondering whether she should flag him, anyway.

Then she discovered that it wasn't necessary. The car, an old Chevy, was slowing, stopping.

"What's he doing?" Hob asked, narrowing his gaze.

The driver's side door opened, and a man emerged.

A tall man.

A broad-shouldered man.

The most beautiful man Jorey had ever seen.

He wore a navy down coat, faded jeans, and boots,

and the mane of hair that blew back from his face in the wind was long and tawny and wavy.

"Hi," he called, lifting a gloved hand in a wave. "Everything all right?"

"Yeah, no problem," Hob shouted back. "We're fine."

Jorey shot him a dirty look and quickly informed the stranger before he could leave, "I wrecked my car."

"Where?" He was walking toward them now, thank God.

"Down there." She pointed blindly behind her because she couldn't take her eyes off him.

It wasn't just that he was big and rugged and had an overwhelmingly masculine aura, making her feel even more conscious of her petite stature.

It wasn't even his perfectly chiseled features—wide-set eyes, square jaw, generous mouth—or the golden hair that streamed back from his face, dotted with delicate snowflakes.

No, it was more than just what he looked like.

She felt drawn to this man—and not simply because he would save her from becoming a human popsicle—or being victimized by the unsavory Hob Nixon.

There was something about him, something that told her she had been destined to run her car off the road, and he had been destined to find her there.

The notion was preposterous. And yet . . .

"How'd you do that?" he asked her.

"What?" she asked blankly.

"How'd you wreck your car?" he said, and it took a moment for his words to register.

"Oh . . . I was reaching down to pop out my Soul Asylum CD . . ."

His eyes narrowed.

A prickle of anger flared inside her, dueling with the attraction she suddenly didn't want to feel for this disapproving, almost arrogant stranger. She had never been able to tolerate arrogant, domineering men.

"What?" she demanded. "Why are you looking at me like that?"

"Nothing," he said. "Go on."

She shrugged. "I lost control of the car, and I was on a curve."

"How fast were you going?"

"Not fast," she told him, not liking his tone.

"You must have been going pretty fast to lose control like that. You're lucky you weren't hurt. Or worse."

The stern expression in his eyes—of course they were a clear, vivid blue—made her bristle. Next thing she knew he'd be calling her "young lady."

"Look, are you here to lecture me, or to help?"

"I'll give you a ride back to town," he said with a shrug.

"I'm giving her a ride back to town, Man."

She glanced at Hob, startled by his voice. She'd forgotten he was even there, so mesmerized had she been by her reaction to the newcomer.

"I'll give her a ride," the blond man told Hob firmly.

Part of her resented his attitude, the way he spoke up before she could protest Hob's statement.

Part of her was grateful for his take-charge attitude. He wasn't someone to mess with, and she wondered if Hob would dare try.

"I got here first," Hob said, scowling. "I'm heading back to town anyway, and she said she'd take a ride with me."

"No, I didn't," Jorey interjected.

"Oh, what were you gonna do? Say no?" Hob asked. "You didn't have a choice."

"Well, I do now."

"What'sa matter? You too good to ride in my truck?"

"Yeah, right," Jorey shot back. "Your truck is luxurious compared to what he's driving—sorry, no offense," she added, glancing at the other man.

"None taken." He jammed his gloved hands into the pockets of his down coat and hunched his shoulders against the wind. He said tersely, "Let's go."

She hesitated, still not thrilled with his attitude. He seemed like one of those arrogant, macho, tell-the-little-lady-what's-best types. The last kind of man she should be getting involved with.

Where had *that* thought come from?

She wasn't getting "involved."

She was catching a ride back to town; that was all.

It wasn't until she was beside him in the drafty front seat of the Chevy as he maneuvered the car to turn it around on the narrow road that she remembered something.

He had been headed in the opposite direction.

Why was he so eager to go out of his way to drive a complete stranger back to town in this weather?

As she watched Hob's pickup truck vanish around the bend ahead, she wondered, with a chill, if she'd made the safest choice, after all.

"Can I ask you something?"

Sawyer was startled by the voice beside him. She'd been silent for the past five minutes or so, and he'd been completely focused on managing the big old car on the treacherous road. There was a virtual white-out, so he had to creep along, and the tires kept skidding.

She hadn't flinched, though, or made a sound.

He got the impression that it would take a lot more than a blizzard to throw her.

She was one of those women who thought she was invulnerable. Why else would she have been out driving alone—far too fast, no doubt—in this storm? Everything about her—the Range Rover, the expensive clothing she wore, the Soul Asylum CD she'd mentioned—told him she was young, and impulsive, and wealthy.

A fool, too. She had told him, when he had asked her back there on the road, that she didn't have a coat, or gloves, or boots.

And beautiful—so beautiful he found it almost impossible to keep his eyes from roaming over her exquisite face.

Young, impulsive, wealthy, foolish, and beautiful.

Hardly a terrific combination.

Especially with the way she kept lifting her chin stubbornly, tossing those glossy, black curls of hers, and the way her green eyes flashed at him.

She cleared her throat, and he remembered her question.

"What is it?" he asked reluctantly, wishing she would just keep quiet.

It wasn't just that he needed to concentrate on the road without distraction. He also didn't have the slightest intention of answering any questions.

"Where were you going? When you came along, back there?"

He shrugged.

But that wasn't good enough for her, and he wasn't surprised.

"You were headed in the opposite direction," she persisted. "Why would you turn around and drive all the way back to town?"

"You needed a ride," he said as if it were obvious.

"But Hob Nixon could have given me a ride."

"No," he said quickly. Too quickly.

"Why not? What's wrong with him?"

He glanced sideways at her and saw that there was a gleam in her eyes. Right. As if she didn't know what was wrong with Hob Nixon.

"He's not the most responsible citizen in the world," was all Sawyer said.

"How do you know?"

"Everyone in Blizzard Bay knows that he—"

She made a snorting sound, and he cut himself short. He glanced over at her and saw that she wore a slightly amused expression.

"Sorry," she said, in a tone that told him she wasn't. "I'd just forgotten what small town gossip was like."

He thought about telling her he was hardly a small town gossip. But he couldn't do that. And it wasn't his duty to dispense warnings about Hob Nixon.

All he'd meant to say was, "It's best to stay away from people like that . . ." He couldn't resist adding, knowing it would rankle her, "Especially if you're a woman stranded alone in the middle of nowhere."

Her reaction was immediate. "You know," she retorted, "I resent the way you keep saying that."

"Saying what?" He felt the tires start to lock and gently lifted his foot off the gas pedal to avoid going into a skid.

"The way you say 'woman.' As if you think women are these helpless victims who can't do anything for themselves."

"Did I say that?"

"You might as well have said it. I can read between the lines."

He shrugged.

For a moment, the only sound in the car was the hissing of the semi-warm air coming through the heating vents.

"Are you married?" she asked, startling him again.

"Why do you ask?"

"Because if you are, I feel sorry for your wife."

"Oh."

For some reason he was disappointed. Well, what had he been expecting her to say? *I was wondering if you're married because I'm interested in you. . . .*

No!

The last thing he was going to do was get involved with a woman. Any woman. Not here. Not now.

Not her.

No, he thought with a shudder, his eyes focused straight ahead on the road. *Not her.*

"So . . . are you? Married? Don't worry, I'm not interested in dating you if you're not," she added brazenly.

Had she read his mind? he wondered as he informed her, "I'm not married."

An image flashed through his mind, of a woman, another woman, walking toward him in a wedding dress. Her face was radiant and beautiful—and then smeared with red. Blood.

To shut out the horrible memory, he glanced at the woman beside him.

Their eyes met, and in that brief moment he realized that she had been lying. She *was* interested in him.

Just as he was lying to himself.

But he wasn't going to do anything about it. He had

no business being attracted to her; no business wondering what it would feel like to forget who he was—rather, who he was *supposed* to be—and haul this tiny spitfire of a woman into his arms, crush her stubborn mouth beneath his lips, and . . .

"Can I ask you something?" he asked, to take his mind off of what he *shouldn't* be feeling.

"You can ask. That doesn't mean I'll answer."

Figures, he thought grimly, steering carefully down a steep curve in the road.

"Where are you coming from?"

"New York."

He nodded. Just as he'd figured. She was a rich city girl who probably had little experience driving, particularly on rugged back roads in weather like this.

"Aren't you going to ask me where I'm headed?"

"Didn't you already tell me? Blizzard Bay." Even as he spoke, he realized he was wrong. She hadn't told him.

He had just known. The way he had known someone was out there, stranded, on the road; someone who needed his help. The way he had known other things, terrible things, long ago.

She was watching him carefully. "I didn't tell you where I was going."

"You didn't?"

"No."

"Well, that's where I'm taking you—you knew that. It's the nearest town. So it makes sense."

She nodded.

He could feel her eyes still on him. As if she weren't certain whether she should trust him.

Good, he thought darkly. *You should be suspicious. Don't trust me, pretty lady. Don't trust anyone.*

Chapter Two

The front door of The 1890 House Bed and Breakfast, with its opaque, frosted glass pane, was thrown open before Jorey could knock.

"You're alive!"

"I'm alive," Jorey echoed her friend Gretchen Ekhard, whose tall, bulky frame filled the doorway, towering over Jorey, and whose familiar face was filled with concern.

"My God, get inside. You must be freezing. You're shivering like crazy."

"I am," Jorey agreed, though she wasn't sure how much of her shivering was due to the frigid wind.

There was something about that man. . . .

She glanced back over her shoulder and saw the Chevy pull away from the curb. So he had waited to make sure she would get safely inside, the way a conscientious date would.

Except that he wasn't her date.

She didn't even know his name.

"Sawyer Howland?"

She turned and saw that Gretchen had spotted the car—and, apparently, recognized the driver.

"That's his name?" Jorey asked.

Her friend nodded, and she furrowed her pale brows, watching the car drive away down the street. "What were you doing with him, Jorey?"

"He gave me a ride into town. I . . . I sort of wrecked my car out on Route Sixteen."

"You wrecked your car? Jorey—"

"I'm fine," she said, and gave an exaggerated shiver. "Except that I'm freezing. Can I—?"

"My God, yes. Come in." Gretchen stepped back and held the door wide open, allowing Jorey to enter the big old house.

She stood just inside the door that Gretchen swiftly closed behind her, and looked around in awe. She knew that Gretchen had turned her parents' home into a bed & breakfast after they had died within a year of each other a while back.

Jorey had assumed the transformation had included some degree of renovation to the old house.

But this was like stepping back in time. Nothing had changed. Nothing at all.

There were those ornate moldings and hardwood floors with the dark finish that showed every nick and scar. And there was that wallpaper with its faded gold pattern, faintly water-stained in some spots and peeling away in others. The tall grandfather clock still ticked loudly, looming beside the doorway leading to the back of the house.

To the left was a double archway opening into what Jorey knew was the front parlor, and to the right a rather steep stairway climbed to the second floor, the same green and gold runner centered on the worn treads. The wall along the stairs was lined with the black and white photos Jorey remembered, all of them in ornate Victorian frames, most depicting unsmiling Ekhard ancestors in stiff poses.

"Wow, Gretchen," Jorey said, looking around. "This place hasn't changed at all."

She saw the expression that darted briefly over her friend's round face, and wanted to bite her tongue. Gretchen's white-blond eyelashes fluttered and she looked down at her feet, her fingers reaching up to toy with the end of her long braid. That had been a habit of hers when they were kids, Jorey remembered in surprise. Whenever she was feeling bad about something, she had started to play with her hair.

It was obvious what was bothering her now. Gretchen had always been sensitive about Jorey's money—and her own family's lack of it. She had been born to older, blue-collar parents and dwelled in a world that couldn't have been more different from Jorey's.

Whenever Jorey spent the night in the Ekhards' guest room, Gretchen apologized profusely about the polyester comforter, lack of air-conditioning, and dismal view of the alley separating this house from the one next door.

Jorey, meanwhile, had envied her friend for having grown up in a single house, worn around the edges as it was. The drafty old Victorian might have been in disrepair, but at least Gretchen could call it home. And though her parents were old-fashioned and out-of-touch and had dozens of strict rules, at least they were there for Gretchen, and provided a stable home life.

Jorey wondered now if she had ever told Gretchen

that she had envied her. Probably. But then again, maybe not.

She should tell her now.

"You're so lucky, Gretchen," she began. "You've lived in the same place your whole life, and—"

"Gretchen?" said a voice from the doorway to her left. Jorey fell silent and looked up to see a stranger standing there. He had gray hair and a gray mustache, was of medium height and build, and was wearing a pair of tan corduroys and a flannel shirt.

"I'm sorry to interrupt," he said, "but the fire's about to die and there's no more wood in the box."

"There's some in the back shed," Gretchen told him. "I'll go get it."

"No, *I'll* go. I was about to head home, anyway."

"So soon? But—"

"I have a lot of paperwork to do tonight, Gretchen. But I'll grab the wood for you on my way out. No need for you to go out into the snow. You just stay here with Jorey . . . this *is* Jorey, isn't it?"

Gretchen smiled and nodded, though she looked troubled that he was leaving. She placed her hand on Jorey's arm and said, Jorey, this is Karl. Karl Andersen. He's my . . . uh, boyfriend."

Good Lord. She was actually blushing, her winter-pale freckles getting lost in the flush of pink on her full cheeks. Jorey couldn't help smiling faintly at the sight, touched at the realization that Gretchen was apparently in love—Gretchen, who, as a shy, overweight teenager had suffered one unrequited crush after another.

How sweet that she had found someone, Jorey thought, and glanced at Karl.

But the moment she saw the strained expression on his face she realized that Gretchen's adoration might not be mutual. Or maybe, she told herself, it was just her friend's use of the somewhat awkward word "boyfriend" that was bothering him.

After all, he had to be close to fifty. And there was something a bit ... *adolescent* about the blushing Gretchen, standing there in a pair of denim overalls, with her hair braided, a look of pure infatuation on her round face.

"It's nice to meet you," Karl said, recovering quickly, shaking Jorey's hand. "Gretchen has told me so much about you."

Jorey didn't know what to say to that. Gretchen had told her nothing about him.

Not that she and Gretchen had spoken more than once or twice in the three months since Jorey had last visited Blizzard Bay. And before that brief summer reunion, they hadn't been in touch since the summer they were eighteen.

There was an awkward moment as Jorey struggled to think of something to say.

Gretchen filled the silence then, telling Karl, "Jorey wrecked her car on the way here. Sawyer Howland gave her a ride into town."

"Sawyer Howland?" His gray eyes behind his thick glasses seemed to grow concerned. "Do you know him, Jorey?"

"No, he happened to come along while I was stranded there on the side of the road. I was pretty glad to see him."

She almost brought up Hob Nixon, but decided against it. She didn't want to distract Karl and Gretchen from the subject of Sawyer Howland. Why did they seem so disturbed that she had taken a ride from him?

"You should stay away from him, Jorey," Gretchen

said ominously, hooking her arm through Karl's. "Really. Just stay away from him."

As if she hadn't already decided to do just that. But . . .

"Why?" she found herself asking, almost defiantly. "I mean, he seemed nice enough."

"Why? What did he say to you?"

She shrugged at Gretchen's question. "Not much."

Karl nodded. "He never does."

"What? Say anything?"

"Exactly. Nobody in town knows anything about him," Gretchen told her. "He keeps to himself. And he says he's a mechanic—"

"He *is* a mechanic," Karl interrupted. "He bought the A-1 Auto Body on First Street.

"He runs the garage," Gretchen agreed, "but he doesn't seem like the grease monkey type. Does he look like any mechanic you've ever seen?"

Jorey shrugged. "Actually, I've never met a mechanic before, I don't think."

Gretchen rolled her eyes and told Karl, "Did I mention that Princess Jorey has lived an extremely sheltered life in Manhattan?"

Jorey grinned, relieved her old friend hadn't entirely lost her sense of humor amidst all this dark, suspicious talk about Sawyer Howland.

"Believe me," she told Gretchen, "I'd have made an effort to hang around garages if I'd had any hint that mechanics were strapping, golden gods like the one who just dropped me off."

"Jorey, don't say that," Gretchen said, the twinkle fading from her slate-colored eyes. "You don't want anything to do with Sawyer, no matter what he looks like. Trust me."

"I was just teasing. But . . . what's wrong with him? Other than the fact that he keeps to himself and doesn't look like a mechanic?"

"It's just that most people in town get the feeling that he's hiding something," Karl told her.

"What do you mean?" Jorey decided that small town folks had way too much time on their hands. In Manhattan, nobody cared what anybody else was doing. The less you knew about your neighbors and the more they kept to themselves, the better.

"There's just something about him," Gretchen said. "He's very . . . mysterious."

Jorey nodded despite her misgivings. There *was* something mysterious about the man. But that didn't mean . . .

"And then there was the murder."

Karl's words cut into her thoughts, giving her a jolt. *Murder?*

"What murder, Karl?"

"A woman tourist was stabbed to death at the cottage she was renting," Gretchen informed her. "Actually, Karl knew her. He lives on the lake, and she was renting a place right down the road from his house."

"When was this?"

"It happened in August," Karl said.

"Right after you were here, in fact," Gretchen put in. "The police haven't solved the case yet."

Jorey frowned. "What does that have to do with Sawyer Howland? Is he a suspect?"

"Well, he was never arrested, or anything—"

"Not even questioned," Karl amended. "But he showed up in Blizzard Bay right around the time it happened. Some people think that's too coincidental for comfort."

"And Karl's caught him prowling around the murder scene early in the morning, when he thinks no one is around."

"He hasn't been *prowling*, exactly," Karl amended. "He's been on the beach behind the cabin. It doesn't necessarily mean he's up to something, but there's really no reason to visit that particular spot—it's private property, although the owner lives up in Glens Falls and is hardly ever around."

"If I were you, Jorey," Gretchen told her, "I would make sure I didn't run into Sawyer Howland again."

"That's going to be a little difficult," Jorey said.

"Why?"

"He's towing my car to his garage. He's going to fix it for me."

"Why did you agree to that?" Gretchen asked.

Because I didn't have any choice, Jorey thought.

She had actually resented Sawyer Howland's take-charge attitude when he'd informed her, right before dropping her off, that he would take care of her car for her. She had icily told him not to bother.

But then he had said he owned the only garage in town. And what could she say to that? That she'd leave her car in the ditch for a few days until she could find someone else, *anyone* else, to help her?

No. She had agreed, reluctantly, to let the man fix her Range Rover. It hadn't occurred to her until she was walking up the steps to Gretchen's house that she hadn't even thought to find out his name, though he had mentioned that he ran A-1 Auto Body over on First Street.

Not the smartest thing to do—entrust your car to a total stranger.

Not just your car. All your belongings, too, she realized

belatedly. She hadn't thought to transfer her luggage to his car. She'd have to get in touch with him now, and arrange to pick up her things.

Her situation would make it a little difficult to stay away from him, as Gretchen was warning her.

But that didn't mean she had any intention of getting involved with him in any way—either before, or after, hearing about his questionable circumstances.

Sawyer Howland might be the most incredibly handsome, charismatic man she had ever seen, but something had warned her to stay away from him from the moment they came face-to-face.

And now Gretchen and Karl were echoing the admonitions of her own inner voice.

"It'll be fine," she assured Gretchen, her voice sounding falsely bright. "Don't worry. I'll just pick up my car when it's fixed and I'll never see him again." *After I pick up my clothes and the rest of my stuff later tonight.*

"That won't be easy in a town the size of Blizzard Bay, and especially at this time of year," Karl said, shaking his head. "Just be careful, Jorey."

"I'm a big girl, Karl," she told him, a little piqued. "And I'm always careful."

Even as the words left her mouth, she cringed.

I'm always careful.

Until now, she had lived her life being anything *but.*

Well, it was time to change. Time to stop rushing headlong through life.

From now on, she told herself sternly, *you don't do anything without stopping to think it over first, without weighing the possible consequences. Otherwise, you might find yourself in big, big trouble.*

So what? retorted another part of her. *You've certainly been in trouble before. You've always managed to get out.*

Then she thought of the woman tourist. The one who had been murdered here in Blizzard Bay.

Around the same time Sawyer Howland came to town. A chill slithered down her spine.

The coffee tasted bitter and impossibly stale.

But he had just brewed it.

Sawyer glanced from the Styrofoam cup in his hand to the decrepit Mr. Coffee machine on a shelf in the corner across the garage. He supposed he really should clean it out one of these days. He'd done little more than rinse the carafe in cold water whenever he refilled it, and the glass was cloudy and rimmed with black stains around the bottom.

Little wonder the steaming liquid in his cup tasted as if it belonged in a museum.

He sighed and took another sip of the rancid, black liquid, making a face.

Then he set the cup on the cement floor and turned again to the open hood of the Range Rover.

What a beautiful machine this was, he thought as he got back down to business.

He thought wistfully of his own cars, safely stored in a Detroit garage that protected them from the elements. And of the Chevy he had been driving since his arrival here in upstate New York. He'd bought it just outside of Albany, telling the kid who was selling it that he planned to use it for parts. Not that the kid seemed to care *who* he was or *why* he'd pay good money for a broken down heap of metal. He was just thrilled to pocket the wad of cash Sawyer handed him.

It had taken Sawyer several days to take the old car

apart and put it back together so that it ran pretty well—at least most of the time.

A beat-up old Chevy was a lot less inconspicuous in Blizzard Bay at this time of year than a shiny, loaded Lexus.

And a stranger who came to town to run an already established business attracted far less attention than an idle newcomer who arrived in the off-season.

Getting A-1 Auto Body had been a stroke of luck. The garage happened to be for sale, and Sawyer happened to be in the right place at the right time.

Marty Dern, the owner, was even more grateful to find a buyer for his decades-old business than the kid with the car in Albany had been to sell the Chevy. Dern had asked blessedly few questions, and informed Sawyer he would be using the money from the sale to buy a condo in Fort Walton Beach, where his daughter lived. He was anxious to get out of town before the weather turned cold; Sawyer was equally anxious to settle in. So it had worked out.

So far, so good, Sawyer thought, reaching into the pocket of his coveralls for a wrench.

He had managed to settle into a routine during the few months that he'd been here. He knew people were wary of him in the way small towners were always wary of newcomers, but as far as he was concerned everything had gone according to his plan. No complications, no distractions.

Until now.

He hadn't bargained on the beautiful, wealthy New Yorker who had come barreling into his life this afternoon.

From the moment he had been drawn out onto that snowy highway until he had left her at that faded Victorian monstrosity on Pleasant Street, he had been distinctly uneasy.

Hell, he had been so rattled he hadn't even bothered to ask her name.

Of course, he found it easily enough—along with her New York City address—on the registration and insurance cards inside the unlocked glove compartment.

Jorey Maddock.

A breezy, unique name.

And a posh Park Avenue address.

Both suited her, as did the designer luggage tossed haphazardly in the back. One bag was half unzipped, and a scrap of filmy, black lingerie peeked through the opening.

He fumbled with the bolt he was trying to loosen, nearly dropping his wrench.

He was jittery, too jittery to be working right now. He should take a break, go back to his apartment, try to get his mind off Jorey Maddock.

But he knew he wouldn't be able to forget about her. Not tonight. Not tomorrow. Maybe not ever.

The way he would never be able to forget about . . .

No.

"No!" he said hoarsely, his voice echoing in the empty garage.

He refused to let his mind go to that dark, horrifying place. . . .

He realized the hand holding the wrench was trembling. Slowly, he straightened and backed away from the car. From Jorey Maddock's car.

Why had he volunteered to tow it, to fix it for her? Why hadn't he simply dropped her at her friend's house and left it at that?

Because he couldn't. He had no choice. Now that his path had collided with hers, he would be haunted by the image of her beautiful face—and other images. Dark, terrifying images .

Yes . . . she *terrified* him.

Not just because he was intensely attracted to her.

Because he knew she didn't have long to live.

"Hello, you've reached A-1 Auto Body. No one is here to take your call at the moment. Please leave your name and number at the sound of the tone. Thank you."

Jorey hesitated, for some reason momentarily thrown by the sound of Sawyer Howland's recorded voice. Then she pulled herself together and found her voice.

"Uh, this is Jorey Maddock. You towed my Range Rover to your garage a while ago. I realized that I forgot my luggage in the car. I'd really appreciate it if you could get back to me as soon as possible at five five five, eight seven oh one. Thank you."

She replaced the phone—an old-fashioned wall style with a curly cord—in its cradle beside the olive green refrigerator.

"I figured he wouldn't be there," Gretchen said right behind her, startling her.

Jorey turned and saw her friend pouring steaming water from the teakettle into a chipped, white porcelain teapot.

"The weather's gotten worse. He's probably gone home for the night." Gretchen was looking toward the back door, where the porch light illuminated the still furiously falling snow.

"Well, do you know where he lives?"

"Why? You're not planning to show up on his door-step, are you, Jorey?"

"No, I figured I could track down his number and call him at home."

"And ask him to drive back through this storm to get your luggage from the garage?"

She nodded.

Gretchen shook her head. "All I know is that he lives outside of town someplace. And that there's no way anyone should be on the roads at this point, unless it was an emergency. And Jorey, I don't think that your not having your silk nightie and mink slippers qualifies as an emergency."

Jorey found herself a little taken aback at the sarcasm in Gretchen's tone.

So many things *hadn't* changed—Gretchen's appear-ance, her house, her longing for male companion-ship. . . .

But every once in a while, her friend said or did something that reminded Jorey that this wasn't necessar-ily the incredibly timid teenage girl she had known a decade ago.

The grown-up Gretchen might still have lapses into shyness and insecurity, but she had a sharp, witty tongue, and Jorey found that refreshing. When they were kids— teenagers, especially—there had been times when she felt that Gretchen was uncomfortable with Jorey's irrev-erent sense of humor and straightforward method of blurting things out. How many times had Jorey watched her friend turn red and grow fidgety over something she'd said without stopping to think?

This new Gretchen seemed to have developed a tougher shell. Jorey no longer had the sense that her friend would wither and blush if she said the wrong thing or made an inappropriate comment.

Now Jorey flashed Gretchen a look of mock indignation and said, "Oh, *please*. I don't have a silk nightie. It's cashmere. And my slippers aren't mink. Mink is *so* over."

Gretchen grinned. "Whatever you say, Princess."

"Look, I'll live without my stuff overnight if you think it's not worthwhile to try to track down Sawyer Howland."

"It's not worthwhile. You can borrow a pair of my pajamas—although you'll probably swim in them."

"I'll just roll them up," Jorey said hastily, in case Gretchen was still self-conscious about her height and weight. She had to be nearly a full foot taller than Jorey, and her large frame was generously padded as ever.

Meanwhile, Jorey hadn't grown an inch since she was seventeen, and was naturally slender—thanks to an extraordinary metabolism, rather than her diet. She remembered how Papa May used to call her "Munch" because of her appetite; she was always munching on something.

Gretchen was busy telling her that she could borrow a robe and slippers, too. "And I keep a bunch of new toothbrushes on hand for guests—you'd be surprised how many people forget theirs."

Jorey was reminded again that Gretchen's home was a bed & breakfast. It was easy to forget about that, since there were no guests at this time of year.

When they'd spoken earlier this week, planning Jorey's visit, Gretchen had mentioned that the place was virtually without guests from October until Memorial Day, and there was plenty of room for Jorey to stay.

Jorey had insisted, during their telephone conversation, that she would be a paying guest. Gretchen had tried to decline, saying that it wasn't as though she'd be taking up space that could be rented to a tourist. But Jorey had refused to take no for answer, knowing that Gretchen could probably use the money—and that Gretchen knew she had plenty of it.

The sound of something slamming upstairs caught her by surprise, interrupting her thoughts.

"What was that?" she asked, glancing up to see Gretchen looking unfazed.

"Must have been Roland."

"Roland?"

"My uncle. Actually, he was my father's uncle. I don't know if you ever met him. Probably not."

"I don't think so."

"He never married, and he lived in the midwest with his sister. She died a few years back, so there was no one to look out for him. My parents took him in, and he lives here with me now that they're gone."

"That's really nice of you, to let him stay," Jorey said, thinking it was just like Gretchen to look out for an elderly uncle. When they were children she had always been the type to take in stray cats and nurse birds with broken wings.

"Actually, it helps me out, too. He does handyman stuff around the house. In fact, I'll have to remind him to shovel the walk later. Do you want lemon for your tea?" Gretchen asked, lifting the lid of the old teapot to see if it had steeped sufficiently. Apparently it had, because she removed the old-fashioned strainer and set it in the sink.

"No lemon, but I'll take milk. And sugar."

Gretchen smiled. "You always did have a sweet tooth, Jorey."

"It's worse than ever. I've been known to eat an entire batch of chocolate chip cookies in a single, twenty-four hour period."

"And you're still a skinny little thing. It doesn't seem fair," Gretchen said ruefully, looking down at her own bulk. "I've lost five pounds since I started dating Karl, but I've still got about fifty more to go."

"How long have you been seeing him?" Jorey pulled out a chair and sat at the formica-topped table, remembering it from her childhood days.

"About six months." Gretchen set a sugar bowl in front of her. "I've known him forever, but he's only been divorced a year. You might remember him from when we were younger ... he's always lived here in town."

"I don't think I remember—"

"He works at Knowles Insurance over in Saratoga and he actually remembers your family. He handled some of your grandfather's policies, including your grandfather's life insurance—"

"I wouldn't have known anything about that," Jorey said hastily, not wanting to be reminded of Papa May's sudden death that long ago summer.

"Anyway, we got together at a Fourth of July picnic."

"You didn't say anything about him when we saw each other in August."

"No, I didn't." Gretchen's back was to her as she took a carton of milk from the refrigerator. "I guess I didn't want anyone to know about him until I was sure it was going to last."

"Well, I'm glad that's the case now."

"It is. I'm so happy with him, Jorey." Gretchen came to the table and sat across from her, pushing a steaming

mug of tea in her direction. "It's as though I find something new to love about him every day."

"That's wonderful," Jorey told her, meaning it. She
was sincerely thrilled that her old friend had fallen in
love.

Yet she felt a pang of envy inside. Would she ever
find a man whom she would grow more fond of as time
passed? It didn't seem so. In every relationship she'd
ever had, it was the opposite.

"You said on the phone that you had broken up with
Kurt," Gretchen said. "What happened? You seemed
so excited about him when you were here in August."

"I was, then. But it just didn't work out."

Jorey's mind wandered back to summer, when she
had visited Blizzard Bay. Kurt was temporarily on location in Saratoga Springs for a week, shooting scenes at
the racetrack for his film, and had suggested that she
join him there. When she'd agreed, she hadn't even
considered a side trip to nearby Blizzard Bay.

In the years since her grandfather's death she hadn't
thought much about the summers she had spent there.
The memories were simply too painful; she didn't want
to be reminded of those happy days, or the man—and
the home—that were gone forever.

But when she arrived in Saratoga Springs she had
found herself growing unexpectedly nostalgic. She'd
remembered going to the famed racetrack with Papa
May, who was a huge fan and a big gambler. She remembered strolling among the Victorian era homes and
shops of Broadway, and visiting the famed baths.

She had grown curious about Blizzard Bay, too, so
curious that she finally had Kurt's chauffeur drive her
there one day when she was bored with watching the
movie filming.

She had been startled to find that the small town looked exactly as it had when she'd last seen it—and that all of her childhood friends still lived there.

She'd found them easily, thanks to Mae Driscoll at the Front Street Diner. When Jorey had stopped in for coffee, Mae had recognized her instantly, welcoming her back with a hug—and a torrent of news about the summer friends she had once known.

Mae had told her that Gretchen still lived in her family home on Pleasant Street, which she had transformed into a bed & breakfast.

Bubbly, redheaded Kitty had married her brother's best friend Johnny O'Connor and had four children, bless her, and another on the way.

Meanwhile, earthy, eccentric Clover was still single and ran a New Age boutique in Saratoga.

Snobby, sleek Adrienne—the only one of the bunch who, like Jorey, had spent just summers in Blizzard Bay—had recently moved into her parents' estate year-round. She was divorced and rumored to be dating a wealthy, married state senator.

Jorey had called Kitty from the limo, and just hours later found herself dining with her four old friends in a local pizza parlor. When she returned to New York a few days later, she kept finding herself reliving those precious hours with the women who had been a part of the happiest days of her life.

That was why, after dumping Kurt, she had impulsively called Kitty, with whom she had always been closest, and mentioned that she was thinking of coming back up for a visit.

It was Kitty, whose tiny house was spilling over with kids and toys, who had suggested that she stay with Gretchen. "I'd love to put you up here, Jorey," she'd said, "but we don't have a spare room, and my mother's here from Florida until the baby comes, and she's sleeping on the couch. But I know Gretchen would probably love the company."

Jorey had said she'd think it over.

But Kitty, with her usual unrestrained enthusiasm, had promptly called Gretchen, and five minutes later Jorey's phone was ringing with an invitation to stay at The 1890 House.

Now here she was.

"Forgive me for prying into your personal life, Jorey," Gretchen said, after sipping her steaming tea, "and if you want to you can tell me to shut up and mind my own business—but how could you let go of someone like Kurt Govan?"

Jorey shrugged, dumping several teaspoonsful of sugar into her mug. "He just wasn't my type."

Gretchen looked dubious.

Frustrated, Jorey said, "Just because the man is a big movie star—"

"And gorgeous, and rich, and sexy."

"And gorgeous and rich and sexy," Jorey conceded. "That doesn't mean that he was Mr. Right."

"I guess, but . . . do you know how many women would have loved to have been in your shoes, Jorey? Myself, included."

"I know," she said, noting Gretchen's wistful expression. "But guess what, Gretchen? I'd rather be in your shoes."

Startled, Gretchen said, *"Huh?"*

"You know where you belong—here in Blizzard Bay. You're running your own business. *And* you're in a relationship with someone you love. Your whole life is settled. You know exactly where you'll be tomorrow, and the next day. But me—I don't know where I'm headed, or what I want. I never have. Until now, it's never mattered. But lately . . ."

She trailed off, realizing she was rambling.

Gretchen was silent.

Jorey swallowed some tea.

Then Gretchen said, "I guess I never thought you were unhappy, Jorey. You were always happy-go-lucky, loving life."

"When you knew me, yes. When I was a kid. Especially when I was up here during the summers. But then things changed. I . . . grew up."

It seemed as though it had happened overnight. In fact, it had been over the course of that one last summer here, when her whole world had fallen apart.

And though she had managed to piece things back together so that she could at least stop moping and crying and feeling sorry for herself, nothing had ever been the same again.

Maybe that was why she had grown so restless lately.

Maybe she needed some kind of peace and stability in her life—the kind of peace and stability she had always associated with Blizzard Bay.

But Papa May was gone.

The house was gone.

Her childhood was gone.

She could never recapture the things that were missing.

Maybe coming here had been a mistake.

Or maybe what she sought wasn't her lost childhood, after all. Maybe it was something else, something she had never imagined she needed.

For some reason she thought of Sawyer Howland then, and wished she hadn't. The enigmatic outsider

was exactly the kind of complication she couldn't afford
in her present frame of mind.

She was definitely searching for something, all right—
but *not* a man.

No, was her next thought, *that isn't necessarily true.*

Jorey was acutely aware of her physical need for a
man; of her craving to be held in someone's strong
arms, kissed deeply, and caressed. She realized that she
missed being in a relationship, even a *wrong* relationship, for that reason.

She longed for passion; life without passion was dull,
far too dull for a woman who thrived on unpredictability
and impulse.

She longed for someone to tenderly make love to
her, to tell her he couldn't get enough of her.

You're insatiable, Jorey.

How many times had Kurt—virile Kurt, ladies' man
and international sex symbol—told her that? Others
had said it, too, making her wonder eventually if she
was too demanding, some kind of sex addict.

But the truth was, no man had ever loved her *enough.*
Not physically, and not emotionally. She was always
ready for more—sometimes found herself startled, even
angry, when a lover, looking sleepy and obviously sated,
rolled away and shut her out. *Wait,* she always wanted
to protest, *I still need you. I still need more. . . .*

And it wasn't just physical intimacy she yearned for;
it was far more than that. She desperately wanted—no,
she *needed*—emotional intimacy.

She longed to lie with her head on a man's naked
chest, to feel his hands stroking her hair or her back,
and to tell him things she had never dared reveal to
anyone before. Things that would leave her vulnerable,

only it wouldn't matter, because she would feel safe with him.

Whoever he was.

Who are you? she wondered, feeling a sudden wave of loneliness swoop over her. *Where are you?*

And she realized, as those thoughts crossed her mind, the source of the need she was trying to fill.

She needed to love and be loved—for real.

What she'd felt for Kurt and others before him must have been infatuation. Why else would it have flared so easily, and been extinguished in no time? Real love didn't come and go so effortlessly.

She was ready for real love. It was the one thing that had been missing all her life.

So she *was,* after all, searching for a man.

But most definitely not a man like Sawyer Howland.

No, she knew, beyond a doubt, that the last thing she would ever feel with someone like him was *safe.*

What was he doing here?

He had to be out of his mind, Sawyer thought as he pulled the Chevy to a stop in front of The 1890 House Bed and Breakfast. Pleasant Street was drifted over in snow, and when he opened the door and stepped out, he found that it was knee-deep. Christ. How would he ever get the car out of here? And if the streets were this bad in the village, what would he face on his four mile drive?

He should have gone straight home, and he should have done it hours ago.

But the thought of being alone in his small apartment hadn't appealed to him then, and it didn't now. He suspected that, in his edgy frame of mind, the place might seem more like a cage than a refuge from the storm.

So instead of calling it quits when he should have he had forced himself to stay at the garage, to keep working on the Range Rover, unwilling to let thoughts of its owner distract him from the job at hand.

After all, there was nothing he could do about Jorey Maddock or the grim fate that awaited her. Nothing at all.

But there was something he could do about the car she had entrusted to his care, and the sooner he finished it the sooner he could start trying to forget about her. Right now, it was impossible.

If he'd gone home hours ago the way he should have, he wouldn't have been in the shop to hear that message she'd left about her luggage. He'd let the machine pick it up because his hands were coated in grease, but when he heard her voice he'd been seized by an unreasonable urge to snatch up the receiver.

It was an urge he couldn't resist, and that knowledge had bothered him ever since he'd found himself hurriedly wiping his hands on a rag and dashing for the telephone. But he was too late; his breathless "Hello?" was met by a dial tone.

He'd considered calling her back, then decided against it. She wouldn't know he had been there to hear her message; she'd assume he'd gone home for the night, the way any sensible person would.

It had taken a long time for him to clean the greasy mess from the telephone receiver, and longer still to pace the garage, wondering what to do, stopping every few moments to eye the pile of luggage in the car.

Finally, he reached a decision. The wrong one, no doubt, but at least he was no longer pacing.

No, he was here, about to pop up on her doorstep with this special delivery.

Why?

He had no idea.

It was too late to change his mind.

He slammed the door and trudged through the snow, hating the squeaking noise it made beneath the rubber soles of his boots. The sound had always sent chills down his spine, the way Styrofoam used to bother his younger sister. When they were kids, he had delighted in making her cringe and shriek by deliberately rubbing two chunks of Styrofoam together.

"Mommy!" she'd yelled. "He's doing it again."

But of course, he disposed of the evidence before his mother appeared and pasted an innocent expression on his face, as though he had no idea what the kid was talking about.

Typical big brother/kid sister stuff.

God, those days had been so very long ago.

At the back of the car he paused to brush several inches of new snow from the top of the trunk, then opened it. Jorey Maddock's pile of bags sat there waiting, the rich, brown leather looking distinctly out of place beside his jumper cables and a paper bag full of empty soda cans he kept meaning to bring back to the supermarket.

He picked up two of the biggest bags and closed the trunk so that the rest of them wouldn't get dusted in the snow that was still coming down heavily. Then he began to wade toward the house, huffing under the weight of the suitcases.

How long was she planning to stay here—a *year*? How could she possibly not have brought warm clothes somewhere in all of this luggage?

He could fit every item of clothing he owned in one of her smaller bags. Rather, every item of clothing back at his Blizzard Bay apartment.

It was so easy to forget, sometimes, that he had another home, another life, and that it had very little to do with this one.

He glanced up at the house that loomed above him. It was as big and old and ridiculously formal as the others on the street, with an equal share of gables and fishscale shingles and gingerbread trim, but it seemed to lack their charm. The peeling paint and generally dilapidated appearance didn't help, but none of the neighboring homes were exactly showplaces, either.

It was more than that, and Sawyer knew it. He fought back a shudder, and the disturbing vision that poked at the edge of his consciousness.

Why, he wondered instead, would someone like Jorey have chosen to stay in this particular inn, especially when there were several luxury hotels right over in Saratoga Springs?

Sawyer mounted the uneven wooden steps, noting that someone had recently shoveled them and the walk. Yellow lamplight spilled from the globes on either side of the door, and a sign in the window read Vacancy.

No kidding, he thought wryly. There couldn't be more than a handful of tourists in the entire area this weekend.

So what had brought Jorey Maddock, alone, to this godforsaken spot at this time of year?

It doesn't matter. She isn't your concern.

He set his jaw resolutely, rang the bell, and waited.

A few moments later, a light went on in the entrance hall, and then the door opened.

Gretchen Ekhard stood there. He knew her by sight,

the way he had come to know most year-round residents in the past few months. But they had never met, and now he set down a suitcase and offered his gloved hand in a formal greeting.

"I'm Sawyer Howland," he told her.

She nodded as though she knew that already, and he didn't doubt that she did. There was nothing friendly or welcoming in her steady gaze, nor in the way she gingerly shook his hand.

"Gretchen Eckhard," she replied tersely.

"I towed a car for one of your guests earlier, and—"

"Is that Jorey's luggage?"

He followed her gaze to the two large bags, and nodded, thinking it strange that she was already on a first name basis with her new guest.

"I'll give it to her." Gretchen reached down and, with surprising strength, grabbed the suitcase he'd set on the porch. She lifted it over the threshold, set it on the floor behind her, and gestured for him to hand her the other one.

"I can bring it in for you," he said. "It's pretty heavy."

She seemed about to protest, but he didn't let her. He stepped forward, and she had no choice but to move aside as he carried the bag into the hallway.

"Thank you," she said, and seemed anxious to shoo him out the door.

He should have been just as anxious to leave, but some part of him wouldn't let her get rid of him that easily. The same part that had insisted on getting inside the house.

He knew why. He was hoping for a glimpse of Jorey Maddock.

It was insane, he knew, and yet he couldn't help it. He was suddenly filled with the inexplicable need to see her again—or maybe just to make sure that she was still all right. Still alive.

"Is Jorey—?"

"She's in the other room, resting by the fire. This was a hard day for her, with the accident and everything. I'll tell her you were here."

"Actually, there are a few more bags in my car. I'll go get them."

He left before she could utter another word; anyway, what could she say?

He got the distinct impression that the woman was wary of him. It was the same feeling he had gotten from others in this small village, and he supposed that was fine with him.

He was, after all, an outsider here. He hadn't expected, nor had he wanted, to be welcomed with open arms.

No, he'd wanted only to be left alone to go about his business, and he'd been able to do just that since his arrival.

Of course, running a business in town he couldn't entirely avoid contact with the locals. But he kept things strictly professional with his customers. He evaded the few who dared to ask personal questions, the way he had evaded Jorey's curiosity earlier.

The best thing he could do, he realized as he removed the other bags from the trunk and slammed it closed again, was to drop off the luggage and get the hell out of there. He didn't like Gretchen Eckard's probing stare, and he had already sworn to have nothing more to do with Jorey Maddock.

But when he returned to the house he found her standing in the hallway, and Gretchen nowhere to be seen.

Unexpectedly coming face-to-face with her again left him feeling as though he'd slipped and gone down on an icy sidewalk. He was breathless, the wind positively knocked out of him.

She was as lovely as he remembered, maybe more so.

She suddenly seemed much smaller and infinitely vulnerable. He wondered why, and looked down and saw that she wore only socks. She was several inches shorter than he'd first realized; no bigger than a child, really. And the defiant expression was gone from her big green eyes. Now they were gazing at him with . . . appreciation?

"I heard your voice from the next room and I wanted to thank you for bringing my bags to me," she said as she held the door open for him, obviously expecting him to step inside.

"Well, I got your message, and I figured I might as well just drop them off on my way home."

"I hope you don't have far to go," she said, peering past him at the swirling snow. She shivered, hugging herself, and closed the door.

"I'll make it." He kept his head bent as if against the wind even though he was inside now, just so he wouldn't have to meet her eyes again.

"That's what I thought, too, this afternoon," she pointed out. "And look where I landed. You should probably just stay here for the night."

Startled, he looked right at her, then realized what she meant. This was, after all, a bed and breakfast. There were rooms available. She hadn't meant—

Of course she hadn't.

But she knew what he'd been thinking. He could tell from the sudden quirk of her mouth and the way she flicked her gaze away from his.

"I'm sure Gretchen has vacancies, since I'm the only guest," she said, and cleared her throat.

"I'm sure she does, but I have to get home."

"Why? You don't have a wife waiting for you." Her tone was amused, and he had to grin.

"No, there's no wife."

"Pets who need to be fed? Dog? Cat? Gerbil?"

"Gerbil?"

"Nah. You don't seem the gerbil type. In fact, you don't come across as the kind of person who'd have a pet, either."

"Why is that?"

She tilted her head at him, studying him. "You're not the nurturing type," she declared.

He blinked. "How can you make that kind of judgement about an absolute stranger?"

"I'm very good at judging people."

"Oh, you are?"

"Actually, no," she admitted readily, taking him by surprise. "I'm a terrible judge of character. That's probably why . . ."

"Why . . . what?" he prodded when she trailed off.

She shrugged. "Nothing. Go ahead, then. Get back to your gerbil, or whatever."

He stared at her, liking her, wanting suddenly to stay. Not because of the storm or the roads, but because of her. He wanted to be near her. To keep an eye on her . . .

To protect her from—

"What's the matter?" she asked, watching him watch her.

"What do you mean?"

"You have this look on your face, as if you're thinking of something terrible."

"Oh . . ."

I am.

"I should go," he said abruptly, and moved toward the door. Without so much as a backward glance, he pushed it open and stepped out into the blustery night.

Chapter Three

Jorey couldn't sleep.

She *had* slept, for at least four or five hours. In fact, she'd been so bone-tired that she'd drifted off the moment she climbed into bed. But she'd awakened abruptly in the wee hours and spent hours struggling to recapture the elusive sleep, listening to the wind roar around the big old house.

She had crawled to the foot of the bed to lean over and raise the shade so that she could peer out into the storm. There was nothing to see but white, and the shadowy outline of the house next door.

Now, as the darkness outside was infiltrated with gray dawn, she was able to make out the room around her. It was unfamiliar and familiar at once, being the same room where she had spent so many childhood sleepovers.

This was even the same bed; a white iron antique with towering head and footboards. Jorey wasn't sure if the highboy dresser had been here before, but she remembered the low, boxy nightstand, the padded chair with the curved back, and the tall, wooden coatrack in one corner. The room was small, with a hardwood floor and a lone window overlooking the alley below. The walls had been painted in the years since Jorey had last visited; the pale gold color having been replaced with plain white.

Gretchen had intended to give her one of the other rooms—either the large suite that had once been her parents' master bedroom or the corner room that had been converted from her father's study.

But Jorey, spurred by nostalgia, had insisted on staying in here, where she had spent so many nights long ago. Because her grandparents' estate was so far out of town, she used to sleep over quite often, rather than ride her bike all the way back home after dark. Papa May didn't like her doing that; he worried about traffic and kidnappers.

"Remember, you're a Maddock," he used to tell her. "And this isn't New York, where wealthy people are a dime a dozen. You can be a target here. You need to be careful."

But for all his warnings Jorey had never felt threatened in Blizzard Bay. When she was there she fit in with the local kids, all of whom knew she came from money—more money than Adrienne's family had, even—and that her father was a big financier.

In fact, Adrienne reminded Jorey of her own older sisters, Sonya and Lianne. All were willowy blonds with delicate features, and a cool restraint that suited their station.

Growing up, Jorey had both envied and pitied Sonya

and Lianne. They never seemed to have much fun, yet they didn't seem to mind.

They did resent that she was the apple of their father's eye—it was no secret that Mayville Maddock II adored his youngest child, who had inherited his vibrant personality and impish features.

By contrast, Jorey's mother had held her at arm's length while doting on her older daughters, who were mirror images of herself. It hadn't bothered Jorey much—she found her mother dull and shallow, and hardly regretted that they didn't spend much time together. When she was younger, Jorey had assumed Amanda Maddock was jealous of the attention Mayville lavished on her. Only after her parents' marriage crumbled was it apparent that they had never loved each other. And Jorey realized why her mother had never been able to warm up to her—she reminded her too much of the husband she had, apparently, barely tolerated for twenty-five years.

Still, Jorey's mother continued to go through the motions of being a mother to her. Just a few days ago she had called from the South of France to wish Jorey well on her vacation with Kurt Govan—and to heave a sigh of relief when she found that her daughter had called it off.

Jorey knew that an actor—even a superstar like Kurt—was hardly her mother's idea of husband material. Still, Amanda had urged her to find somebody new, and as soon as possible.

"Jorey, it's time to settle down and stop casting off men like last season's handbag," Amanda had said. "Otherwise, you'll spend your life as a single woman."

"What would be so horrible about that?" Jorey retorted.

And her mother, who had promptly married an English lord who was far wealthier than the Maddocks the moment her divorce from Mayville was finalized, rattled off a number of reasons Jorey shouldn't remain unattached.

None of them involved love.

No wonder her marriage, and Jorey's sisters' marriages, seemed so stiff and unfulfilling. Both Sonya and Lianne had married men who were handpicked for them by Amanda. Crisp, dry-cleaned men with side parts and blue blood and stable professions.

A vision of Sawyer Howland drifted into Jorey's mind, unbidden and yet a welcome contrast to the buttoned-up images of her brothers-in-law.

With his long, unruly blond hair, his rugged outdoorsy clothing, and his handsome face tinged by a pronounced five o'clock shadow—not to mention his dubious character—he was exactly the kind of man who would horrify her mother and her sisters. Jorey's lips curved into a faint smile at the thought of what her mother would say if Jorey presented Sawyer Howland as her future son-in-law.

Not that that would ever happen in a trillion years, she amended hastily. She had no intention of becoming captured by Sawyer's enigmatic allure. The man was too arrogant—and, perhaps, too dangerous.

For a few moments, as she bantered with him in the hallway last evening, finding herself drawn to his undeniable charisma, she had forgotten Gretchen and Karl's warnings about him. But then he had changed suddenly, become withdrawn, scurrying off into the night without another word. Suddenly, it was easy to imagine that he might be connected to the dark and sinister murder that had haunted Blizzard Bay for the past few months.

Still . . .

Would a cold-blooded killer go out of his way to bring a stranger her luggage in this treacherous weather?

Intellectually, Jorey knew that anything was possible. That Sawyer Howland's mesmerizing blue eyes might conceal the soul of a bloodthirsty criminal.

But in her lonely and maybe naive heart, she wanted to believe that he was just a man.

Just a man . . .

Jorey yawned and rolled over in bed, finally allowing sleep to steal in and claim her. But instead of sweet dreams she encountered nightmares.

In them, she was running frantically through a snowy, barren forest, running for her life because someone was chasing her. And though she never saw him, she sensed Sawyer Howland's presence looming all around her, and heard his deep voice calling, "You can run, but you can't hide, Jorey. No matter how you try to get away, you'll never be able to hide . . ."

Sawyer gave up trying to sleep. It was past six, anyway, officially morning, and he had never been one to lie in bed very late.

He got up, fumbled through a pile of clothes on a chair, and pulled a long-sleeved T-shirt over the plaid, flannel boxer shorts he'd worn to bed. He'd never been one to sleep in pajamas, not even in this drafty room with freezing temperatures outside. He didn't like being encumbered by buttons and sleeves and drawstrings when he slept.

Nor did he like feeling constricted by day. He had always favored comfortable clothes—baggy sweaters and loose-fitting jeans and untucked flannel shirts. It wasn't that he had anything to conceal; his body was lean and hard and muscular—a fact that had surprised and thrilled many a woman the first time he undressed in front of her.

He wondered, fleetingly, whether Jorey had imagined what he looked like beneath the layers of warm clothes he'd had on yesterday. He had certainly found himself fantasizing about her petite form, particularly after their second encounter last night.

She was tiny and compactly built, yet not scrawny or boyish. Rather, she had exquisite curves and an aura of provocative femininity, and he couldn't stop imagining what it would be like to scoop her into his strong arms and cradle her against his broad chest.

He felt himself stirring now at the thought and pushed it out of his head, crossing over to the dormer window to gaze out at the still furious storm.

Instead, he found himself remembering how guileless she had seemed, standing there in her stocking feet, grateful that he'd brought her bags and worried about him getting home in the blizzard. So different from the stubborn, defensive woman he'd first glimpsed out there on the highway.

The Jorey he'd met last night hadn't just filled him with forbidden longing. She somehow made him want to take care of her.

He had no doubt that the prickly, independent streak he had glimpsed earlier existed, nor that she would resent the idea of any man stepping into her life to safeguard her. Yet ultimately she was vulnerable, whether she knew it or not.

And only Sawyer could protect her, because only he knew what was going to happen to her.

Just as he had known the last time. . . .

He turned abruptly away from the window and crossed to the fireplace across the room. Opening a built-in cupboard beside it, he reached up inside until his fingers found a high shelf off to the side, against the brick.

He'd discovered the secret cubbyhole not long after moving in. The first time he'd felt his way along the shelf he had encountered something soft and furry and had swiftly withdrawn his fingers, thinking it was some long-dead animal.

Later, when he'd poked his head up there and investigated with a flashlight, he'd discovered that it wasn't a dead animal but a stuffed one. A stuffed dog, to be exact, with soft, brown fur and big, floppy ears, and glass eyes that looked incredibly real.

The toy was well-worn, as though some child had once loved it dearly, and Sawyer had found himself wondering how it had come to be tucked away, forgotten, in that musty cupboard. He had rescued the stuffed dog and washed the cobwebs and dust from its polyester fur, and it now sat on top of the bookcase beneath the sloping ceiling in an alcove across the room.

And on the secret shelf in the cupboard was a large, flat, black, leather-bound scrapbook.

He lifted it out now, with trembling hands, and carried it over to the sagging, beige couch opposite the fireplace. There, he sat for a long time, just holding it on his lap, remembering.

Finally, with a deep, steadying breath he opened the first page and stared at the headline of the carefully mounted clipping from a local newspaper.

"Young Female Tourist Slain in Lakeside Cottage"

* * *

". . . and remember the day we were trying to catch that frog and we fell into the lake with our dresses on?" Kitty asked, giggling.

"How could I forget?" Jorey grinned at the memory. "We showed up at Adrienne's birthday party soaking wet. I'll never forget the look on her mother's face."

"Well, can you blame her?" Adrienne asked, not nearly as amused as they were. "She had invited the governor's granddaughters—"

"They thought it was hilarious," Kitty cut in. "Remember? They were nothing like I expected them to be. The older one was a real hoot. That was the best party you ever had, Adrienne. How old were you that year? Ten?"

"Thirteen. And so were you," Adrienne said pointedly.

"Thirteen? That old?" Kitty raised her reddish eyebrows. "What were we doing chasing frogs at the lake, Jorey?"

"Guess we matured later than everyone else," Jorey said with a shrug and a grin.

"You and Kitty were always getting into some kind of trouble," Clover said in her quiet way.

"I don't know about Jorey, but I still am." Kitty deliberately rubbed her enormous belly, and they all laughed. "I never thought I'd wind up having *five* children, believe me."

"Maybe you need to have a little talk with Johnny," Jorey suggested.

"Or some advice from Planned Parenthood," Adrienne put in.

"Oh, they were all planned," Kitty told them. "I love having babies. Honestly."

"Then maybe you should see a shrink, because you're out of your mind," Adrienne said.

"Adrienne! That's terrible."

"Relax, Clover, I'm just kidding. It's just that the thought of what women go through to give birth . . . ugh." Adrienne gave a delicate little shudder.

"Well, I think it's a beautiful thing," Clover retorted. "It's miraculous."

The two of them were so different, Jorey thought, gazing from Clover's serious, bespectable face to Adrienne's meticulously made-up one. How had they ever become such close friends—any of them, really?

Was it any surprise that they hadn't remained that way over the years? Even the four who lived in Blizzard Bay had gone their separate ways in the past decade, rarely seeing each other except by chance, according to Kitty.

But this afternoon they had all come together again, in honor of Jorey's visit. Gretchen had invited everyone to lunch at the bed and breakfast for the second reunion in the past few months, and the weather had cooperated, the storm having tapered off to flurries by late morning.

Everyone was able to get here, even Adrienne, who was living at her estate several miles out of town.

When they'd met back in August they had spent most of their time together catching up on each other's lives. But today, as they sat around the large table in Gretchen's dining room, a fire blazing cozily on the hearth and classical music playing in the background, the conversation seemed to keep drifting back to the past.

Gretchen came into the room, carrying a coffeepot and a plate of cookies.

"You can put those right between me and Jorey," Kitty said promptly. "I'm eating for two these days—and lord knows Jorey's always eaten for two. Or three."

The others laughed and Jorey helped herself to the plate, smiling at how well these women knew her even though they'd been apart for so many years, save the brief reunion last summer.

"What are these?" Kitty asked Gretchen, examining a cookie.

"Clover brought them."

"I made them. They're organic fruit jumbles," Clover said, the stack of bangles on her forearm clanking as she reached for one.

"They're pretty good," Jorey complimented her around a mouthful. "Even if they are healthy."

"Oh, God, I just thought of something—remember when Hob Nixon sent you those cookies from the bakery on Second Street?" Kitty asked, rolling her eyes.

"What bakery on Second Street?" Adrienne wanted to know.

"The one with the purple awning—it burned down a few years a ago," Gretchen said.

"Remember how Jorey ate the whole box before she found out who'd sent them?"

Jorey frowned. "He sent them to *me*?" She'd assumed Kitty was talking about one of the others.

"Who else?" Kitty asked. "You were the one he was in love with."

Huh? "No way! I don't remember that."

"How could you forget?" Adrienne wanted to know. "He was practically stalking you. Following you around, calling you and hanging up—"

"And when you found out the cookies were from him, you threw up immediately," Kitty told her. "Remember?

You stuck your finger down your throat right there on the sidewalk. You thought he might have poisoned them."

"Or put some kind of herbal love potion in them," Clover said matter-of-factly.

"Nobody thought *that* but you," Adrienne said.

"Well, I never believed he was such a horrible person," Clover said. "He has a cat. People who have cats can't be all bad."

"Oh, please," Adrienne said.

"How do you know he has a cat?" Kitty asked.

"Because it wandered away from his trailer and wound up on my property last winter, and he came around looking for it. I had been feeding it, and he thanked me."

"You didn't let him into your house, did you?" Adrienne looked horrified.

"Into the kitchen. It wasn't a big deal. Gretchen's let him into her house, too."

They all turned to Gretchen, who shrugged and looked uncomfortable. "I hired him to do some painting last spring, when Uncle Roland got the flu for a week. That's all."

"Listen, he's a human being, no matter what he looks like and how he lives."

"Oh, Clover, come off it. There was a time when you were just as grossed out by him as the rest of us were," Kitty said. "When he was all over Jorey, you weren't exactly encouraging her to date him. None of us were. We all thought he was a creep."

"I can't believe I don't remember any of this," Jorey said, looking from one friend to another. She searched her memory, trying to recall the incident, but came up blank. "When was this?"

"I don't know . . . we were probably about sixteen or so," Adrienne told her.

"No, we were eighteen. At least, I was. It was the summer after high school graduation," Kitty corrected her. "I remember, because I had gone to the senior prom with Johnny that June, and then he ignored me all summer because he had a crush on Jorey, and I thought Hob Nixon was jealous and that he was going to kill Johnny or something, he was such a psycho."

"*Johnny* had a crush on me?" Jorey blinked. "He did not."

"Sure he did. Ask him. I was teasing him about it when you called to say you were in town that day. He remembers, too."

"Huh," Jorey said, mystified. "I had no idea about that."

"Yes, you did," Gretchen spoke up. "You told me you thought Johnny was cute, but that you knew Kitty liked him so you weren't going to do anything about it."

Jorey pondered that, but couldn't recall it—or, more disturbingly, anything about Hob Nixon having had a crush on her when they were young.

She almost brought up the fact that he'd come along and offered her a ride yesterday afternoon when she was stranded, but kept it to herself. That topic would lead naturally to the subject of Sawyer Howland, and he was the last person she wanted to talk—or even think—about right now.

"Speaking of Johnny," Adrienne said. "What ever happened to that freaky cousin of his? The one with all the tattoos and the Mohawk hairstyle?"

"The one Clover dated?" Kitty asked.

"He wasn't freaky," Clover said defensively. "He was a punk rocker."

"He was freaky, and he still is," Kitty informed her. "Last we heard, he was travelling around Europe with some cult that believes the world is coming to an end at the millennium."

"Cullen," Jorey said. "Cullen O'Connor. That was his name."

"Right," Kitty agreed. "That's him."

Relieved, Jorey told her, "For a second there, I thought I was losing my mind—or at least, my memory. I have, like, total amnesia about this whole Hob Nixon thing with the cookies—"

"Well, who wouldn't want to wipe *that* out?" Adrienne asked with a shudder. "I don't blame you for trying to forget. Actually, I heard that creep was arrested for a rape case not long ago. The thought of it makes me sick."

"And *I* heard that the police are considering him a suspect in that murder," Kitty said.

The others murmured that they'd heard that, too.

"The one last August?" Jorey asked.

"What other murder is there?" Kitty replied. "It was the first homicide this town has seen in years."

"And Hob Nixon is a suspect? Why?"

"*Why?* Come on, Jorey. That guy was born to be a serial killer," Adrienne declared.

"Well, *that* might be extreme, but there *was* always something suspicious about him," Kitty said.

Jorey couldn't argue with that. She remembered what Sawyer had said about Nixon—how he'd warned her to steer clear of him. Did he know something about the murder—maybe about Hob's being involved? Was he actually one of the good guys?

Or was *he* the bad guy, trying to throw suspicion off himself, Jorey wondered.

Somehow, neither scenario seemed all that far-fetched, and Jorey spent the rest of the afternoon with Sawyer Howland squarely on her mind, unable to ignore a vague sense of relief that maybe—just *maybe*—he had nothing to do with the murder after all.

Then again, maybe he did—and the possibility continued to fill her with dread.

Chapter Four

"Hello? Is anybody here?"

Sawyer straightened at the sound of a voice in the doorway of the garage. An already familiar voice . . .

Sure enough, Jorey Maddock was standing there.

She was a breathtaking sight, vividly framed against the snowy street behind her with the piercing, blue sky as a backdrop. She wore faded blue jeans, some ridiculous, high-heeled boots, and a bulky red sweater and a red beret perched jauntily on her mop of black curls. Her cheeks were flushed and her breath was frosty in the November chill, puffing through lips that were meticulously lined in the same shade of red as her sweater and cap. A brown leather bag was slung over her shoulder, the kind of expensive, oversized bag a woman would carry down a busy Manhattan street—not here in the North Country in the dead of winter.

That was where she belonged—in the city. Not here.

Not here, where danger lurked. Why hadn't she stayed in the city?

"Hello?" she called again, blinking her long, black lashes as though to adjust her vision to the dim interior of the garage.

Sawyer found his voice and called, "Hi," as if she were just any customer. He moved slowly away from the open hood of a pickup he'd been working on, reaching into the pocket of his coveralls for a rag to wipe his greasy hands.

She took a few steps into the garage, still holding the door open with one hand, obviously reluctant to seal herself off from the street, as though contact with the outside world offered some measure of protection.

From him?

Did she feel that he was some sort of threat?

"I was just wondering," she said, "if you'd fixed my car yet."

"Actually, I needed a part. It'll be here tomorrow. So—"

"Okay . . ."

She paused, cleared her throat just as he did.

"What was wrong with it?" she asked, and he had the impression that she really didn't care about the specifics. She was just struggling to make conversation, to make the awkward tension between them go away.

Why was *she* tense? he wondered. His reason was obvious; he knew something about her, something dark and frightening and inescapable. . . .

And then, beyond that, there was the fact that he was hopelessly attracted to her.

He was reluctant to admit it, even to himself, and yet he couldn't deny it. Not with her standing here in front of him, and his heart throbbing so loudly in his chest that she must be able to hear it.

Now he wondered whether her hesitation stemmed from some instinct that she was in danger, or from her own attraction to him, an attraction she was fighting as fervently as he was.

He began to speak, to tell her in great technical detail exactly what had been wrong with her car.

She listened intently—or at least, she pretended to. Her eyes were focused on his face, her head tilted slightly, nodding every so often as if to say she understood what he was saying.

Finally, he stopped talking.

She took a deep breath and slapped her palms against her thighs. "Well," she said, "it sounds pretty complicated, but as long as it can be fixed—"

"It can be."

"Good."

"You didn't have to come all the way down here to find out. I was actually going to call you at the bed and breakfast and tell you what was going on," he said, and it was the truth. He had, however, been putting it off, reluctant to initiate further contact with the woman who had been on his mind for the past forty-eight hours.

"It's all right. I couldn't stand being cooped up inside for another minute," she said. "I'm meeting Gretchen for lunch in a little while—"

"Gretchen?"

"Eckhard—she runs The 1890 House."

"I knew who you meant. I didn't realize you knew each other well enough to meet for lunch."

"We've known each other for years. Anyway, I decided to take my time walking over, so that I could do a little sightseeing along the way. I happened to pass right by here, so . . ."

He nodded, then said, "So you're checking out the local sights?"

"More or less."

"There's not much to see, is there?"

She shrugged. "That depends on how you look at it. I spent a lot of time here when I was growing up, so to me it's an interesting place. I'm curious about how things have changed, and what's remained the same."

"You spent time here in the past?"

"My grandparents had an . . . a house. Outside of town, on Fieldstone Road. I spent every summer here with them."

"I live on Fieldstone Road." He had spoken before he realized what he was doing; had offered information about himself to a virtual stranger. What had gotten into him? He had learned, over the past few months, not to give away the details of his personal life, lest someone in Blizzard Bay suspect that he was not what he appeared to be.

"Which house?" she asked, raising two perfectly arched brows at him.

"It's just . . . an apartment house."

"An apartment house?"

He could practically see her mind working. And as he watched her, he wondered if . . .

No.

That would be far too great a coincidence.

"There aren't really any apartment houses out that way," she said. "Just a lot of summer estates. But I recently found out that my grandparents' old house was converted into apartments when they sold it. To be honest, the thought of that . . . well, it made me sick."

He watched her wordlessly, his mind racing.

"Which house do you live in?" she asked then. "It isn't, by any chance, a big stone mansion—three stories, with a wraparound porch?"

Her words slammed into him, leaving him momentarily speechless.

She had described the one house on Fieldstone Road that fit that description.

His house.

So he was living in her childhood summer home. Could that coincidence possibly explain, somehow, what had been happening to him ever since she'd arrived in town?

"That's the house, isn't it, Sawyer? I can tell by the look on your face," she said.

He couldn't lie. He nodded slowly, hearing in his mind the echo of his name on her lips. She had uttered it with a note of familiarity that seemed incongruous with their status as virtual strangers.

Yet . . .

He lived in her house.

He had been driven out into a raging blizzard to find her.

He hadn't been able to get her out of his mind.

He knew things about her. . . .

Things he couldn't possibly know; didn't *want* to know.

But this isn't the first time it's happened to you, he reminded himself, struggling to deny any exceptional link to Jorey Maddock. *You're no stranger to this kind of thing. You knew. . . .*

He flinched at the memory that threatened to barge into his consciousness, forcing it away out of habit.

"What's wrong?" Jorey asked, watching him closely. "Are you all right?"

"I'm fine. I just ..." He rubbed his temple. "I just—"

"You just smeared grime all over your head," she said, smiling faintly, when he trailed off.

"Oh ..." He looked down at his still greasy hand. "Oops. I forgot." He pulled out a rag and began rubbing at his hand.

"So you live in my grandparents' house," she said, making another forward movement, this time letting the door close behind her to shut out the scraping rumble of a snowplow on the street outside.

They were alone together in the silent garage. He lowered the rag and worked it in his hand, intently focused on looking for an unsoiled spot to use on his head.

She took a few more steps toward him, until they were only a few feet apart. "What's it like?" she asked. "The house, I mean. I've been wondering about it for so long. Is it rundown and shabby? Is there laundry hanging on the porch, and are there fire escape ladders on the outside?"

He glanced at her, amused despite himself. "No," he told her. "It's actually fairly respectable looking."

"I'm sorry." She smiled slightly. "I just keep picturing it turned into a tenement or something. All kinds of sloppy strangers living in this place that was once so special to me. My grandfather used to take such good care of that house ..."

There was a faraway look in her green eyes, as if she were lost in her memories.

"It's still in good shape, Jorey," Sawyer told her

almost gently. "The owners seem to take good care of it. If you want to, you can come by and see for yourself."

As soon as he'd spoken the words that sounded suspiciously like an invitation, he wanted to take them back. What had gotten into him? He was supposed to be trying to stay away from her, not asking her to visit him at his home.

But he didn't have to worry. She was shaking her head rapidly, as though equally repelled by the idea.

"No," she told him hastily, "I couldn't do that. I really don't want to see the house . . . not after so many years. I guess I'd rather just remember it the way it used to be, with my grandfather there."

"He died?"

She nodded. "The summer I turned eighteen. Dropped dead of a heart attack while we were fishing together in the pond on his property. One minute, he was showing me how to tie a fly, and the next, he was just lying there . . ."

He saw tears glistening in her eyes, and found himself longing to comfort her somehow. Without stopping to think, he reached out to touch her arm.

Then he remembered the grease that still coated his fingers, and he retracted his hand reluctantly.

But she had seen his gesture and she looked up at him, wearing a grateful expression. Grateful that he had started to reach out to her, or grateful that he had stopped?

She frowned slightly and said, "You still have dirt all over your head. Here . . ."

She reached into her enormous leather bag and rummaged around, then pulled out a handkerchief. It was white, with lace-scalloped edges, the last thing he would ever expect a woman like Jorey Maddock to be carrying around.

"Don't," he said, as she moved closer and reached toward him with it. "You'll ruin it with grease."

"As if I mind," she said carelessly. "I have hundreds of these. My mother always insisted that I carry a clean handkerchief around with me. That's what ladies do, you know." Her tone was mocking.

"And old habits die hard?" He felt her begin to stroke his hand with the soft fabric and did his best not to flinch, or pull away.

He didn't want her to know how her tender touch affected him; how profoundly intimate he found the contact, even though her fingertips barely brushed against his skin.

"Old habits die hard," she echoed, nodding, still stroking his hand.

Her movements stirred the air in front of his nostrils and he could smell her perfume—a fresh scent that reminded him of a mountain breeze—and it took him by surprise. He wouldn't expect a woman like Jorey to remind him of the outdoors—of pine trees and sunshine and the wind on his face.

She was a New Yorker. Brash and fashionable, as utterly out of place in this tiny rural town as caviar at a potluck supper.

But what about you? an inner voice nagged him. *Where do you fit in? You're an outsider yourself, more so even than she is. This town was a part of her past.*

"Why did you come back here?" he heard himself asking her.

There was silence, and her hand stopped moving on his temple.

He pulled back slightly and saw her clutching the

handkerchief in midair, a bemused expression on her face.

"I don't know," she said after a long pause. "To tell you the truth, I just don't know. It's strange. I just felt I needed to come back."

He tried to look away, but couldn't. Instead, he stared down at her upturned face, fascinated by the distant look in her eyes. She seemed almost oblivious to his presence for a moment—while his entire body tingled with absolute awareness of her.

Then her gaze shifted and her eyes collided with his. He actually heard her breath catch in her throat at that instant.

He knew that she felt it, too. Felt the unbridled magnetism between them, and the sudden, urgent need to do something about it. He knew that if he dared to move, dared to take a breath or blink an eye, he would give in to the temptation that swept over him.

He stayed motionless for as long as he could, then leaned forward all at once, bending over her. He moved his big hands behind her head, tangling his fingers in the thick curls and tilting her face back so that her slender throat arched and her red beret tumbled to the floor behind her.

Poised above her, he held her like that, his eyes still locked on hers, both of them knowing what he was going to do. She didn't resist, nor did her eyelids flutter closed in delicate, feminine anticipation of his kiss.

And when he brought his lips down to crush hers he found her responding as readily as if she had been the one to initiate the contact. Her mouth opened beneath his, and her arms swiftly found their way up to his neck, where at last her fingertips stroked his bare skin. He could feel her clutching him tightly to her, and heard the faint moan in her throat when he deepened the kiss, sliding his tongue past her teeth to stroke the tender flesh beyond.

He was lost, lost, no conscious thought intruding— only pure sensation as he embraced this forbidden woman at last.

He lifted his mouth from hers to brush his lips along her taut, graceful throat, moving downward until he found the hollow between her jutting collarbones, pushing aside the soft cashmere of her sweater so that he could nuzzle her there.

She groaned his name, and it was then that reality descended upon him, instantly shattering the mood.

"Sawyer . . ."

Sawyer.

Yes.

The truth swooped over him, as numbing and effective as a cold shower.

He was Sawyer Howland to her—to everyone in this godforsaken town.

He had a mission here, one that demanded his utmost concentration.

He couldn't afford to be distracted, nor could he allow anyone—not even her—into his carefully manufactured existence here.

He lifted his head abruptly, saw the startled look on Jorey's face, and felt her body stiffen in his arms.

But she recovered swiftly, pulling back even before he could release her.

"We shouldn't have done that," she said, her tone almost chiding.

"No," he agreed, "we shouldn't have."

"I'm glad you agree."

He nodded, noting the straightforward way in which

she was looking at him, her chin lifted defiantly, not a trace of chagrin green eyes. She was gutsy, yet he'd had a fleeting glimpse of her vulnerability only moments before, when she'd yielded so readily to his passion.

He corrected himself. She hadn't *yielded*. She had met him halfway. Jorey Maddock was no fair maiden helplessly surrendering herself to the wanton desires of a man; she had given and she had taken, just as he had.

Still, he sensed that she was vulnerable—if not on a physical level, then on an emotional one. She had needs.

Needs that he might be able to fulfill.

Again, just as he had been when he last saw her, he was seized by a powerful urge to protect her. He couldn't let her fall victim to the grim destiny that awaited her in Blizzard Bay.

It was up to him to save her, because he alone knew her fate.

Because you failed her before . . .

This is your second chance, he thought, even as he became momentarily confused.

Then his thoughts cleared, and he realized the truth.

That wasn't Jorey. He hadn't failed to save Jorey.

No, Jorey was still alive, standing right here in front of him, her tousled hair and slightly smeared red lipstick the only evidence of the passion that had claimed them both only seconds before.

It wasn't too late to save Jorey.

He could try.

He *would* try.

The decision came easily, not really a decision at all. Not when the only other option was to sit by and watch this exquisitely alluring creature go blindly to her death.

There's no guarantee that you can save her.

Yet he had to try. It was his duty, perhaps his *destiny*, to try.

What he wouldn't do was let her into his life—or give her any more information about himself than she already had.

Nor could he permit himself to care about her. To love her.

Because when you loved someone, there was far too much at risk.

And Sawyer Howland had learned—the hard way— not to take those kinds of risks.

The Front Street Diner was virtually empty when Jorey stepped inside, and for a moment she was taken aback, wondering if something was wrong.

Then she realized that she had never been here in the off-season. The place was always filled to capacity during the summer; the crowd waiting for a table had spilled over onto the street when she had been here last August.

But today, there was just a lone policeman sitting on one of the round vinyl and chrome stools that lined the counter, and only one booth was occupied; the farthest from the door.

As she made her way back to greet her friend, she saw that Gretchen was apparently not alone. There was a man's coat hanging from the hook at the side of the booth.

Sure enough, Karl emerged from the nearby men's room just as Jorey arrived at the table.

"I hope you don't mind if Karl joins us," Gretchen

said. "He's in town on his lunch hour investigating a claim, and I invited him along."

"No problem. Hi, Karl," Jorey said cheerfully, masking her disappointment.

It wasn't that she didn't like her friend's boyfriend —although something about him did prevent her from warming to him completely. That might be simply because he was so much older. Or perhaps because she somehow resented his warnings about Sawyer Howland.

No, she told herself, *that would be ridiculous. You like Karl just fine. Any other time, you'd be happy to have him join you and Gretchen for lunch. The more the merrier, and all that.*

It was just that today, after what had just happened between her and Sawyer, she wasn't in the mood to make the kind of forced conversation that was necessary in the company of someone she didn't know very well.

"Don't you have a coat?" Karl asked her, eyeing her red sweater as she slid into the booth across from Gretchen.

He seemed to hesitate slightly before slipping into the bench beside Gretchen, and Jorey was struck by the sense that he might have been planning to sit where she was.

She supposed it wasn't so odd, considering that Gretchen was a large woman and there wasn't much room on the seat beside her for a man of Karl's size. Still . . .

"You must have been freezing out there," Karl said, casting a meaningful look at her sweater, and she remembered that he'd asked her about a coat.

"I have thermals on underneath this," she said. "And it's not that cold out. The snow's melting."

"It's cold enough to make your cheeks all red," Karl said, peering across the table at her. "Almost like you're blushing. Very charming."

"Where's your hat?" Gretchen asked. "Weren't you wearing one when you left the house earlier?"

Jorey's hand flew up to her hair and she vaguely remembered that Sawyer had knocked the beret from her head when he grabbed her to kiss her. She felt her cheeks flaming at the memory, then wondered guiltily if Karl and Gretchen could somehow tell what she had been up to. They would undoubtedly be horrified if they knew, considering the way they felt about Sawyer.

But despite their apprehension, Jorey had almost decided that there was no reason to be suspicious of him.

In fact, she *had* decided. Her gut had told her, as she stood in his garage chatting with him about her grandparents' house, that there was nothing sinister about this man.

She'd only had the slightest hint of any misgiving when he'd ended their kiss and brusquely told her he had to get back to work. His about-face seemed rather sudden, although she'd done her best to take it in stride. In fact, she was almost thankful that he'd been the one to interrupt the clinch and bring them both back to the real world. She should have done it herself.

But she hadn't.

The fact that he had didn't mean there was any reason to doubt his character. Just because he seemed able to turn his emotions on and off like he was flicking a butane lighter.

Just because one moment he was making love to her

with his mouth and tongue and hands, and the next he was all business, as impersonal as if they were perfect strangers.

Well, we are strangers, an inner voice pointed out. *We barely know each other.*

Why was it so impossible to remember that when she was with him?

Why—

"Jorey?"

"Hmm?"

"Your hat?" Gretchen asked in a tone that told Jorey she'd missed something.

"Oh, my hat. I guess it must have blown off my head while I was walking," Jorey said, careful not to glance out the window at the perfectly still afternoon.

She could feel their eyes on her, and she knew that both Gretchen and Karl were wondering what she had been up to. Lest they suspect, or ask, she reached for the stack of laminated menus propped between the wall and the silver-topped, glass sugar dispenser.

"We should order. I'm starved," she said, pushing two menus across the table at them and opening the third. "What's good here?"

"Everything," Gretchen said. "Same as always."

"The tuna melt is especially good, though," Karl suggested.

"I'll keep that in mind," Jorey said pleasantly.

She hated tuna.

She tried to keep her mind on food, intently scanning the list of burgers and club sandwiches and breakfast items as though searching diligently for something she'd never find there, like mussels marinara or Beef Wellington.

She remembered when she'd first started coming

here as a child, and how surprised she'd been at the difference between upstate diners and those in the city. Back in New York, some restaurants referred to as "diners" had twelve page menus, foods of many nationalities, and exotic, five-course meals.

But here at the Front Street Diner in Blizzard Bay, it was egg salad, meatloaf, and blueberry pie a la mode, same as it always had been.

There was something comforting about that, and about Mae's familiar grin as she appeared to take their order.

"Jorey Maddock!" she exclaimed, her white eyebrows bobbing up beneath her curled white bangs. "You're back *again*. What a wonderful surprise. How long are you staying?"

"I'm not sure," Jorey told her. "Probably about a week."

Suddenly, the thought of leaving depressed her. There was nothing to go back to in New York City.

That's not true. You have Daddy—and your apartment— and your friends. . . .

But her father, though he adored her, was caught up in his business, same as always.

Her newly decorated apartment—on the top of an exclusive doorman building—was lovely, with its sweeping views of the skyline and the river. But it didn't feel any more like home than any of her parents' impeccably appointed apartments ever had.

As for her friends, she had a broad social circle, and her calendar typically revolved around brunches and gallery openings and nightclubs and parties.

But she didn't miss any of that. Not yet.

She'd supposed that after a week in deserted Blizzard

Bay she would be craving Manhattan, but this small town adventure was still so new. . . .

And then there was Sawyer.

Sawyer Howland, who should have nothing to do with how long she stayed in this remote, snow-covered village—but whose presence here was rapidly taking on increasing significance now that he had kissed her.

"So what would you like?" Mae was asking, order pad poised.

What would I like?

I would like Sawyer Howland to sweep me into those strong arms and hold me against that broad chest and carry me off to his bed. I want him to lay me down and gently peel off my clothes and then rip off his own, and I want him to finish what he started.

Jorey looked up at Mae, swallowed hard, and said lamely, "I'll have the tuna melt."

The snow was almost thawed by evening, leaving behind only patches of slushy residue that promised to vanish overnight, with temperatures predicted to rise into the forties.

Jorey found herself almost disappointed as she looked out the window before bed at the world that was once again green and gray. She listened to the steady dripping of melting ice from the eaves and she wondered whether it would snow again while she was there. She hoped so.

The blizzard had been a novelty for her, and so had the local reaction. New York City would come to an utter standstill if it were socked by a storm like the one this village had just weathered. But up here people simply dug out and went on, seeming to take it in stride.

Well, they don't call it Blizzard Bay for nothing, Jorey

reminded herself, dropping the curtain and crawling into bed. She reached out to turn off the bedside lamp, then froze with her hand on the switch.

She was certain she'd just heard a footstep outside her door.

Not footsteps, as though someone had walked by on their way down the hall.

No, *a* footstep. As if someone were lurking on the other side of her door.

It was nearly midnight. And she hadn't heard Gretchen come home from her movie date with Karl.

Silently, Jorey stood and made her way across the short distance to the door. There was no lock; until now, that hadn't bothered her.

Now, even as she reached for the knob she wondered how she, a jaded city dweller, could have even considered sleeping in a room without a lock.

In one swift movement she grasped the knob, turned it, and threw the door open.

She let out a little scream at the sight of a man standing in the hallway.

He turned toward her, looking as startled as she did.

He was elderly, perhaps in his early seventies, with a shock of gray hair, weathered skin, and thick glasses perched on his nose. He wore a tool belt around his waist and held a lightbulb in his hand.

This had to be Gretchen's Uncle Roland. Jorey hadn't met him yet, but she knew he had a room on the third floor and that he did handyman chores around the house.

Why would he be sneaking around outside her room in the middle of the night?

"What are you doing?" Jorey demanded, even though it was obvious. He was changing a bulb in the wall sconce outside her door. She had noticed that it was burned out earlier, and saw that he had already removed the glass globe to start the job.

He didn't reply, just looked at her and shook his head. Then he went back to changing the lightbulb.

Jorey watched him for a moment, taken aback.

Then, because she didn't know what else to do, she stepped back into her room and closed the door. She leaned against it for a moment, her heart still beating from the scare.

Then she looked around for something to wedge beneath the knob. If she couldn't lock herself in, at least she could make it difficult for someone to get in and . . .

What?

Kill her, the way someone had butchered that female tourist by the lake last summer?

She told herself not to let her imagination run away with her. Just because Gretchen's uncle had given her a scare . . .

But who *wouldn't* be frightened at finding someone sneaking around at this hour? Why hadn't she seen him before now? Why would a handyman choose midnight to change a lightbulb? And why hadn't he spoken to her when she'd asked what he was doing?

Jorey decided that there was something creepy about Gretchen's uncle, and made a mental note to ask Gretchen about him tomorrow.

She waited until she'd heard his footsteps fade away down the hall a few moments later. Then she dragged the only chair across the room and shoved it beneath the doorknob the way she'd seen people do in movies.

It seemed utterly ineffective, perhaps because it was padded, or because the back was curved.

Still, she left it there and stacked two suitcases on it for good measure, figuring that if anyone tried to sneak in while she was asleep, the racket of everything falling would wake her up.

When Jorey went to bed—leaving the light on—a sexy, blond-haired mechanic was the furthest thing from her mind.

She dreamed of him anyway, though.

A graphic, erotic dream in which she and Sawyer were lying naked in the snow, which somehow wasn't cold— rather, it was warm and fluffy as a featherbed.

Sawyer was doing to her all the things that she had scarcely dared to imagine when he'd kissed her so passionately that morning.

The dream was so real, so captivating, that when Jorey woke in the wee hours, squirming, panting, and drenched in sweat, she had forgotten all about the handyman in the hallway and the booby trap chair in front of the door.

She had forgotten everything, for the moment, but the seductive, mysterious man who had somehow found his way into her subconscious and made her tremble at the realization that she would actually be seeing him again tomorrow.

Chapter Five

Sawyer stood on the narrow strip of rocky beach, his hands jammed into the front pockets of his jeans against the morning chill as he watched the sun come up over the lake. It cast a shimmering, golden path along the November-gray water, a path that stretched from the shore to the horizon—and, he figured, beyond. . . .

Are you out there, somewhere? he asked silently, kicking the toes of his boots into the pebbles, staring at the brightening sky. *Can you hear me? If you can, I want you to know that I'm still here. And I swear that I'm still trying. . . .*

He pulled his hand out of his pocket and swiped it across his tear-filled eyes, then turned away from the water. Slowly, head bent, he began to head back toward the deserted road, where his car waited.

He could imagine what this lakefront neighborhood was like during the tourist season, when the rustic, waterfront cottages were occupied and traffic meandered along the winding, tree-lined road. If he closed his eyes he could almost hear squeaky screen doors slamming, radios playing, and gleeful children splashing on the beach.

But at this time of year there was only an aura of desolation, despite the few year-round residents who braved winters on the lake's icy shore.

He picked his way up the pebbly incline leading away from the beach, and stepped onto the muddy grass of a small yard. He made himself keep walking toward the boarded-up cottage that stood between there and the road, but couldn't bring himself to look up at it.

He knew it by heart, anyway; had spent long hours sitting in front of it, staring at it, memorizing it, so that the details often haunted him in his sleep.

He knew the exact spots where the faded, forest green paint was peeling, knew that the porch railing was missing the fourth slat over from the slanted steps, that the tattered remains of yellow, police crime scene tape were still stuck to the lamppost beside the door.

The wind stirred the trees above his head, and it was a mournful, sighing sound that mingled with the lapping of the water and the crunch of his footsteps through the piles of dead, brown leaves that no one had bothered to rake away.

Then he heard the sound of wood banging against wood in the distance, and saw that the door of the cabin down the road had been thrown open and carried by a gust of wind to slam against its shingled wall. The figure of a man stood there, his back turned away from Sawyer.

He couldn't see his face but he knew that it was Karl Andersen, and that he was waiting for his dog to come in.

He heard a shrill whistle from the man's lips, and then the jingling of the animal's collar as the large sheepdog came bounding up from the beach. The animal's fur, Sawyer knew, would be gray and matted with lake water; he would shake himself off before venturing up to the porch and disappearing inside the house.

It was the same routine every morning.

Sawyer wondered sometimes if Andersen ever saw him, or noticed the old Chevy parked a short distance down the road. He didn't think so, because the man never lingered long in the doorway, or seemed to glance in his direction.

Sawyer certainly didn't want to be seen, but he couldn't seem to keep from coming here. Most days, he woke before dawn and was compelled to visit the deserted cabin, to walk the beach behind it, and to contemplate the tragedy that had taken place there only a few months ago—the bloody event that had changed his life forever.

He had reached his car now, and took one last glance over his shoulder before getting in and driving away, toward town.

"I think I met your uncle last night," Jorey announced to Gretchen, who glanced up from the cup of coffee she had just poured.

"You *think* you met him?"

"There was an old man in the hallway outside my room, fixing the wall sconce there."

Gretchen nodded, pulling her chair toward the table across from Jorey. "That was Uncle Roland. I told him that the bulb had burned out."

"Does he always, uh, *work* at midnight?" Jorey asked,

reaching for a second piece of toast from the plate in the middle of the kitchen table.

"Mostly," Gretchen told her. "Which is why you haven't met him before now. I forgot to tell you Uncle Roland prowls around at odd hours. He spent years on the night shift at a factory, and after he retired he couldn't get used to sleeping at night and being up all day. And why should he? It doesn't matter to me when he changes a lightbulb or fixes a sink."

Jorey shrugged, dumping a generous dollop of strawberry jam on her toast and spreading it. "I guess not. But when I asked him what he was doing, he just looked at me. Maybe he doesn't like having someone around at this time of year."

"Oh . . ." Gretchen shook her head. "That's not it. I can't believe I didn't mention to you that Uncle Roland is deaf. And mute."

"I can't believe you didn't mention it, either," Jorey muttered. "Geez, Gretchen, I was thinking there was something wrong with him, that he was some kind of creep, sneaking around in the dead of night, not responding when I spoke to him. You could have filled me in."

"Don't worry. He's harmless, Jorey," Gretchen said, sipping her coffee. "I know I should have told you about him, but I've had other things on my mind these days, I guess . . ."

"It's all right." She bit into her toast, watching her friend's face.

There were dark circles under Gretchen's eyes, accentuated by her pale complexion and blond lashes. And her hair, usually worn in a tight braid down her back, was loose and uncombed this morning, as though she hadn't had the energy to bother with it yet.

"Are you okay?" Jorey asked her. "I mean, you seem preoccupied. If you want to talk about anything—Karl, or anything else—I'd be glad to—"

"No," Gretchen said quickly. Too quickly. "No, everything's fine with Karl. You know, I'm going to be working on the third floor front bedroom all day today. Painting all the trim. I did the wallpaper last month, and I finally managed to buy the paint for the woodwork. Want to lend me a hand, if you have nothing else to do?"

"I'd love to," Jorey lied, "but actually, I do have some things I have to do. I'm going over to Kitty's— she invited me for lunch so that I can meet her kids— and I have to pick up my car at the garage. It'll be ready by noon, Sawyer said."

"Sawyer?" Gretchen made a face. "Sounds like you're on awfully familiar terms with him, Jorey."

"Not exactly. I just—what am I supposed to call him? 'Mr. Howland'?"

"No, but . . . just watch your step, okay? You don't know anything about him."

"Neither do you," she said defensively, before she could stop herself.

"That's the trouble," Gretchen replied in an even tone, but she set her coffee cup down so hard that the black liquid splashed over the rim. "Nobody in Blizzard Bay knows anything about him. There *was* an unsolved murder here, and people are saying he might have something to do with it. I just don't want to see you get hurt."

"Gretchen," Jorey said patiently, "I'm picking up my car from Sawyer Howland's garage. How is that going to hurt me?"

"Forget I said anything."

"I will," she said, and then remembered something. "Do you mind if I use the phone? I have to make a few calls to New York."

"That's fine," Gretchen said, looking hesitant.

"I'm planning to put them on my credit card," Jorey added hastily.

"No problem," Gretchen told her. "Listen, Jorey . . . if you don't mind my asking . . . I've been wondering . . ."

"What?" she prodded when her friend hesitated.

"What do you *do?*"

"What do I do?" Jorey echoed blankly.

"I mean, do you have a job back in the city, or . . . ?"

Oh. *That* old question.

Jorey sighed and wished the subject of her employment—or lack thereof—hadn't come up.

Here was Gretchen, obviously struggling to make ends meet and keep this vast old house from falling apart. Not that she wasn't aware that Jorey's family had always had money, but . . .

How would she react to the fact that Jorey lived off the comfortable trust fund her grandfather had left her? That her father had bought and furnished her Park Avenue apartment? That her mother sent monthly checks for "extras," courtesy of her wealthy, aristocratic second husband?

"Actually," Jorey said carefully, "I'm in between careers right now."

"Oh?" Gretchen was obviously waiting for her to go on.

"I haven't quite decided what I'm going to do next."

"What did you do before?"

"After college?"

I travelled around the world. Lived in Europe with Mom

and Reginald until they drove me crazy. Spent a year in L.A. mingling with the celebs.

"I did a little bit of everything," Jorey said truthfully. "When I settled down in New York eventually, I thought I would go into the family business. My father hired me as a buyer, but I wasn't terrific with the nine to five stuff."

Aside from getting great seats at all the designer shows and travelling to Paris and Milan, fashion was too boring . . . at least, as a career.

"So then, I went back to school for creative writing."

I took a screenplay writing night course—three two hour sessions in a church basement with a frustrated Woody Allen wannabe.

"But I decided that I wasn't talented enough."

Sitting alone in front of a computer isn't my idea of being creative.

"I still want to be my own boss and do something that's personally rewarding. Lately, I've been toying with the idea of opening my own business."

Daddy says he doesn't want me to be bored, which I am, and that if I can just figure out what I want to do he'll buy it for me.

"But I'm not quite sure what kind of business it should be. And that's about it," Jorey told Gretchen, who had been listening intently.

"Your own business? You mean, like a store, or something?"

"Not a store. I mean, my family is already in retail. That would be kind of redundant. I was thinking about something more along the lines of . . ."

Actually, I wasn't thinking along any particular lines.

"You could run an inn, like I do," Gretchen suggested.

"I could."

Except that I've never been the domestic type.

"Although I can't really see you doing that," Gretchen continued, eyeing her.

She bristled at the expression on her friend's face. "What do you mean?"

"You're just not the domestic type."

"Oh." She could hardly argue with that.

"Don't worry," she told Gretchen. "I'm sure I'll figure something out sooner or later. It's not as though I'm going to just do *nothing* for the rest of my life."

The way my mother and sisters, and my grandmothers before them, have always done.

But the thing was, nobody had ever told Jorey that she should be preparing for the future. Nobody had suggested that she should have any goal in life beyond landing a suitable husband.

Not even Papa May, by far the most sensible person in her family, had ever said that she should have a career. Rather, he used to tell her how fortunate she was that she would never have to slave away the way his widowed mother had.

Great-grandmother Maddock had taken in laundry and sewing; anything to provide for her son after her husband died when the child was an infant. And Papa May had sworn that when he grew up he would become rich so that his mother—and the other women in his family—would never have to work again.

So, here she was—a third generation Maddock, wealthy enough to spend the rest of her life . . . doing nothing.

Absolutely nothing.

Doing it alone.

She stood abruptly, turning away from Gretchen in

case her face betrayed the sudden sense of desolation that had come over her. "I'm going to use the phone now, if that's all right," she said.

"It's fine . . . you can use the one in the front parlor if you want."

She nodded and left the kitchen, making her way through the dining room to the parlor. As she went, she noticed a handknit, blue wool cardigan draped over the back of a chair. She remembered that Clover had been wearing it when they'd had lunch on Sunday. She must have forgotten it. Jorey made a mental note to mention it to Gretchen.

In the parlor, she perched on a chair and dialed her home phone number, intending to check her messages.

There were several—all of them from acquaintances, all of them calling to tell her about upcoming parties and get-togethers.

So my life isn't that lonely, Jorey told herself, hanging up the receiver. *I have plenty of things to do. All that's missing is a career.*

And a man.

On the heels of that thought, of course, came the image of Sawyer Howland leaning down to kiss her.

It figured, Jorey thought, that the one man she found remotely interesting—well, far from *remotely*—was more unsuitable than anyone she'd ever known in her life.

She banished him—and his kisses—from her mind and dialed the number of her father's office.

"It's Jorey, Helen," she told his secretary when she answered.

"Jorey! How are you, Dear?"

"I'm . . ."

Frustrated. Sexually frustrated.

". . . just fine," Jorey murmured. "Is Daddy in?"

"He's in a board meeting this morning, Jorey. Can I have him return the call?"

"No, just tell him that everything's fine and I'll be in touch again soon."

She thanked Helen and hung up, trying to ignore the hollow feeling in the pit of her stomach.

Why, all of the sudden, did her entire life seem to lack meaning? She had come up here to Blizzard Bay because she was feeling restless and nostalgic—maybe even to "find herself," like the heroine of some seventies feminist novel.

But all she had found was a village that hadn't changed and old friends who had moved on, and a hell of a lot of snow.

And temptation, in the form of a strapping mechanic who, for all she knew, might be the devil himself.

So.

She had come here to find herself, but never in her life had Jorey felt more lost and alone.

Today, when Jorey showed up in the doorway of his garage Sawyer was waiting for her. Actually, he had been keeping one eye on the clock and the other on the door all morning.

Still, when she appeared he felt caught off guard. His heart leapt and his hands trembled slightly, and he forgot whatever it was that he'd been planning to say— some casual greeting that would show her he had forgotten all about what had happened between them twenty-four hours ago in this same spot.

"Am I early?" she asked, this time walking right in and allowing the door to close behind her.

"No, you're not early. The car's all set, and I parked

it outside," he told her, going over to the drawer where he kept the keys and paperwork.

"I saw it there. So that means you got the part with no problem? And it's running all right?"

"Everything's fine. I took it for a test drive a little while ago."

He didn't say that he'd driven it further than was necessary, just so he could keep inhaling the scent of her that still clung to the car's interior.

Or that the longer he'd sat there, in her car, breathing her scent, the more urgently he'd felt the need to see her again.

And not just to see her. To ensure that she was all right, that nothing terrible had happened to her.

He stared at her, standing in his doorway wearing black corduroys that hugged her slim figure and an oversized leather jacket that made her look smaller and more delicate than she was. And he noted something in her eyes, something that had changed since yesterday.

Did she sense that she was in danger?

Or . . . had something happened to frighten her?

Was that why some of the light seemed to have gone out of her gaze?

Something clearly weighed on her mind. Even her movements, as she walked toward him, were less jaunty than they had been.

He pretended to be busy figuring out the invoice for the repairs, but his brain wasn't functioning properly. He found himself adding the same column of figures three times, and coming up with three different totals.

She didn't even seem to notice. He saw when he glanced up at her that she was preoccupied, staring off into space.

"Is everything okay, Jorey?" he asked impulsively.

Her eyes flicked to his face, and he half-expected her to say breezily, *Everything's fine,* or even, *What's it to you?*

But she didn't. She said, "I don't know."

"What do you mean?"

She shrugged. "I'm just . . . I don't know."

"Did something happen?" he probed, worried.

"No. It's just that I'm kind of feeling down, I guess. I'm sure I'll snap out of it."

He nodded, then heard himself say, "Do you have any plans for the afternoon?"

She hesitated. "I was supposed to go and visit a friend of mine. But she called just before I left and asked if I could come tonight, instead. So . . . no. No, I don't have plans. Why?"

He had no idea why he'd asked. He'd simply blurted out the question, just as he blurted out the next thing out of his mouth.

"I was thinking that if you wanted to, we could do something."

She looked startled. "Together?"

He nodded, realizing he had no choice but to finish what he'd started.

"Don't you have to work?" she asked.

He shook his head. "Business is slow. I can take a few hours off with no problem."

"And do what?" she asked.

"We could drive over to Saratoga Springs and have lunch."

She smiled faintly. "That sounds like fun. I love Saratoga."

Still, he could see that she was hesitating. Maybe she would tell him that she couldn't go, and that would be the end of it.

But she didn't. She paused only a moment longer,

clearly weighing her decision, before saying, "All right. I'll go with you. And I'll drive."

He was about to protest when she looked him in the eye and added, "I want to see how it runs. After all, I did quite a bit of damage when I wrecked it."

He couldn't argue with that.

Her take-charge attitude shouldn't really surprise him. He'd only known her a few days, but he already was well aware that Jorey Maddock didn't appreciate being told what to do, and wouldn't take kindly to a man who treated her like a fragile female.

Which would make protecting her trickier than he had anticipated.

It was going to be complicated enough, considering that he didn't plan to spend much time with her if he could help it.

You're off to a terrific start, here, he thought wryly, realizing he would be at her side for the remainder of the afternoon, on what seemed suspiciously like a date.

At least he'd be able to keep an eye on her.

And, hopefully, his hands *off* her.

Jorey's spirits lifted as she steered the Range Rover down Broadway in Saratoga Springs, taking in the familiar sights along the famed, charming street.

They passed City Center and the sprawling Collamer Building on the left, and the stately Adirondack Trust Company and grand Rip Van Dam Hotel on the right.

How many times had Jorey and Papa May strolled past these buildings on hot summer days, poking in and out of the specialty boutiques and always stopping so that he could treat her to an ice cream sundae?

Sawyer's voice interrupted her reverie, asking, "Do you know where the Spa State Park is?"

She nodded and pointed. "Straight ahead, a ways down. Why?"

"I was thinking we could eat at the Gideon Putnam."

"The Gideon Putnam?" she echoed, picturing the magnificent Victorian hotel in the middle of the 2000 acre park down the road. That wasn't exactly what she'd had in mind when he'd suggested lunch in Saratoga.

"What's the matter?" he asked, and she could feel his eyes on her.

"It's just . . . I figured we could eat at Hattie's."

"Hattie's?"

"Hattie's Chicken Shack." She glanced at him, and saw his brows go up.

"It's my favorite place to eat in town," she explained, remembering how she and Papa May would sneak off to Hattie's whenever he said, in a fake Southern accent, "I've got a hankerin' for some home cookin', Chile."

They sat on mismatched chairs at a rickety table covered in checkered vinyl, and they gorged themselves on fried chicken and rich mashed potatoes and pecan pie—all forbidden treats for Papa May, as far as Grandmother was concerned. She was always nagging him to watch what he ate—with good reason, Jorey thought sadly now, not without a flicker of guilt. All that sinful food they'd shared couldn't have done his heart any good, and she tried to banish an image of her beloved grandfather thrashing on the ground, making horrible gasping sounds as he clutched his chest—

Sawyer broke into her thoughts once again, and this time she was grateful. "Are you sure you wouldn't rather eat at the Gideon Putnam?"

"I'm positive," she said firmly, wondering if he was

trying to impress her by suggesting one of the finest restaurants in town. He didn't seem the type to frequent upscale dining establishments, and they certainly weren't dressed for a fancy date.

Then again, he had scrubbed and changed his clothes before they'd left the garage, emerging from the back room in a pair of slightly rumpled khaki pants and a bulky, oatmeal-colored, textured sweater. He looked as if he'd stepped out of an ad for J. Crew, so handsome she had to keep sneaking glances at him as they walked out to her car.

Now, she kept her eyes focused on the red traffic light straight ahead as she told him simply, "Let's go to Hattie's. Okay?"

"Okay."

She had half-expected an argument, just as she had when she'd informed him earlier that she would drive to Saratoga. If he had protested then, she would have flatly refused to go. In fact, that was basically what she'd had in mind, once she'd shocked herself by agreeing to go with him. Her next thought had been, *How do I get out of this?*

Now she was glad she hadn't.

Why not throw caution to the winds and simply enjoy an afternoon with Sawyer—even if he *wasn't* her soul mate and the answer to all her problems?

"You were right," Sawyer told Jorey as they stepped out onto the quiet side street an hour and a half later after a meal of chicken and catfish, black-eyed peas, cornbread, and sweet potato pie—the most delicious food he had ever eaten in his life.

"I was right about what?" She zipped her leather coat

against the wind, which had picked up while they were inside. The sun had disappeared behind a bank of ominously gray clouds moving in from the west.

"You were right about Hattie's Chicken Shack. That place was perfect."

"I told you so."

He grinned at her choice of words.

"What?" she asked, catching him. "What's so funny?"

"I would have pegged you as an 'I told you so' type. You like to be right, don't you."

She shrugged. "Who doesn't? Anyway, I pretty much always am."

He raised an eyebrow at that and saw that she was smiling, but he sensed that she wasn't entirely kidding.

"What should we do now?" he asked her, buttoning his corduroy barn coat against the chill.

"I don't know . . . head back?"

"Head back?" He consulted his watch. "But it's only . . . two thirty. What time are you meeting your friend?"

"At seven," she admitted.

"We can go back if you want to," he told her, trying to ignore the flicker of disappointment at the thought of ending their afternoon.

"Or we can stay and walk around a little," she said, taking him by surprise. "If you want to," she added, and he saw that her cheeks were flushed.

"Since we're here, we might as well," he agreed. "For a while, at least. It would be fun to see what's here."

"Have you spent much time getting to know the area since you moved to Blizzard Bay?" she asked.

His guard shot up.

The whole time they had been in the restaurant, their conversation had revolved around impersonal topics—

the food, the eclectic decor, the framed photos of various celebrities on the walls. Not even once had he thought about who he was supposed to be, or his reason for leaving his real life behind and coming to the North Country.

But now, reality came at him like a freight train, and he paused before answering her question.

"I haven't spent much time here, no," he replied. "It's getting colder—"

"Where did you live before Blizzard Bay?"

"The midwest," he said tersely. "Did you happen to hear a weather report this morning?"

"Me? Uh-uh. I never check the weather reports."

"Why not?" he asked, partly to keep the conversation steered in a safe direction, and partly out of curiosity.

She shrugged. "Because there's nothing you can do to change it, anyway. And if you don't know it's going to rain, you can wake up every morning and hope for sun."

He considered that. She had no idea the irony her words held for him. No idea at all.

"Although," she added, "some people might think I was a fool for not checking the weather reports before I headed up here on Saturday, right into a major blizzard."

"If you had known there was going to be a snowstorm, would you have postponed your trip?"

"No," she said promptly. "I would have come anyway. I would have figured I could handle it. And I did."

"With a little help," he couldn't resist pointing out.

"With a little help. Thank you, by the way . . . did I ever thank you? If you hadn't come along, I would have been stuck taking a ride from Hob Nixon."

"I thought that was fine with you," he said, remembering her attitude that afternoon as he'd driven her into town.

She flushed again, a habit he found charming and inconsistent with the brasher aspects of her personality.

"Actually, I didn't want a ride from him. That was before I remembered that he once, uh, had a thing for me, too. When we were kids."

"I take it the attraction was one-sided."

"Of course. In fact, I was so horrified that I had apparently wiped the whole thing out of my mind."

"But now you remember it?"

She hesitated. "Not exactly. It's strange. I don't remember other things about that summer, either. It's as if I have a huge memory blank. Maybe because it was a really rough time for me—"

"How so?"

"It was the summer before I went away to college. My parents told me they were splitting up on the night I graduated from high school. I don't think they thought I would care much—it wasn't as if we had an all-American family life."

"But it bothered you?" he asked quietly.

"It did. A lot. I loved my father—he was always my ally. And their divorce meant he was moving out. Oh, I was moving out, too—going to Bennington and all. But I figured that when I came home, he'd be there."

"And he wasn't?"

She shrugged. "He got a place across town. I spent as much time with him as I did with my mother and sisters. More, once my mother remarried—and it didn't take her long. But you know, it didn't matter as much as I thought it would—the fact that they were divorced. Because once I left home, I hardly ever came back. I spent school breaks and summers travelling and visiting my friends."

"And coming to Blizzard Bay?"

"No," she said, a melancholy expression in her green eyes. "Until this year, I never came back here again after that summer. My papa—my grandfather—died in July. I told you about that."

He nodded, remembering what she'd said yesterday, in his garage. That her grandfather had dropped dead of a heart attack, and she was with him when it happened. He remembered her tears . . . and how he'd reached out to comfort her. And how that had led to kissing her.

Something stirred deep inside of him, in a place he would rather not acknowledge.

"Then what?" he asked her, thinking that if she just kept talking and they kept walking he could ignore the memory of what had happened between them.

She obliged, telling him, "After my grandfather was gone, my grandmother put the house on the market. It seemed as if she did it the next day, but I know it couldn't have been that soon. We all went back to New York for the funeral. All I know is that the moment she listed it, it sold. And she had packed it up and handed over the keys before racing season was over that August. I never set foot in the house again after the day we drove away behind the hearse, heading back to New York for the funeral."

"So you never got to say good-bye."

"Not to the house, no. And maybe, in a way, not to him," she added suddenly, as though the thought had just struck her. "Maybe I've always felt as though he was still there, somehow. As though I had left him

behind when I left. Maybe that's part of the reason I've
never been able to let go of this place."

"Is it why you came back now?"

"I don't know," she said softly.

He glanced at her, and then at their surroundings,
realizing they had left Phila Street and were back on
bustling Broadway, the main drag. They were in front
of a newsstand, and he caught a glimpse of a headline
in the local paper.

"Look," he said, nudging Jorey's arm and pointing.

" 'Area Prepares for Second Snowstorm This Week,' "
she read. "Oh, good."

"Good?"

"I love snow. We don't get much in the city. Not
compared to here. And not at this time of year."

"Well, if it's going to snow you need warm clothes,
Jorey. A jacket. Gloves. A hat—"

"Hey, I *had* a hat. You didn't happen to find it in
your garage, did you? It fell off my head when—"

She broke off there, and he knew what she was thinking. He could see it in her eyes, and they were focused
directly on his face. On his lips.

She was remembering how he had grabbed her and
kissed her yesterday, so recklessly that he had knocked
her hat to the cement floor. He'd found it there after
she'd gone. For a long time he had held it to his face,
breathing her scent and remembering what it had been
like to hold her. Then he had forced himself to shove
it into a drawer, where he wouldn't be reminded.

"I have it," he told her now, and his voice sounded
hoarse and unfamiliar to his ears. He cleared his throat
and said, "I'll drop it off for you . . . or you can pick it
up."

"It's no big deal." She started walking again, her

arms now folded in front of her and her pace slower than it had been before.

"You'll need it," he said, falling into step with her. "It's going to snow, remember? You need a coat, too. Let me buy you a coat. And gloves."

"Gloves?"

"Mittens?" he suggested instead, and was rewarded when she smiled.

"I haven't worn mittens since I was a little kid."

"Let me buy them for you, Jorey. And a coat."

She tried to sound indignant, but he could tell she was secretly pleased when she said, "You don't have to do that. I can buy myself a coat and . . . and mittens. I mean, you don't have to take care of me, Sawyer."

Oh, but I do, he thought grimly. *I do have to take care of you, Jorey. Your life depends on it.*

He thought of what she'd said earlier. *If you don't know it's going to rain, you can wake up every morning and hope for sun.*

And he wondered what it would be like to live like that—how it would feel not to always sense dark clouds looming . . . even before they were on the horizon.

Chapter Six

"Jorey Maddock! If you don't look exactly the same—"

"Hi, Johnny," she greeted Kitty's husband.

She couldn't say the same about him. If she hadn't known who he was she never would have recognized him. He'd lost most of his reddish hair and had gained a considerable amount of weight in the past ten years.

She recalled what Kitty had said about Johnny having a crush on her that last summer, and tried again to remember the details. But she drew a blank.

How could she have forgotten something like that? Kitty had been one of her closest friends, and as her older brother's best friend, Johnny had been a part of their summer crowd since they were all children.

Now, knowing he'd once had feelings for her, Jorey found herself feeling slightly uncomfortable as she and Johnny looked each other over.

"Who is she, Daddy?"

Jorey looked down to see a pint-sized version of Kitty peeking out from behind her father's legs.

"This is Mommy's old friend Jorey, Maureen. What do you say to her?"

"Thank you," the little girl responded promptly.

Johnny grinned and told Jorey, "We've been working on manners lately. No, Maureen, I meant, what do you say when you meet someone new?"

"Oh. Pleased to meet you."

Charmed, Jorey bent over so she was on eye level with the child, whose mop of red hair was the same shade as her mother's. She wondered what it would be like to see so much of herself in another human being, and felt a pang, wondering if she would ever know. She had never really imagined herself as a mother; had never had more than a passing thought about having children.

Now, suddenly, she was acutely aware that she wanted a child. Someday.

She did. Yes. She wanted to be someone's mommy.

With that knowledge came speculation about what kind of father a man like Sawyer would make.

Before today, she might have found herself utterly unable to imagine a man like that with a child. But she had seen a side of him this afternoon that had startled her.

There was a nurturing, tender side to the man who all too often seemed to be trying to maintain a gruff, detached exterior. He had, for a little while, seemed like someone she could count on—someone who would take care of her.

If she wanted to be taken care of.

Not that Jorey did. She was perfectly self-sufficient; had always prided herself on that. She didn't need to be taken care of, and never would.

Still . . .

It had been nice to feel Sawyer's concern, to have him insist that she try on warm winter coats in a clothing store on Broadway. He had bought one for her; a Black Watch plaid pea coat made of soft wool. It was more casual than anything she owned, perfect for these Adirondack villages, and hardly inexpensive.

Sawyer had insisted on paying for it. He had paid cash, removing several hundred dollar bills from his wallet—a wallet he seemed to keep carefully shielded from her, as if he knew she'd be curious, trying to sneak a peek at anything personal that might be revealed by it.

If Kurt, or one of the other men she'd dated, had spent that kind of money on her she wouldn't have blinked. But she had never dated a small town mechanic, and she knew that for Sawyer this was a major purchase. It had to be. How much could he make, owning an auto body repair shop in a resort town?

When she'd questioned him about it, he had brushed her off, saying business had been good lately.

"Look, Daddy," Kitty's daughter was saying. "Jorey's wearing mittens like mine. I wear mittens, too, Jorey. Only mine are red."

"I like red mittens, too," Jorey said, taking off the dark green, fuzzy ones Sawyer had bought her to go with the coat. "How old are you, Maureen?"

"Three. I'm three." Maureen held up three fingers and waved them at Jorey. "Next month I'll be four. Four. This many."

"Wow! What a big girl you are!"

"I see you've met our chatterbox."

Jorey looked up to see Kitty balancing a flame-haired

toddler on what would have been her hip if she weren't so enormously big and round.

"Thanks for not minding that I had to change our plans this afternoon, Jorey," Kitty said. "I had completely forgotten that it was my day to be lunchroom monitor at Patrick's kindergarten."

"I'm Patrick," piped a voice from above, and Jorey saw a little boy wearing only a pair of light blue underpants perched at the top of the banister on the stairway.

"Don't you dare slide down that banister," Johnny called. "Don't even think about it."

The child pretended he was about to, then grinned, hopped off, and bounded down the stairs. Toward the bottom, he pretended to trip and lose his balance, then flashed another grin at his mother and said, "Fooled ya."

Kitty rolled her eyes and looked at Jorey. "Never a dull moment."

No sooner had she spoken than a voice called, "Kitty? Can you come up here? Kathleen has a rash all over her stomach!"

Kitty sighed and told Jorey, "That's my mother. She's supposed to be in charge of bath time. Johnny, grab Maureen and bring her up and get her undressed. And Patrick, get back up there and let Grandma put you into the tub. Move it. Be right back, Jorey."

"No problem."

"Actually, here . . . you hold Sean while I go. You don't mind, do you?"

Before Jorey could reply, Kitty had handed over the child she was carrying, placing him in Jorey's arms and taking off up the stairs, trailed by her husband and the other two children.

Jorey looked down at the little boy, who was drooling

profusely and gnawing on some kind of round, brightly colored plastic thing.

"Hi," she said tentatively.

The child took the plastic ring out of his mouth and smiled up at her.

She melted.

Oh, yes. She wanted to be a mom someday. She wanted . . . this?

She wandered dubiously around Kitty and Johnny's tiny house, noticing the scuff marks on the walls and the toys scattered across the worn carpet and the folding gates blocking most doorways. A cup of milk had tipped over on the coffee table, the sink was filled with dishes, and in the tiny family room adjacent to the kitchen a Barney video blared from the television set.

She could hear splashing and a child shrieking upstairs and footsteps, and several adult voices raised above the noise, shouting things like, "Get back here!" and "Cut that out!"

Chaos.

Pure chaos.

Yet . . . there was something appealing about it.

She leaned against the counter, looked down at the child in her arms, closed her eyes briefly, and imagined that he was hers. Hers . . .

And Sawyer's.

Knowing it was preposterous she envisioned them as parents, anyway, as a married couple living together in a house like this one; a regular house set close to the other houses on a brick-paved, small town street, a house with a porch light and too few bedrooms, and crayoned pictures stuck to the refrigerator with magnets.

She imagined herself lugging a child around, and being a lunchroom monitor.

She saw herself pregnant, as enormously pregnant as Kitty was, and she imagined what she and Sawyer had done to make her that way, and she was so overcome by longing that she suddenly actually *ached*.

The little boy in her arms babbled something and she opened her eyes and glanced at him. He looked nothing like her and nothing like Sawyer; he wasn't hers, and this wasn't her life.

Her life was a world away.

"You look wistful."

Startled, she saw that Kitty was back, reaching out to take the little boy from her and placing him in front of the Barney video.

"I know what you're thinking," Kitty said.

"What?"

"That you can't wait to get out of this zoo and back to New York for some peace and quiet. And I don't blame you. Have a seat," she added, pulling a vinyl-backed chair away from the table and brushing some crumbs into her hand.

Jorey smiled and sat down, wondering how Kitty would react if she knew Jorey had actually been thinking the opposite. She said, "Most people don't think of New York as being peaceful or quiet, you know."

"Are you kidding? Do you know what I would give for one night alone in that glamorous city?"

"Alone? What about Johnny?"

Kitty dismissed that notion with a wave of her hand. "When you've been married as long as we have, a break is sometimes better than togetherness. Besides, he says he can't go away and leave his plumbing business—even if you ask me, though, he just doesn't like the idea of travelling. But I'd love to stay in some cushy hotel room with a view, and to get all dressed up in designer clothes and take a cab to some fabulous restaurant and eat a gourmet dinner—mind you, without grubby, sticky little hands grabbing food from my plate and spitting things out into my napkin."

"Ugh," Jorey said, because she knew Kitty expected it.

But she was thinking about her life in New York, which was pretty much the way Kitty had described it—about her elegant, professionally decorated apartment, and her designer wardrobe and her sophisticated friends, and the posh restaurants and clubs they went to.

Why did it suddenly seem so sterile? So . . . empty?

Because you've suddenly decided you want to marry a long-haired mechanic and settle down in the boondocks to have a bunch of kids.

Though it was exactly what she had been imagining, the idea caught her completely off guard.

Marry Sawyer?

Have his babies?

Stay here in Blizzard Bay?

"Jorey?" Kitty was asking, running water at the sink. "Do you want coffee?"

"Coffee? No. No thanks . . ." Caffeine would only keep her up all night, and if she couldn't sleep she would find herself thinking more absurd thoughts about Sawyer.

"A Coke, then? Or a glass of wine?"

She could use a glass of wine. Wine would relax her. Wine would make her forget these crazy images that kept flitting through her mind.

"Wine would be good," she told Kitty.

"Great. I'll live vicariously through you, since I'm forced to be on the wagon until this kid decides to put in an appearance—which could be any day now. I think he's already trying to tunnel his way out," she said, rubbing her bulging belly with one hand while she leaned back against the other, which was propped in the small of her back.

"What does it feel like?" Jorey found herself asking, staring at Kitty's stomach.

"It feels like there's a fully-grown human being trying to jam its feet into my lungs and its head into my crotch. Which, incidentally, is exactly what's going on. Why so curious? Are you thinking of having a baby?"

"Me? No. God, no. At least, not for a long time."

"So there's no special man in your life these days, now that Mr. Movie Star is history?"

"Nope, nobody in my life," Jorey said quickly.

Kitty handed her a bottle of merlot and a corkscrew. "You do this while I get the glass," she said, then turned to a cupboard and asked, "What about Sawyer Howland?"

Jorey, about to poke the pointed end of the corkscrew into the cork, missed and jabbed it into her hand instead. She clutched it, the pain mingling with her shock at Kitty's question.

"Sawyer Howland?" she managed to ask. "What about him?"

"Clover saw you walk by her shop with him this afternoon. She was busy with a customer, so she couldn't run out and say hello."

Belatedly, Jorey remembered that their friend owned a New Age Boutique in Saratoga Springs. How could she have forgotten about that?

Because you were distracted by Sawyer. That's why.

"How do you know that?" she asked Kitty.

"Jorey, you can't keep anything a secret in a small

town. Johnny bumped into Clover at the mini-mart on his way home from work, and she mentioned it to him."

"Oh." She busied herself opening the wine.

"So . . . you and Sawyer Howland?"

"We were . . . just walking."

"On a date?" Kitty set a stemmed glass on the table in front of her.

"No. We had lunch. That was all."

"Lunch can be a date."

"Well, it wasn't."

"Jorey, do you know that people are saying he might have had something to do with that murder?"

She must have been out of her mind, thinking she could settle down in a place like Blizzard Bay, where everybody knew everybody else's business and nobody seemed to hesitate to spread gossip.

"I really don't think Sawyer Howland is a murderer, Kitty," she said coolly, pouring wine into her glass and then taking a long sip.

"But how well do you know him?"

"Well enough."

Well enough to just have been fantasizing about bearing his children.

"Jorey, I just don't want anything to happen to you. The woman who was killed . . . she wasn't from here, either. Johnny met her a few days before she died; there was a leak in her kitchen faucet. He said she was quiet and withdrawn, and seemed to be the type who wanted to keep to herself. There was nobody around to tell her to stay away from certain people."

"Like Sawyer Howland," Jorey said flatly.

"Or Hob Nixon."

"What woman in her right mind wouldn't want to stay away from Hob Nixon?" Jorey drank more wine.

Kitty shrugged. "Hey, you never know."

"No," Jorey agreed. "You never do."

Sawyer paced across the floor of his apartment, and then back again, and raked a hand through his hair.

Something was wrong.

He could feel it.

He moved to the window, lifted the curtain, and looked out into the night.

His room looked out over the side of the house, where the rolling lawn gradually gave way to a steep, wooded incline. During the day, the silhouette of the mountains in the distance could be seen. But tonight, there was only blackness.

And white.

Swirling white snow. The storm that had been predicted had arrived and it was starting to fall in earnest now, driven by a powerfully gusting wind that rattled the glass.

Sawyer turned abruptly and crossed back over to the bed. Reaching down, he picked up a soft, red object, raising it to his face. Eyes closed, he took a deep breath, inhaling Jorey's scent that still clung to her beret.

Where are you? he wondered. *Are you out in this storm? Are you in trouble?*

Clutching the hat, he returned to the window and stared into the night, searching for answers.

But all he found was a growing sense of trepidation— and an inability to block out the dark memories that had haunted him since August.

So he let them come, bracing himself for the torture of reliving that horrible, violent death—and knowing that he was responsible.

* * *

"Gretchen?"

"In here."

Jorey poked her head into the parlor and saw her friend sitting on the uncomfortable-looking Victorian sofa, *Country Living* magazine open on her lap.

"You're still up? It's almost midnight."

"I just finished doing a last coat on the trim in the third floor bedroom," Gretchen said, stretching. "I wanted to unwind before bed."

Jorey felt a stab of guilt. When Kitty had called to postpone their get-together she had considered spending the afternoon helping Gretchen paint. After all, it seemed the least she could do since Gretchen was putting her up—not that she didn't intend to pay for her room.

But when Sawyer had suggested lunch in Saratoga, she had somehow been unable to turn him down.

Now she wondered whether Gretchen, like Kitty, had heard about how she spent her afternoon. She knew Karl worked in Saratoga Springs. Had he, too, seen her with Sawyer? Or had he bumped into Clover there and gotten an earful of gossip?

"Uh, have you talked to Clover at all today?" she asked Gretchen.

"Clover? No. But I sent Uncle Roland over to her house earlier tonight to drop off her sweater. She left it here on Sunday. Why do you ask?"

So Gretchen didn't know about her date with Sawyer.

Not *date,* she corrected herself. *Lunch.* Her *lunch* with Sawyer.

"Actually, that's why I asked. Because of the sweater.

I noticed it earlier, and I figured I would see if you wanted me to bring it by.''

"Well, Uncle Roland already did," Gretchen said again, turning a page of her magazine.

And Jorey sensed a sudden tension in the room.

Maybe Gretchen had heard, through someone else, that she had spent the day with Sawyer. Was she angry that Jorey had seemingly ignored her and Karl's warnings about him?

Or was she upset that Jorey had chosen to enjoy herself rather than pitching in and helping with her remodelling project?

Or maybe it was something else entirely.

Maybe Gretchen and Karl were having problems, and her friend was brooding about him. Again, Jorey was struck by the sense that something wasn't quite right between them.

That Gretchen wasn't revealing everything though she claimed to be happy relationship.

Jorey made a vow to spend more time with her friend for the duration of her visit.

"Do you have any plans for tomorrow, Gretchen?" she asked, slipping out of her coat and sitting on the edge of a chair to pull off her boots.

She had almost stopped by the door to take them off there, but then had seen wet footprints leading across the wooden floor toward the stairs, as though someone else had recently come in. She figured Gretchen must not be that fussy about the battered hardwoods. Besides, it was only snow.

"Tomorrow?" Gretchen echoed. "I was just going to drive to Glens Falls to pick up more paint so I can start working on the upstairs hall."

"More trim to be done?"

Gretchen nodded.

"Doesn't your uncle do all the handyman stuff around here?"

"He's good at fixing appliances and running errands, that sort of thing. But I do a lot of the cosmetic stuff— I actually kind of enjoy it. Anyway, it keeps me busy. Gives me something to do with myself."

Jorey nodded, struck by this evidence of Gretchen's lonely, solitary life. "If you want company driving to Glens Falls, I'll be happy to tag along, Gretchen."

"Really?"

But her friend didn't seem as pleased as she had anticipated.

"If you want me to come," Jorey added.

"Sure, I do. I . . . I was going to ask Karl, but you and I could go instead."

"No, I didn't mean to horn in on your plans with your boyfriend. You two can go ahead," Jorey said hastily. "There are lots of other things I can do."

Like trying to keep myself from dropping by Sawyer's garage, she thought grimly.

"No, it's all right. He'll probably be busy with work, anyway. It's hard for him to get away from the office, although once in a while, we meet for lunch. You and I will go, Jorey. Thanks for offering."

"Are you sure?"

"I'm positive."

Jorey studied her friend's round, earnest face. "Gretchen," she said, "is everything all right between you two?"

"Between me and Karl? Sure . . . why wouldn't every-thing be all right?" Her voice was higher-pitched than usual.

"I was just wondering." Now Jorey knew that she

hadn't imagined it. Gretchen was definitely fretting about her relationship.

A day or two ago, Jorey might have pried further. But now, she let the subject drop.

After all, she could understand how someone would want to protect her privacy when it came to discussing the man in her life.

She certainly hadn't appreciated Kitty's questions about what she had been up to with Sawyer, or the fact that Clover had spread the news so eagerly.

"Is that a new coat?" Gretchen asked suddenly.

Jorey looked down at it in her lap, and nodded. "I heard it was going to snow again, and I needed something warm to wear," she said simply.

"It's nice."

"Thanks. I think I'll go to bed. Are you coming up?"

"Later," Gretchen told her. "I'm not tired yet."

"Goodnight."

Yawning, Jorey made her way up the creaky staircase and along the shadowy hall as the storm outside unleashed its full fury on the small, lakefront village.

Chapter Seven

The snow continued to fall steadily the next morning, and Gretchen told Jorey that she had decided against driving to Glens Falls.

"We can go tomorrow," she said over coffee in the kitchen. "I'm in no rush to paint the hall, and it's not a good idea to take chances on these roads in weather like this."

Jorey knew she was right—look what had happened to her on Saturday.

Still, as she drifted around the old house after breakfast she found herself struck by cabin fever.

Gretchen had decided to clean out her bedroom closet, and insisted to Jorey that she didn't need help, that she should just relax.

So she tried to read a book—a murder mystery she found on the built-in shelves beside the fireplace in the parlor—but couldn't concentrate.

Then she turned on the television and watched half

of a morning talk show. She turned it off when the host mentioned that an upcoming guest would be the actress Lacey Stearns—who, Jorey knew, happened to be co-starring with Kurt Govan in his about-to-be-released new movie.

She didn't want to be reminded of Kurt right now—and not because it hurt to realize that they were no longer together. It didn't. Rather, she didn't want to think about the life she had left behind in the city, a life that had revolved around Kurt and people like him.

Here in Blizzard Bay she was removed from that world, and the longer she stayed the more reluctant she was to go back.

But what was there to keep her here?

What had brought her here in the first place?

She didn't know the answers to those questions . . . or maybe, suddenly, she was afraid to contemplate them.

Restlessly, Jorey made her way into the kitchen, and her eye fell on a row of glass canisters lining the vinyl countertop. Flour, sugar, salt . . .

She was struck by a memory.

There had been similar canisters in the kitchen at her grandparents' house. She had never seen anyone use their contents other than Edwina, the housekeeper.

Until one night that last summer in that house, when she had awakened thirsty and come down to the kitchen for a glass of water. She had been startled to see the light on, and to smell the faint scent of natural gas, which meant someone was heating the big, old-fashioned oven.

"Papa May?" she had asked, startled, finding him wearing an apron over his pajamas and mixing something in a bowl at the counter. "What are you doing?"

"Baking blueberry muffins," he told her. "My mother's old recipe. Edwina never gets it right. If you want something done, Munch, don't be afraid to do it yourself. Don't ever forget that."

"But . . . I didn't know you knew how to cook."

"I know how to do a lot of things that a man in my position will never have to do if he doesn't want to. Come on, you can help me pick through the berries."

She still remembered how those muffins had tasted, crumbly and piping hot out of the oven, sweet and tart at the same time. She and Papa May had eaten a half-dozen between them with butter before the sun came up and they scurried hastily off to bed—only after hiding the evidence so that grandmother wouldn't know what they had been up to.

That was the first and last time that Jorey had ever baked muffins . . . or anything else.

But she *could* bake something, if she wanted to. All she had to do was follow a recipe.

There was a row of cookbooks on the shelf above the sink. The spines were worn. They must have belonged to Gretchen's mother, Jorey figured. She walked over and took one down, flipping through the musty-smelling pages with pictures of good things to eat—cookies and breads and cakes.

Suddenly, Jorey was filled with an intense craving, and she realized that it wasn't for food.

She remembered those intimate, cozy, pre-dawn hours spent with Papa May in the sweet-smelling kitchen and she wanted more than anything to recapture that innocent time before her world had shattered.

But she couldn't go back.

No matter how Jorey searched for what she had lost, she could never recover it.

It wasn't just Papa May, or the house, or her childhood that had been taken away from her that summer.

It was a sense of belonging.

A sense of security.

A sense of peace.

She had experienced fleeting remnants of that long-lost warmth just now, when she'd suddenly remembered baking muffins with Papa May in the kitchen that last summer.

She wondered what other memories were locked away in her mind.

She closed the cookbook and replaced it on the shelf, then glanced toward the window. The snow was still falling, but the wind had died down. Instead of a white blur, she saw drifting flakes that had coated the trees and the slats of the back fence and lay in pristine white drifts on the ground.

Suddenly, the walls of the silent old house seemed to be closing in on her, and she needed to be out there, out in that pristine landscape and invigorating wind.

It occurred to her that she could ask Gretchen if she felt like going for a walk, but she realized just as quickly that she didn't want company. She didn't want to walk. She wanted to be alone with her thoughts, and she wanted to drive out over the country roads that led away from town.

Roads that led to the one place that might trigger more memories of the happy, elusive days of her past.

She dashed up the stairs to grab her coat and keys, and then down again and out the front door before she could stop to change her mind.

*   *   *

His breath puffing as frosty white as the flakes falling gently all around him, Sawyer stepped over a snow-covered bump and saw that it was a log that had fallen to the forest floor.

He continued to make his way purposefully through the barren trees, keenly aware of the crunching of his footsteps in the snow-muffled silence of the forest.

He had been walking out here for hours, having waded more than a mile through the deepening snow out to the edge of the property, where the woodland rose steeply into the foothills of the Adirondack wilderness.

Now, with his gloved fingers numb and his toes stiff and cold in his boots, he knew it was time to make his way back.

He was reluctant to return, though, uncertain of what he would find there.

Something, he knew, was wrong. Something terrible had happened somewhere, to someone, during the sleepless night.

He was terrified that it had happened to Jorey.

Several times as he tossed and turned in his bed he had reached for the telephone, wanting to call her, to make sure she was all right.

But how could he call the bed and breakfast in the dead of night and ask to speak to a woman he barely knew—a woman who continued to hold him at arm's length though she had obviously welcomed his passionate kiss just days ago?

Wasn't he trying to keep his distance from her, as she so obviously was from him? At least, emotionally?

Every moment spent with her yesterday had intensified his longing to take her into his arms and kiss her again. But he wouldn't let himself. He wasn't supposed to want her that way.

He had promised himself that he would give her protection, but nothing more.

Protection—and how had he protected her last night, when he had so strongly felt the presence of danger lurking nearby?

He hadn't.

He couldn't bring himself to contact her, not then, and not this morning. All because of a stubborn unwillingness to subject himself to temptation again.

Falling in love with Jorey Maddock would only lead to heartache, and Sawyer Howland had lived through more than his share of that.

He had disappeared into the snowy woods this morning in an effort to escape the emotional turmoil—the incessant wondering how, or even if, he could possibly protect Jorey, and himself. Her life was at risk; his heart was at risk.

He had reached the edge of the woods, and the big, stone house came into view across a broad expanse of snow-blanketed lawn. As he began to cross it, he felt a sudden prickle of foreboding that made him stop short and stand utterly still, waiting.

Moments later, he heard the sirens in the distance.

Jorey slowed the Range Rover as she rounded a curve in the narrow, country road and saw flashing red lights ahead.

Had some fool actually been speeding on this icy road in this weather? she wondered. Even *she* was taking the drive slowly and cautiously, still haunted by the memory of how it had felt to go careening off the road to land upside down in a ditch in the middle of nowhere.

But she saw, as she neared the flashing lights, that the police car hadn't pulled over another car. It was, instead, parked in front of a small, red, ranch house with black shutters. Curious, Jorey glanced at the house as she passed and saw that two police officers were standing by the front door with a woman who appeared distraught, waving her hands in the air.

Jorey wondered idly what had happened. Maybe the woman's dog was lost in the storm, or maybe she'd had a fight with a threatening boyfriend.

A short distance down the highway she turned onto Fieldstone Road and was struck by the landscape, familiar though she'd never seen it at this time of year, in the snow.

She passed the narrow lane that had led to Hob Nixon's rundown trailer, noticed houses that hadn't changed in a decade, and saw, jutting above the snow, the crumbling remains of the old stone wall that lined the road. She crossed the bridge over a briskly moving creek, one of the special spots where she used to fish with Papa May.

She was drawing nearer to the house now, and wondered what she would do when she arrived.

The house wouldn't be visible from the road, and if she wanted to see it she would have to venture past the stone pillars at the foot of the driveway. Would she drive only far enough to see the house?

Or would she get closer, hoping to find . . .

Sawyer?

He wasn't the reason she had driven out here. At least, she hadn't believed that he was.

She had thought that she simply wanted to glimpse

the place where she had spent the happiest days of her childhood. But somehow, the closer she got the more Sawyer had become tangled up in her thoughts, until she couldn't tell *what* she wanted.

Up ahead, on the right, she spotted the fence that marked the beginning of her grandparents' former estate. She kept going until she reached the stone pillars, and hesitated only a moment before turning into the driveway.

It had been plowed at some point, and there were tire tracks in the snow that covered the surface. It was odd to think of strangers living there, coming and going as though it were *theirs,* odd to realize that Sawyer was one of those strangers, and that *she* was the outsider.

Jorey passed the clump of evergreens that meant she was almost in view and took a deep breath, steeling herself for her first sight of the home she had visited so often in her memory these past several years.

Then it was there, in front of her, looking from that distance exactly as it had the last time she saw it, except for the coating of white on the roof.

She slowed the car and let out a shaky breath as she drew to a stop. She stared at the familiar house, noting the gables and the wraparound porch and the big, double front doors with arched, stained glass panels. The shutters were still painted forest green; the porch trim white.

There was no sign from the outside that a decade had passed and the house no longer belonged to the Maddocks.

A movement, a sudden blur of color against the white backdrop in the distance, caught the corner of her eye, and Jorey turned to see a figure out on the lawn, trudging through the snow toward the house.

It was a man, bundled against the weather, and she couldn't see his features through the screen of lightly falling snow.

Even so, she knew without a doubt that it was Sawyer Howland.

For a moment she sat with her hands poised on the wheel, ready to turn the car around and leave before he could spot her and wonder what she was up to.

Then she realized he would see her, anyway, and it would be better to offer some sort of explanation than to let him think she'd come here looking for him.

Because she hadn't.

Even though she found her heart pounding in anticipation at the sight of him now.

Jorey turned off the engine, shoved the keys into her pocket, and opened the car door, becoming instantly aware of the hush in the frigid air. The wind rustled the evergreen boughs above, and the snowflakes seemed to make a soft swishing sound as they fell, but other than that, there was nothing.

She sat and absorbed the tranquility until the far-off sound of footsteps crunching through snow reached her ears.

Then she buttoned the top button of her coat—the coat Sawyer had bought her just yesterday—and stepped out into the falling snow.

She could feel his eyes on her as he drew nearer, and saw that he hastened his pace until he practically seemed to be running toward her.

"Jorey!" he called, sounding breathless.

"Sawyer?" She was puzzled by his urgency, by the eagerness in his voice.

Then he reached her, and she found herself pulled into his arms, held against his chest. They wore so many layers of clothing that there should have been no intimacy in the contact, yet Jorey felt herself begin to tremble, felt her insides become molten.

She didn't dare lift her face to see what was in his eyes. He gave her no choice, though, reaching between them to tap a gloved forefinger beneath her chin and raise her head toward his. She saw an expression of wonder and relief in that blue gaze, as though he was stunned.

But why?

"You're okay," he said then, and for a moment she had no idea what he meant.

"I'm fine," she replied, puzzled. "Why wouldn't I be?"

"I heard sirens. I thought—"

"But why would you think—"

"I don't know. Never mind. I'm just glad you're okay."

Her vague confusion gave way to something else entirely then, as he bent his head and she realized what he was going to do. She gasped in surprise in the instant before he gently touched his mouth to hers.

Then Jorey was utterly lost in the kiss, allowing her eyes to flutter closed and her mittened hands to reach up around his neck to caress the hair that poked from beneath the woolen cap he wore.

She longed to take off his hat and her mittens and more, and she pressed her body against his, frustrated, feeling only the cushioning layers of clothing between them.

He opened his lips against hers and she was struck by how hot his mouth was in contrast to the chill in the air. She welcomed his warm tongue as it stroked the tender flesh against her teeth, and the exquisite sensation evoked other, more provocative images that sent molten quivers through her.

She squirmed against him, as though she could somehow get past the thick down and wool and flannel that obscured the evidence of his arousal. He groaned and moved, pulling her closer with his big gloved hands splayed against the small of her back, and she could feel that he, too, wanted desperately to shed the fabric barriers between them.

She dragged her mouth from his and murmured his name, catching herself just short of asking him to take her inside and make love to her. She didn't dare say it, terrified that if she did, it would happen . . . or that it wouldn't.

The sound of her voice seemed to snap him back to reality, and he opened his eyes and slowly released his hold on her.

They were both panting raggedly, their frosty breath mingling visibly in the air between them as they stared at each other, motionless.

"I won't say that I'm sorry that happened," he said finally, his blue eyes boring into hers.

"I'm not sorry, either."

"But it shouldn't happen again."

She pondered that, then asked boldly, "Why shouldn't it?"

He blinked and, for the first time since she had known him, seemed to waver, only momentarily. Then his eyes narrowed slightly and his chin lifted, and he said, "Because we both know where it's leading. And we barely know each other."

She shrugged. Even as she wondered what she was doing, she said defiantly, "So? Can't we get to know each other?"

He just looked at her.

"Do you have something to hide, Sawyer? Some reason you don't want me to know you?"

Her words hit home with him. She could see it in his face even before he turned his head away from her, to look off across the frozen field.

"What are you hiding?" she asked.

"I'm not hiding, I just don't want . . . this." He looked directly at her, motioning back and forth between them with his hand.

"You could have fooled me a minute ago."

"Don't get me wrong, Jorey. You're a beautiful woman. I'm not numb to that. Any man would want you in his bed. But I'm not available for anything more than that. And I know you well enough to know that you would demand more."

"You don't know me at all," she shot back, though he was telling the truth. "If you knew me you'd be aware that I've never wanted to get bogged down in anything complicated."

"Until now," he said simply, and she was inflamed by the utter arrogance in that statement and the undeniable validity of it.

"Don't flatter yourself, Sawyer," she bit out, and turned to go.

He caught her by the shoulders, and his next words came in a vastly different tone.

"Jorey, wait," he said softly, almost tenderly. "Please, wait."

She waited, but she didn't turn back to him.

"I want that, too. What you want."

"You don't know what I—"

"No," he interrupted, "I do know. I could feel it when I kissed you, and even before, and after. We both want it. But it can't happen. It shouldn't happen. And I can't tell you why."

"Because you don't know?"

"Because I can't tell you. I'm sorry."

Slowly, she turned toward him. In his eyes she saw stark honesty.

And pain.

"What is it?" she asked, her voice a mere whisper. "Please, Sawyer, whatever it is, you can—"

"No," he said. "No. No, I can't. So. I guess you were right, Jorey. I am hiding something. But not in the way you think."

"I don't know what I think about you." She studied his face. "But you're not dangerous. That, I know. Not dangerous in the way that they think."

"Who?"

"Only the whole damn town. I've been warned about you—told to stay away from you."

He seemed to ponder that, then nodded. "It's just as well that they think that," he said cryptically. "And I'm not surprised. But . . . you didn't listen to the warnings."

"No."

"Why not?"

She tilted her head. "I don't like being told what to do. I'd rather draw my own conclusions about things."

He grinned. "So you're a rebel."

She smiled faintly. "When I was a kid spending summers up here my grandmother used to warn me about the pond in the woods—not far from here, on this property—have you seen it?"

He shook his head.

She wanted to tell him she'd show him sometime, but that would make it sound like she was planning a future for them, and she wasn't. No matter what he thought.

Instead, she went on, "I went fishing there with my grandfather pretty often. It was one of our special places, you know? But my grandmother always told me that the pond was dangerous, and that if I ever went there alone and fell in, nobody would ever find me or know what happened to me—as if the water would just swallow me up, you know?"

Something dark flickered in his eyes and was gone before she could question it.

She cleared her throat and focused on the distant trees that marked the edge of the woods that concealed the pond. "But I used to go there anyway, without my grandfather. I sneaked away sometimes in the afternoon, when he was busy with his paperwork in his study and my grandmother wasn't around, and I went there. I was always a little bit scared, because of what my grandmother said. I looked at the water and I saw it as being murky and dark and threatening. Then one day, one sweltering, humid day, I was walking on a log near the edge and I fell in."

"What happened?"

"At first I was caught off guard because the water was really deep—at first, I thought it was over my head. But then I found my footing, and came up for air, and . . . it was perfect. I was so hot and sweaty, and it was refreshing and clear and beautiful. So I swam around. And it didn't swallow me up as my grandmother had said it would."

She flicked her gaze back to his and saw that he was watching her carefully. She wondered why she had told him that story, and wished that she hadn't.

"Sometimes when people warn you about things, Jorey, there's a good reason."

She shrugged. "And sometimes, there's not. I'm not afraid of you, Sawyer. If that's what you're getting at."

No, she wasn't afraid of him. Just afraid of what he made her feel . . . of what he made her want.

"I should be getting home," she said abruptly.

"Don't you want to come inside with me?"

Startled, she looked up at him and saw him grow flustered as he realized what she was thinking.

"I mean, come inside so that you can take a look at the house. I thought you wanted to see it."

She glanced at the big stone mansion and shook her head. "No, thanks. At least, not yet. It looks exactly the same on the outside. For a while, I think I just want to remember the rest of it the way it was."

"That makes sense. But if you change your mind . . ."

"Maybe I will."

"So, I'll see you, Jorey."

"Maybe you will."

He frowned slightly. "What does that mean?"

"It means I don't live around here. I'm only visiting. Sooner or later, I'll be going back home to New York."

He seemed to hesitate, then said, "That might be the best thing you could do."

Taken aback, she took her car keys from her pocket and spun on her heel, tossing a brittle, "Good-bye, Sawyer," over her shoulder as she left.

If Jorey went back to New York, she would be safe.

That made sense to Sawyer. He was fairly sure that whatever danger she was in stemmed from being here, in Blizzard Bay.

Then again, maybe he'd been wrong, after all. Maybe his emotions had become so frazzled during these past few months that he had begun imagining things. Like last night—when he had been so certain that something terrible was going to happen.

When he'd heard those sirens in the distance his stomach had turned over, and he had braced himself for the realization that Jorey had met a terrible fate.

Then, miraculously, she was *there,* standing in front of him. She had come to him, almost as if she knew he'd been thinking of her.

That was why he had gotten so carried away, why he had grabbed her and kissed her, driven by the passion he sensed in her response. It had taken every ounce of willpower he possessed not to scoop her tiny body into his arms and carry her into the house and up the stairs to his bed.

Now, as he sat on the couch to pull off his boots, he glanced at the bed, still rumpled from the restless night he had spent there. He imagined being there with Jorey, being able to feel the naked length of her body against his at last.

He turned away, busying himself with taking off his boots and both layers of damp socks. He pulled on a dry pair and stood, deciding to make himself a can of soup. He hadn't eaten anything all day.

He was on his way to the kitchen area tucked into one corner when a far-off sound caught his attention.

Sirens.

Again.

Jorey.

No.

She had just left him, not more than five minutes ago. He couldn't start believing that something had happened to her every time he heard a siren's wail. Yet . . .

Jorey came to a stop in the road, peering through the snow at the cluster of flashing lights up ahead. For a moment she thought there had been an accident. Then she realized that this was the house she had passed earlier, with the lady and the cop on the front steps. Apparently, something was really wrong. There were several police cars now, nearly blocking the road ahead.

She crept forward until she reached the roadblock, where a uniformed officer was gesturing her forward, pointing for her to steer around the cars in the road.

She rolled down her window and stuck her head out. "Did something happen, Officer?" she asked stupidly, glancing at the activity up at the house. The woman she'd seen earlier was gone, but there were several policemen on the lawn, and the front door was being held open by another.

Obviously something happened, you idiot, she told herself. *These cops aren't swarming all over this house because they're paying a friendly visit.*

The traffic cop ignored her question, saying only, "Please proceed slowly, Ma'am. The road is icy and there's not much room to go around."

She rolled up the window against the chill and kept going, glancing uneasily in her rearview mirror as she left the house behind.

Then her thoughts returned to Sawyer, something

she'd been trying unsuccessfully to avoid since she'd
left him.

Cursing, she reached out and turned on the radio as
a distraction, pressing the SEEK button until she found
a Beck song she liked. And she began to sing. Loudly.
As though she hadn't a care in the world.

Chapter Eight

Besides the diner, Cafe Jolie was the only decent restaurant in Blizzard Bay, and it was crowded that night. The maître d' informed Gretchen and Jorey that the wait for a table would be at least forty-five minutes.

"Do you want to go someplace else?" Jorey asked Gretchen, as they stepped toward the jammed bar area off to the side.

"There is no place else," Gretchen said ruefully. "Unless you want fast food."

"I wouldn't mind a Big Mac," Jorey admitted, her stomach rumbling. "But the seafood special on the chalkboard out front sounded awfully tempting."

"Let's just wait," Gretchen told her. "Maybe it won't be as long as they said. I was here with Karl one night and they told us it would be a half hour, and it wasn't more than ten minutes."

Jorey thought there was something wistful about the

way Gretchen said her boyfriend's name. "Where is Karl tonight?" she asked. "Didn't he want to join us?"

"Actually, I asked. He had other plans."

"Oh." Jorey waited for something more, but Gretchen offered nothing, so she said, "I'll go to the bar and get us drinks while we wait. What would you like?"

"Oh . . . just a Seven-Up. I don't drink," Gretchen added, as though sensing Jorey was about to protest.

"Ever? Why not?"

"I don't like the feeling of not being in control."

Jorey thought of her own wanton behavior this afternoon with Sawyer, of the heady, exhilarating loss of control she'd experienced in his arms.

"There's something to be said for not always being in control," she told Gretchen before stepping toward the bar, where she ordered Gretchen's soda and a glass of merlot for herself. As she waited for the bartender to bring the drinks she spotted a familiar, blond head at a dark table in the far corner.

"Isn't that Adrienne?" she asked when she returned to Gretchen.

"Where?"

"There. With that man, sitting in the corner."

Gretchen looked, then nodded. "It looks like her. And that's Jack Carpenter with her."

"Who's he?"

"A state senator. Very wealthy. And married."

"Figures," Jorey said, shaking her head slightly, not surprised. When it came to morals, Adrienne had never made any pretenses.

"His wife is dying of cancer," Gretchen went on. "At least, that's what I heard."

"It never ceases to amaze me that everyone in this town knows everything about everyone else," Jorey said.

"Actually, Jack Carpenter lives over in Hadley. But I know what you mean—oh, Adrienne's spotted us."

Jorey lifted a hand and waved at their friend, who waved back without looking the least bit embarrassed to be seen in public with a married man. In fact, she eagerly motioned the two of them over to the table.

"I guess she's not that concerned about hiding it," Jorey told Gretchen as they made their way through the crowd.

"You know Adrienne. She's not concerned about anything. Ever. Never has been."

Adrienne was impeccably dressed in a brown wool suit with a black velvet collar and buttons, with gold jewelry that was somehow tasteful yet extravagant at the same time. Her face was expertly made up and there wasn't a blond hair out of place on her head despite the brisk wind outside.

"Jorey! It's wonderful to see you again," she said when they arrived at her table. Belatedly, she added, "Oh, you, too, Gretchen."

Then she turned to her companion and said, "Jack, this is my old friend I was telling you about. Jorey Maddock, from New York. Her family owns the department store. Jorey, this is my friend, Senator Jack Carpenter— Oh, and Jack, this is Gretchen Eckhard, another old pal."

The senator, an older, well-dressed man with graying temples, smiled and shook hands with them, although he looked distinctly uncomfortable. His gaze kept shifting over their shoulders, as if he were trying to make sure he hadn't been recognized by anyone in the bar.

"We had no idea this place would be so crowded

tonight," Adrienne said, placing a manicured hand on his arm.

"It almost always is," Gretchen said pointedly, and Jorey suspected that Adrienne had been aware of that, and actually wanted to be seen around town with the senator.

Adrienne discarded Gretchen's comment with a wave of her hand, then turned her attention back to Jorey. She smiled meaningfully over the rim of her martini glass as she said, "I hear you've been keeping busy all week."

Jorey's guard went up as she noticed the glint in Adrienne's eyes. "What do you mean?" she asked.

"Oh, a little bird told me you've been spending time in Saratoga with Sawyer Howland."

"Was that little bird named Clover?" Jorey asked, conscious of Gretchen's startled glance, but ignoring it.

"No, that little bird was actually a Kitty," Adrienne said. "I ran into her at the doctor's office this morning. I was picking up a prescription, and she was getting checked to see if she was in labor, poor thing."

"Was she?"

"Not yet. But she looks like she's ready to pop. She told me that you had been over last night and that you told her all about you and Sawyer—"

"I didn't tell her all about me and Sawyer, because there's nothing to tell."

"She said you'd had lunch together in Saratoga."

"We did. He towed my car and fixed it for me. I was grateful, so—"

"So you took him to lunch."

"Basically."

Except that he had paid the check. *And* bought her a coat. And mittens.

"Clover thought the two of you looked pretty cozy together when she saw you."

"I'm going to kill Clover when I see her," Jorey said through clenched teeth.

"Jorey!" Gretchen looked disapproving. "You shouldn't talk like that."

"Well, doesn't she have anything better to do than spread rumors about me?"

"Actually, Clover has plenty to do these days," Adrienne piped up, raising her perfectly arched, skillfully darkened brows. "Her business partner, Sheryl Frampton, has been trying to buy out her half of the store for over a year now. Clover doesn't want to sell, but Sheryl's really pressuring her."

"Well, anyway," Jorey muttered, "I resent the fact that she's going around town discussing my personal life with everyone she meets."

"Relax, Jorey. She only told Johnny, and he told Kitty—"

"And Kitty told you."

"Exactly. If you don't have anything to hide and things are so innocent between you and Sawyer Howland, then why are you so worked up?"

"It's not that. I just . . . I'm not used to being the subject of small town gossip."

She let the subject drop, then, while Adrienne chattered on about the sofa she was having reupholstered and the custom-made curtains she'd just ordered for the arched, floor-to-ceiling windows of the music room, and how Jorey really did have to come over and visit while she was in town.

"It's such a shame, Jorey, that your grandparents'

old place has been turned over to *renters*," Adrienne said, shaking her head and telling Jack, "It was the most beautiful estate. But once it left the family . . . you know how these things happen."

"Actually," Jorey said, "I was out there today, and the house is still in good shape. In fact, it pretty much looks just as it did when my grandparents had it."

Then, in case one of them figured out that Sawyer Howland happened to live there, she hastily changed the subject, saying, "You know, on the way back to town I passed a big commotion at a house on Brookway Road. There were about a dozen cops there."

"Which house was it?" Gretchen asked.

"A red ranch not far from the intersection with Fieldstone. Why?"

"Doesn't Clover live in a red ranch on Brookway Road?" Adrienne asked, turning to Gretchen, who nodded.

Jorey felt a sudden chill. "Does it have a white, split rail fence out front?"

"I think so. Why?" Gretchen asked. "Was that the house where you saw the police?"

She nodded slowly. "I hope everything's all right. Maybe one of us should call her and check to make sure."

"I'll do it," Gretchen said, pulling some change out of her pocket and adding pointedly, "After all, Jorey, you just said you wanted to kill Clover. You're probably not in the mood to chat with her right now."

"I only meant—"

But Gretchen was gone, heading for a pay phone on the back wall.

"Sometimes she can be such a bitch," Adrienne said. "I was telling Jack earlier that I can't figure out why we ever spent so much time with her when we were younger. We had absolutely nothing in common.''

"I've always liked Gretchen," Jorey said protectively, but she knew that Gretchen wasn't thrilled to have learned that she had ignored her warnings about Sawyer Howland. With her cautious, conservative nature she'd never understand how Jorey could fail to heed what people had told her about him.

And Jorey would never be able to convince Gretchen that he wasn't dangerous—at least, not in the way that she and Karl and the others thought.

He *was* fiercely protective of his privacy. He had even admitted that he was hiding something. He had all but told her to stay out of his life, to go back to New York where she belonged.

Jorey would be a fool not to take his advice. After all, he didn't want her here. And there was nothing else keeping her in Blizzard Bay; not really.

She decided, as Adrienne went on and on about some benefit ballet performance she and Jack had attended the night before, that she had no choice but to leave in the morning. To just go, and never look back.

She had come here searching for some key to her past, or maybe to her future, and she hadn't found it. She had obviously been wrong to think that revisiting Blizzard Bay would prove to be a turning point in her life.

The sooner you get out of town, and away from Sawyer Howland, the better, she told herself firmly, having made up her mind.

Then Gretchen returned to the table, clearly shaken, her face looking far more pale than usual.

"For God's sake, what happened to you?" Adrienne asked, cutting herself off in mid-chatter.

"It's Clover," Gretchen said, sinking into a chair and shaking her head incredulously. "She's been murdered."

Sawyer stood at the edge of the crowd that had gathered in front of the low, red, ranch house on Brookway Road. It had been several hours since darkness had fallen, and freezing gusts kicked up the powdery snow that had fallen earlier, but still they came: the curious, the morbid, the gossips, and perhaps a few mourners, as occasional muffled sobs could be heard above the wind.

A handful of people in the crowd were members of the press, and it was easy to tell the television reporters from the rest of the bystanders. They wore long, cloth, dress coats and thin, leather shoes or pumps, and their perfectly coiffed heads were bare, while the locals were in down parkas and rubber-soled boots and knit hats.

There were news vans parked along the road, and camera crews mingled on the lawn, testing lighting and angles. Grim-faced police officers came and went, ignoring the reporters except to keep them, and the rest of the crowd, well behind the yellow, crime scene tape that cordoned off the house.

Sawyer watched the scene through narrowed eyes, wondering if this was what it had been like on that humid August night at the cabin by the lake, after a Federal Express delivery man had discovered the mutilated body lying on the floor just inside the door.

Had people heard the news and come tumbling out of their houses to stand and watch and wait for something else to happen?

What was it that they were waiting for, he wondered

with a flicker of ire, looking at the expectant faces all around him.

Did they think they might be able to catch a glimpse of a bloodied corpse? Or that the crazed murderer would suddenly stagger out of the bushes, clutching a dripping dagger?

They were ghouls, all of them, the bystanders and the reporters who hovered at the murder scene, eyes fixated on the house.

For all anyone knows, you're one of them, Sawyer reminded himself. *For all they know, you're here because you, like them, turned on your television or radio or answered your telephone after supper and found out that a second woman had been murdered in Blizzard Bay.*

But that wasn't how it had happened. Not for him.

He closed his eyes and took an involuntary step back from the crowd, as if that could further separate him, somehow, from the rest of them.

After Jorey had left him this afternoon, he had found himself pacing his small apartment, agitated, a growing edge of panic building within him.

He hadn't been able to forget the earlier sound of the sirens, or shake the nagging feeling that something was wrong. He had just seen Jorey, had just held her and kissed her and reassured himself that she was safe. But the foreboding hadn't gone away. As darkness settled over the house he had found himself pulling on his coat and hat and boots, heading out into the blustery night to find . . .

Jorey?

He supposed he'd had a vague notion of heading toward town and the bed & breakfast when he'd turned his car onto Brookway Road, though he had no idea what he would have done when he actually got there.

Not after he'd all but told her to get out of town. She wouldn't know why he'd said it. To her, it would have come across as a command to stay away from him.

All I want is to keep you near, to keep you with me, and safe.

Would he have told her that, if he had reached the bed & breakfast tonight?

He would never know.

No sooner had he turned onto Brookway than he'd spotted the commotion. With a sickening realization, he'd braked and come to a stop at the side of the road, understanding that this was what he'd been meant to find. This was the reason he had left his home and headed down this road.

From the conversations all around him, Sawyer had gradually learned the details. That the woman—the one who lay dead inside the small house not fifty feet from where he stood—was named Clover Hartdale. She had been in her twenties, and attractive, and single.

Just like the first victim, people murmured, shaking their heads knowingly, their words searing his mind with haunting memories and unwelcome comparisons.

And just like Jorey.

Clover Hartdale had been stabbed repeatedly with a knife that had been taken from her own kitchen; there was an empty slot in the wooden block stand on the counter.

He had heard that bit of information solemnly relayed by a woman who said her husband was one of the investigating officers on the scene.

"Jimmy told me it's an absolute blood bath in there," the woman had told everyone in earshot. "Just a mess. She was chased all over the house by the killer, obviously trying to escape, poor thing. They found her in the bedroom at the back of the house. And she had white wall-to-wall carpeting in there," she added, as if that made it all the more tragic.

Sawyer opened his eyes and his gaze fell on a familiar figure hovering, as he did, at the edge of the crowd, a few feet away. It was Hob Nixon, his hands jammed into the pockets of his dingy, camouflage cloth coat, his gaze focused straight ahead from beneath the brim of his dirty, tattered cap.

Sawyer watched him for a few minutes, searching for some movement, some indication of what the man was thinking.

As though he sensed that he was under scrutiny, Nixon slowly turned his head, his black eyes looking directly into Sawyer's. For a moment he just stared. Then he seemed to smirk, and reached slowly into the top pocket of his coat.

Sawyer found himself flinching involuntarily as he watched, waiting to see what Nixon was going to do.

He removed a cigarette and a package of matches, and Sawyer quietly exhaled, turning away as the man lit his cigarette.

His eyes fell again on scene before him, on the yellow crime scene tape. He was seeing not a red ranch house, but a weathered cottage by the lake.

So it had happened again.

This, he now realized, was what he had subconsciously been waiting for since arriving in town several months ago.

Waiting for death to strike again.

On some level, he felt a numbing sense of relief that it hadn't been Jorey.

Yet.

Now that there had been a second murder, he stood

firm in his conviction that she was in danger here in Blizzard Bay. That whoever had killed the woman whose blood had spilled all over the white wall-to-wall carpeting would strike again.

Next time—like the first time—the victim might not be a stranger to Sawyer.

"Did you reach Karl this time?" Jorey asked Gretchen, who returned to the small sitting room off the kitchen clutching a mug she had just refilled with steaming coffee in her clenched, trembling hands.

"Yes, I reached him. He said he just got home." Gretchen sank onto the couch beside Jorey and put her cup on the coffee table in front of them. One of the legs had moved off the edge of the area rug; the table wobbled slightly, sloshing dark liquid onto the worn cherry surface.

Gretchen didn't seem to notice.

Jorey leaned forward and wiped up the spatters with a tissue from her pocket.

"Did you tell him about Clover?" she asked Gretchen, who nodded.

"Is he coming over, then?"

"He said he can't. He has a report to get ready for a meeting at work tomorrow."

Jorey frowned. "Doesn't he know that you and Clover were friends?"

"Of course he knows that. He had met her a few times himself, actually . . . her boutique in Saratoga is a few doors down from his office."

"Well, did you tell him that we're nervous about spending the night alone in the house?"

Gretchen shook her head. "I didn't want to make

him feel bad. He has to do that report. Anyway, we won't be alone. Uncle Roland's here."

Now there's a comforting thought.

Jorey couldn't shake the knowledge that Gretchen's uncle had gone to Clover's house last night to return the sweater she had left behind.

Gretchen had called the police and told them about it as soon as she and Jorey got home. The officer who had answered had said they would plan to question him, since he might have been the last person to see Clover alive.

But Jorey wondered if perhaps they would consider him something more than just a witness. If they thought that the elderly handyman might actually have had something to do with Clover's death.

She hadn't voiced the thought to Gretchen, who was already distraught over what had happened.

"Is your uncle still asleep?" Jorey asked Gretchen, who had ventured upstairs before trying to call Karl again.

"He must be. His door was closed."

"Did you knock?" Jorey asked stupidly, before remembering that it would be a useless gesture. Roland Eckhard was deaf.

And mute.

And, according to Gretchen, completely illiterate. He didn't even know sign language or how to read lips.

Jorey knew Gretchen communicated with him through a series of hand movements, and sometimes by drawing pictures on a pad of paper. That was how she let him know what needed to be done around the house.

But how were the police going to question him about the murder?

What, if anything, did he know?

The details of what had happened to Clover were still sketchy. Apparently, nobody had seen her since Johnny O'Connor had bumped into her at the mini-mart on her way home from work last night.

Kitty, who had called Gretchen and Jorey a short time ago, was beside herself over Clover's death. She said that the convenience store clerk had told the police that Johnny had been with Clover in the store, and that Johnny had been summoned by detectives for questioning.

"He wasn't with her. He ran into her. But they're acting as though he might know something," Kitty had said, upset, "and all he did was chat with her when he saw her. He doesn't know any more than anyone else about what she did or who she saw after she left the store."

Kitty had added that when Clover hadn't shown up at the boutique this morning her partner, Sheryl Frampton, had assumed it was because of the weather. But she had grown concerned after trying repeatedly to call Clover at home, and had driven over to make sure everything was all right.

She was the one who had discovered Clover's body—and she, presumably, had been the distraught woman Jorey had glimpsed outside the house with the police when she'd driven by this afternoon.

Jorey watched Gretchen tap her fingers distractedly on the arm of the sofa and wondered if her friend thought Karl was just making up excuses about why he couldn't come over tonight.

Jorey certainly thought so. After all, two woman had been murdered in Blizzard Bay—one a close friend of Gretchen's—and the killer was on the loose. Wouldn't he feel obliged to at least come by and comfort his girlfriend, if not spend the night? And if he was so worried about doing his report, why would he have stayed out so late? Where could he have been?

Gretchen glanced at Jorey, as though she sensed she was watching her.

"You look tired, Jorey," she said. "You should go to bed. It's almost midnight."

Jorey stifled a yawn and realized it was true. She *was* tired. Exhausted—mentally, emotionally, and physically.

"Jorey," Gretchen said, and then hesitated.

"What?"

"It's probably nothing, but . . . I just . . ." Gretchen paused, then lowered her voice.

"What is it, Gretchen?"

"It's Uncle Roland. I can't help wondering—"

"Wondering what?" Jorey prodded, seeing the troubled look in Gretchen's pale eyes.

"Nothing. Never mind. Forget I said anything."

Jorey sat, wanting to ask Gretchen what she'd been about to say, but knowing better than to push her. If Gretchen wanted to talk, she would.

Finally, she stood and asked Gretchen, "Are you coming up?"

"Not yet. I'm too upset to sleep."

"Do you want me to stay with you?"

Gretchen shook her head. "I'll be fine. Go ahead."

Jorey sensed that her friend wanted to be alone. Though she knew Gretchen was disturbed by Clover's death, she wondered if she suspected her uncle had been involved.

Maybe, Jorey realized, Karl was part of the reason

she was so troubled. The fact that he wouldn't come to her seemed to indicate where he stood.

Jorey didn't dare ask. Gretchen had made it clear that she didn't intend to discuss her relationship, and Jorey wasn't surprised. Gretchen had never been the type who talked about things that were bothering her.

Anyway, Jorey had other things on her mind. As she made her way up to the second floor hall she thought about Sawyer, about what he'd said today when she'd threatened to go back to New York.

That might be the best thing you could do.

At the time she had been infuriated, certain he just wanted to be rid of her.

Now, she wasn't so sure. There had been something in his tone, something that made her wonder. . . .

And the way he had run toward her, so happy to see her, exhilarated, even, the way he had grabbed her and kissed her and held her.

Why would he welcome her so demonstratively one moment, and turn her away the next? It didn't make sense.

Clearly, he didn't want to care about her, but couldn't help himself.

Which was exactly how she felt about him.

Now, with Clover's death having rattled her—and temporarily changed her plans to leave town—Jorey found herself needing him.

She heard a footstep creaking overhead, and hesitated in the hallway outside the closed door to her room.

She could get into her lonely bed, barricade her door, and lie awake for hours, wondering about Roland.

Or she could leave.

But where will you go?

As if she didn't know.

This is insane. You can't.

But she had to.

Before she had a chance to think better of the decision, she slipped into her room.

For a moment, she considered stopping to change out of the dressy skirt and sweater she had worn to the restaurant. But if she hesitated, even for a few minutes, she knew she wouldn't go through with it.

So she grabbed her coat and her keys, then crept quietly and swiftly back down the stairs and out into the night.

Chapter Nine

"Jorey?" Sawyer held the door open and peered out into the night. "What are you doing here?"

"I'm not . . . I don't know," came a voice from somewhere in the shadows. Then she stepped forward, and he saw her clearly in the glow of the moon reflecting off the snow-covered yard. She wore the coat he had given her, and a long skirt with high-heeled leather boots. She was hatless, her dark curls tumbling to her shoulders. Her expression was haunted.

"My friend was killed."

"Clover Hartdale was your friend?"

Jorey nodded. "I hadn't seen her in ten years, but we were together once this summer and again on Sunday afternoon, and—my God. Who would slaughter an innocent woman?"

He stared at her face, at her eyes, which suddenly looked enormous.

"Do you want to come in?" he asked, holding the

door open wider and gesturing at the stairway behind him.

She ignored the question, asking, "How did you know I was here?"

Because it was another sleepless night and he had been brooding, looking out the window, staring into the night, when he had seen a pair of headlights coming up the driveway. He had known, even before the Range Rover came into view, that it would be Jorey.

He shrugged. "I heard a car. It's past midnight, so I looked out to see who it was."

"I'm sorry that I woke you up."

"You didn't. Come in, Jorey."

She looked at the doorway behind him, then met his gaze. "I don't know if I should."

"Why else are you here?"

"I just . . . something made me come. I guess it's the house—maybe I thought that being in a familiar place could offer some level of comfort after what happened."

"Or maybe you thought that *I* could," he said quietly, taking a step forward and reaching out to lay a hand on the sleeve of her coat.

She looked down at his hand, then up at his face. "Maybe you were part of the reason I came here. But—"

"But you're fighting it," he said softly. "I know, Jorey. We both are."

She studied him. "There are probably people in this town who are going to say that you killed Clover. But I know that you didn't."

"How do you know that?"

"I just know."

The wind stirred the pine trees at the edge of the

steps, blowing powdery snow around them. "Come inside, Jorey."

"Who are you, Sawyer?"

He tensed at the question. He was prepared to give her anything she needed—a shoulder to cry on, words of solace. Anything but the truth.

"Who do you think I am?"

She shrugged. "I don't know . . . and maybe I don't care, tonight."

"Maybe I don't either, tonight."

He tightened his grip on her arm, pulling slightly so that she took a step toward him. He could see that she was trembling all over.

"Come inside, Jorey," he said, his voice suddenly sounding hoarse to his own ears. "Let me help you warm up."

"I'm not cold."

"You're shivering."

Her eyes met his and he knew that it wasn't the cold that was making her quake. He felt it, too, building within him—a barely contained desire that rocked his very soul.

He leaned toward her and brushed his lips against hers, lightly, briefly, so that they barely touched. But the slight, sweet contact made him shudder and he had to take a step back to keep himself from claiming her then and there with his mouth and his hands and his aching masculine arousal.

She seemed startled, first by his spontaneous kiss, and then by his retreat.

"What was that?" she asked him in her straight-forward way, clasping a mittened hand to her mouth.

"What do you think it was?"

She shook her head, watching him, and then said, as

though she'd just resolved some inner struggle, "I'll come inside."

He nodded and stepped back to let her in. She stomped the snow from her boots and looked around the small vestibule, lined with three closed doors, then up at the staircase leading to the second floor.

"This wasn't all closed in when I lived here," she said. "It was a big foyer, and there was a fireplace and a balcony looking down from above. Which floor do you live on?"

"The third." He closed the door behind them, shutting out the wind and making the small hallway seem even smaller.

"My room was on the third floor," she told him. "I used to pretend it was a tree house because the windows were surrounded by branches and when I looked out I couldn't see anything but leaves and the sky."

They began climbing the stairs, and at the second floor landing, where there were more closed doors leading to more apartments, they turned toward another staircase leading upward.

The house was hushed with the slumber of the residents in their beds behind those doors, and he didn't bother to turn on a light.

"It's so strange," she commented, her voice barely above a whisper. "This stairway was here, too, but it was open. They've chopped things up with all these walls and doors."

He led her up to the third floor, which was divided into only two apartments. The one across the hall was empty; a young couple had vacated it shortly after Sawyer had moved in.

His door was standing open, the way he had left it. He gestured and told Jorey, "This is my apartment."

She had already turned toward the doorway expectantly, and he saw that she was nodding. "This was my room."

Then it made sense to him, the connection that had drawn him to her since before they had even met. Not only was he dwelling under the roof of the house where she had spent her childhood summers, but his spacious studio apartment under the eaves had been her bedroom for all those years.

She had undoubtedly left some part of herself behind; he had sensed her very essence, so that when he met her she'd seemed strangely familiar, as though she was already a part of his life.

She walked into the room and stood, turning slowly around, in the middle of the floor. He hadn't left a light on; he had spent this night, like so many others, brooding in the dark. The snow and the moonlight illuminated the room through the uncovered dormer windows, though, outlining the silhouettes of furniture and the sloping angles of the ceiling.

"This was my room," she breathed, continuing to spin as if in slow motion, like a music box ballerina winding down, "and it looks the same. Exactly the same. Except . . ."

She moved to the window and gazed out. "You couldn't see anything then. The trees . . ."

"The branches are bare, now," he told her, coming up behind her and looking out over the frozen field below. "But when I first came, the leaves covered the view. Just like you said."

"Sawyer . . ." She turned toward him, her face only inches from his. "I'm glad you're the one living in this room. I always thought of it as belonging to me, and I've hated the thought of sharing it."

"But not with me?"

"No, it's all right to share it with you," she said softly. "I have no idea why that is. But it just is."

He nodded, thinking that he hadn't wanted, hadn't planned, to share any part of his life in Blizzard Bay with anybody, and yet here he was inviting her into his private world, needing her there, and knowing, somehow, that it, too, was all right.

Now that she was here he desperately needed to forget everything else, forget the months of lonely torment. He was seized by a fervent inner demand for emotional and physical release.

"Why don't you take off your coat?" he asked in a low voice, reaching out to unfasten the top button for her.

"I shouldn't . . . stay."

"Why shouldn't you?"

"You don't want me here."

"Yes I do, Jorey." He gently slipped another button from its hole, careful not to let his hands brush against the rounded swell of her breasts beneath her thick, cotton sweater as the coat fell open.

"This afternoon you told me to leave."

"I didn't mean it." He unfastened another button, then the last, and carefully slid his hands beneath the shoulders of the coat, pushing it away, and down her arms. It fell to the floor behind her.

"If you didn't mean it, why did you say it?"

"Don't you ever say things you don't mean? Things you wish you could take back?"

She seemed to consider that, then shrugged.

She still wore her mittens, and he reached out and took the wrist of her right hand, pulling the mitten and then lifting her fingers to his mouth. He kissed her hand tenderly, as tenderly as he had earlier kissed her lips, barely brushing her flesh with his mouth when he longed to take it greedily. He removed her other mitten and stood facing her, clasping each of her small, icy hands in each of his own.

"What now?" she asked softly, searching his face. "What do you want?"

"I think you know. I think you want the same thing."

His breath caught in his throat at the revealing glint in her eyes. He didn't dare exhale, didn't dare move, because if he did the moment might shatter and he would be left alone with this fierce, hollow ache.

She was the one who exhaled, her breath a sweet sigh that stirred his hair so that it tickled his cheek. She was the one who moved, taking a step closer to him, and then another, bending her arms so that their clasped hands came up between them to form a last barrier.

He let his breath out raggedly, could feel the uncomfortable tightening of his flesh, felt himself grazing the fleecy lining at the front of the gray sweatpants he wore.

She slipped her hands from his grasp then and moved her arms up around his neck, and there was nothing between their bodies now except the flimsy layers of their clothing—his sweats and her skirt and sweater and whatever she had on underneath. He imagined only narrow wisps of lace and satin shielding the most provocative parts of her bare skin and felt his arousal grow even more taut, straining now against the confines of the soft, cotton fabric.

He was consumed by the craving for contact, and, as though she sensed what was happening to him, Jorey took the final step forward that closed the gap between their bodies. His erection throbbed against the soft indentation of her stomach and he reached behind her and pulled her even more tightly against him.

She squirmed slightly and he realized that she wanted more intimate contact than the difference in their heights allowed. In a swift movement he lifted her easily and sat her on the wide windowsill at her back, so that their hips were at the same level. Now he stood between her open legs, the cottony gauze of her skirt draped between them, and pressed himself into the yielding flesh there, and she let out a high-pitched gasp that was cut short when his mouth descended hungrily over hers.

He held her head, tilting her back, and kissed her passionately, allowing his tongue the intimate entry that his masculinity so boldly desired. She sucked gently on his tongue and moaned and moved against him, and then he felt her cold fingertips slip beneath the waistband at the back of his sweatpants. She stroked the bare skin at the base of his spine, then pulled him closer, clasping his body to hers.

He moaned, knowing that he was dangerously close to the release he sought, and that it was too soon. He lifted his mouth from Jorey's and eased his hips back, putting distance between them and causing her to protest with a soft, "No!"

"Not yet, Jorey," he said into her ear, raking his lips through her hair. "Not like this. Let's go to the bed . . ."

"No," she said again, and moved her hands from the back of his waistband to the front. He looked down and saw the evidence of his arousal protruding from beneath the folds of thick fabric, and felt her tugging on the drawstring.

She loosened the waist and pulled his sweatpants down over his hips so that he sprang free, and he shuddered when he felt her hand on him. Tension was building rapidly within him, and he closed his eyes and clenched his jaw with the effort to control it.

"Let me . . ." she said, and made a movement to get down from the windowsill, bending her head toward him so that he had no doubt what she had in mind.

"No," he bit out, "I can't hold back. I can't—"

"Then don't," she crooned.

That was all the invitation he needed. He reached out and swiftly pulled her skirt up, realizing with pleasure that she wasn't wearing stockings. The seductive sight of her bare legs in those high boots drove him wild, and he ran his hands up her firm, bare thighs, raising her skirt as he went. Where her legs met he found what he had expected; a silky band of lace-edged material. He assumed that it was panties and went to pull them down, but she reached out and stopped him.

"No, it's a teddy," she said, smiling, and quickly unfastened the snaps between her legs. Then she raised the satin fabric and the skirt around her waist and leaned back slightly against the window, pulling him toward her, guiding him into her.

He groaned as he sank his hard flesh into her warm, wet core, burying his face in her neck. She wrapped her legs around his waist and he braced his arms against the window frame as he pumped deeply into her.

"It's all right," she whispered, stroking his face when, just moments later, panting and straining, he could no longer hold back and exploded with great tremors. He cried out her name and she held him to her until he had stopped shaking.

"I'm sorry," he told her when he could finally speak. He bent and pulled his sweatpants up, fumbling with the waistband.

"Why?"

"It's been a long time since I . . . it was over before it started."

"We have all night," was her remarkable reply, and she led him to his bed.

Jorey lay with her ear against Sawyer's heartbeat, feeling his arms around her, his fingertips playing lightly up and down her spine.

She ached for more than that, longed to remove his clothes and her own and make love here in his bed.

But for all she knew, he was spent and drifting off to sleep.

For all she knew, he would push her away if she made a move, so she simply lay there with him, fully dressed, realizing that the frenzied intercourse they had shared had done nothing to sate her appetite for him.

If anything, she was more frustrated than she had been before.

"Jorey?"

The sound of his voice startled her, and she lifted her head and looked at him.

She couldn't see his expression there in the shadows, away from the window; he might as well have been wearing a mask.

She said nothing, only waited, and then she felt his fingers brushing her hair away from her face. He lifted his head and kissed her, a long, searching kiss that sent any conscious thoughts careening away.

His arms were around her and, with his lips still on hers, he rolled so that she was on her back and he was on his side, the length of his body against her.

He moved one hand along her sweater, over her stomach and then over her breasts, stroking them through the thick layer of wool. She felt her nipples harden in anticipation as he slipped his hand beneath the sweater and moved it upward. He pulled it expertly over her head, then moved aside the narrow shoulder straps of the champagne-colored satin teddy, pulling them down along her arms until she was naked from the waist up.

He ran a thumb over one of her swollen nipples and then the other, then dipped his head to her. She felt his mouth on her breast, at first merely kissing and licking the soft mound, then sucking at the desire-shriveled tip, creating an unbearably exquisite pressure that made her arch her back and thrash her head from side to side on the pillow behind her.

She clutched his head and tangled her fingers in his hair, holding him to her, then, wanting him naked against her, moved her hands down over his neck to grab at the collar of his gray sweatshirt.

"Take this off," she told him, pulling at it. "Please, Sawyer . . ."

He obliged, sitting up and yanking it over his head. He tossed it aside, then stood and slid the sweatpants down over his hips.

She could see him in the moonlight, standing beside the bed, and she was stunned at the contours of his body. Muscles bulged in his arms and broad chest, tapering to a lean stomach and strong thighs. A wave of yearning swept over her as she stared at his magnificent build, and she needed to be in his arms, to feel his skin against her skin.

As though he sensed what she was thinking, he leaned over her and slowly slid her skirt down the length of her body. He set it aside, draping it with care over the footboard of the bed. Then he unzipped her high leather boots, tossing first one and then the other aside.

He peeled off the silk trouser socks she wore beneath them.

It occurred to her that she should have been wearing stockings and a garter belt; something sexier and more appropriate for the moment. But she couldn't stand the confinement of stockings, or even tights or panty-hose. And anyway, he didn't seem to mind now, and hadn't earlier, that her legs were bare.

She was naked, now, and so was he. He lay beside her again, his head propped on his elbow as he trailed a hand down along her waist, over the curve of her hip, to her thigh.

She quivered when he rested it there, and wished that she could see his face. But it was hidden now that he was back in the shadows. There was no telling what he was thinking, what he wanted.

"What is it that you need, Jorey?" he asked her in a low voice. "Where do you want me to touch you?"

She didn't dare reply. She felt his hand stroking the side of her thigh and then the top of it, and she wondered whether he could feel the goosebumps that promptly formed on her skin in response.

His fingers drifted upward again, passing up over her hip bone to the soft swell of her belly just beneath her navel. He lifted his head and she held her breath as he brought it down, sighing in pleasure as she felt his lips against her stomach. He rained light kisses there, and then she squirmed, wanting him to go lower, struggling against the primitive urge to reach down and guide his head to her most intimate place.

But she didn't need to urge him; a moment later she felt his fingers fluttering between her legs, separating the moist folds of flesh. He began to stroke her expertly and she clamped her thighs around him, rocking against his hand.

After a few moments, he gently forced her legs to open, and then she felt the intense, velvety pressure of his mouth and tongue on her. She was lost then, writhing on the bed, terrified that he would stop what he was doing to her. But he didn't; he kept up the rhythmic strokes, driving her closer and closer and closer to the edge. She moaned low in her throat and clenched her fists and tossed her head, and then finally, *finally*, felt herself beginning to tremble.

She let go with a high-pitched cry and gave in to the waves of pure sensation that swept through her, certain that she was melting from the inside out.

He held her when it was over, and she was still. He ran his hand over her hair as her head lay once again on his chest, and she allowed her fingertips to drift over the warm, hard muscles beneath her.

They didn't speak; for once, there was nothing to say. Jorey let the silence wrap around her like the safety of his arms, and gradually, sated, she allowed herself to drift off to sleep.

Sawyer woke at dawn, finding himself entwined with the sleeping woman whose body warmed his bed. Carefully, not wanting to wake her, he untangled his limbs from hers and moved to the edge of the mattress. He pushed back the covers and swung his bare legs into the chilly room, shivering as he fumbled on the floor for the sweatshirt and sweatpants he'd tossed there earlier. He dressed swiftly, then went to the window.

Staring out into the misty gray light, he pondered what had happened last night between him and Jorey.

It had merely been hot, raw sex—purely physical.

Yes. And you're just a mechanic who came to Blizzard Bay to get away from it all.

Who was he trying to kid? That hadn't been purely physical at all. There had been an undercurrent of emotion between them, a need that went well beyond their bodies' primal instincts to mate.

He looked over at the bed and saw Jorey huddled beneath the quilt, her curls glossy black against the white pillowcase, her lips parted slightly in slumber.

Here, with him, she was safe. That was why he had managed to get a few solid hours of sleep for the first time in many nights. He didn't have to pace his small apartment and wonder where she was, whether she was all right.

What if he left Blizzard Bay, and took her with him, so that he could always keep her safe?

The notion was so tempting that for a moment he actually considered it. Then he came to his senses.

There was no guarantee that he could keep her safe, that the peril that stalked her here wouldn't follow her wherever she tried to escape.

If she was marked for death, then death would claim her.

Christ, Sawyer thought, swallowing over the enormous lump that rose in his throat.

He couldn't leave Blizzard Bay. Not yet. Not until he had accomplished what he had come here to do.

Anyway, Jorey might be safe with him now, but *he* was in danger. If he fell in love with her, and he lost her, he couldn't bear it. He just . . . couldn't bear it.

Not again.

He closed his eyes and glimpsed a casket being lowered into the ground, and jerked them open again. He couldn't allow those disturbing images to come back to haunt him.

Nor could he lose sight of the reason he was in this town, living a life of lies.

But what about Jorey? You swore to yourself that you would protect her.

Protect her, yes. But not . . . *this.*

His gaze fell on her, sleeping in his bed, naked beneath the comforter.

This was what he had promised himself wouldn't happen. And he couldn't—*wouldn't*—let it happen again.

Jorey was in the woods near her grandparents' house, running from something. Her friends were with her; she could hear their giggles and shouts rippling through the trees, though she couldn't see them. Everyone thought something was funny, so very funny. Everyone but Jorey.

She was disturbed; kept calling them to stop, that it wasn't nice, what they were doing.

But they kept giggling, ignoring her, and she couldn't catch up with them.

I'll tell Papa May what happened, Jorey thought. *He'll know what to do about it.*

"*Papa May!*" she called, her voice echoing through the woods. "*Papa May, I need you!*"

But there was no answer.

So she kept calling, then shouting, then shrieking his name, as the sounds of her friends' voices faded away and she found herself alone.

Alone . . .

With a start, Jorey woke up.

When she opened her eyes, she found herself staring

at the sloping ceiling above the bed, tracing with her eyes the familiar network of faint cracks in the white paint.

For a moment—a most haunting, fleeting moment— she was back in the past, lying in her old bed in her grandparents' summer house. It was summertime, and Papa May was downstairs on the porch in a green-painted Adirondack chair with his coffee and his pipe, waiting for her. And she knew she had to hurry down and talk to him about the disturbing thing that had happened at the pond in the woods with her friends. . . .

Then she realized that it was bleak November and Papa May was gone, and she was a grown woman and so were her friends, and she was in this bed because she had made love with Sawyer Howland last night, and he lived here now.

My God.

Shaken, she tried to shove the dream out of her head, along with the vague notion that there was something she should be remembering, something important.

She turned her head and glimpsed, in morning's grey light, what she hadn't been able to see last night. There was the exposed brick wall beside the door, and the windowed alcove with the built-in seat where she used to read, and the double doors leading to the walk-in closet.

Some things, of course, were different. One end of the room had been converted to a kitchenette, with an apartment-sized stove and refrigerator and a small, round table with a single chair. And of course, her posters were gone from the walls, and her books weren't on the shelves over there, tucked beneath the sloping ceiling.

Then she realized, with a start, that some of the furni-

ture was the same—She recognized the bookcase and
the rocker by the fireplace, though its oak finish was
hidden now beneath a coat of white paint, and that
standing lamp in the corner—the shade was different,
but the wrought-iron scrollwork of the base was familiar.

And, good Lord, this bed, this white iron bed, was
her childhood bed. She felt her face growing hot at the
memory of what she and Sawyer had done here only
hours before, and turned to look at him, wondering
whether he was still asleep, and almost hoping that he
was. She wasn't yet ready to face him, or the memories
of what had happened between them.

But the pillow beside hers was empty.

She heard water running, then, from somewhere
nearby.

She frowned, looking around, and realized it was coming from behind the closet door. She slipped out of
bed, puzzled, and wrapped the quilt around her naked
body, shivering in the morning chill. Then she crossed
the room and opened the door to find that the walk-
in closet had been transformed into a small bathroom.

A bathroom that contained a shower stall where the
water was running.

Sawyer was in that shower, his nude form visible
amidst a cloud of steam behind the semi-see-through
glass doors.

Jorey stood and stared for a moment, unable to help
herself, imagining his glistening, soap-slicked, muscular
body and water streaming in his golden hair. She felt
something stir in the pit of her stomach, or lower, and
she half-considered tossing the quilt aside and joining
him beneath the pounding spray.

Then she came to her senses, thanks to a series of
words and images that flitted through her mind.

Sawyer's voice saying, "Sometimes when people warn you about things, Jorey, there's a good reason."

Gretchen's disapproving expression when she'd found out Jorey had been spending time with him.

The police cars clustered around Clover's house, where she lay dead.

And the nagging sense that there was something she should be noticing, or remembering, something that had to do with the dream she'd just had . . . a dream that was already fading away.

Jorey swiftly but quietly closed the bathroom door, her heart pounding.

Somehow, though she hadn't even come face-to-face with him yet, in the light of day Sawyer seemed like a stranger to her again. It was almost as though the stolen midnight interlude had never happened, and she knew she didn't belong there, that she didn't want to confront him.

It wasn't that she was afraid . . . was it?

She didn't believe he had murdered Clover any more than she believed he had murdered the woman tourist back in August.

Or maybe she didn't want to.

Maybe that was the elusive thought she couldn't quite seem to grasp—something that had to do with Sawyer, and the murder.

Shaken, Jorey put the quilt back on the bed and hurriedly got dressed, shivering her way into the suddenly uncomfortable skirt and sweater, socks, and boots. She crumpled the silk teddy into a wadded ball and shoved it into her coat pocket.

Then she went over to the cheval mirror in the corner to see if she looked presentable.

Not really.

She looked as if she were wearing last night's clothing; her hair was a tangled mess of curls and her face a palate of smudged makeup.

It struck her that she looked exactly like what she was—a woman who was making a hurried escape after a night of forbidden passion, underwear in her pocket and all.

She heard the old pipes creak and groan as the sound of running water suddenly stopped.

Hastily and silently, Jorey grabbed her coat and mittens and left, dashing down the two flights of stairs and out into the frozen November morning.

Sawyer sat at the small table, the morning edition of the local newspaper in front of him.

"Second Woman Slain in Blizzard Bay," screamed the front page headline.

The article, which he had read at least a dozen times, went on to give the details about the murder of Clover Hartdale.

According to the press there were no known suspects, but the police were working on a number of leads. There were similarities between this case and the one involving Rebecca Latimer, who had been killed in August. Both women had been living alone; both died of multiple stab wounds from weapons that were not recovered. In Clover Hartdale's case, a knife was missing from the kitchen; in Rebecca Latimer's, the presumed weapon was a pair of scissors that had been kept out in plain view in a cup on a desk in the living room.

The piece noted that Rebecca Latimer had been twenty-three and spending the summer in Blizzard Bay;

that she was from Chicago; that her murder remained unsolved.

Anyone with information about either case was asked to contact a special hot line that had been set up by the Blizzard Bay Police Department.

Sawyer got up and went to the drawer beside the sink in the kitchenette, jerking it open and removing a pair of scissors. He clutched them for a moment in his trembling hand, staring at the sharp metal blades.

Then he returned to the table, picked up the newspaper, and began carefully clipping out the article about the most recent murder.

Chapter Ten

"Are you all right?" Jorey asked Kitty as she returned from her third bathroom trip in the past hour or so since they had gathered in the sitting room of the bed & breakfast.

"If you mean am I in labor, the answer is no," Kitty said, grunting and clutching the arms of the wingback chair as she leaned backward and lowered her bulky frame into it again. "I just drank too much coffee this morning, and the baby is crushing my bladder, so . . ." She shrugged.

"If Clover were here," Jorey said, "she'd probably tell you that coffee isn't healthy for pregnant women."

"If Clover were here, I would have gotten at least some sleep last night, and I wouldn't have had to drink all that coffee," Kitty replied, shaking her head.

They were quiet then, all four of them, and the only sound in the sitting room was the ticking of the mantel clock. Outside, the scraping sound of a neighbor's shovel could be heard.

It was early afternoon, and a chilly sun shone brightly on the snow-covered world.

But inside the big Victorian house the blinds were drawn and the mood was somber.

It was Kitty who broke the silence. "I can't believe she's gone."

"I can't, either," Adrienne said. "Of all people . . . she was a quiet little mouse. My God—why would anyone have a reason to kill Clover?"

Gretchen spoke up. "Psychotic killers don't need a reason, Adrienne. It could have just been some stranger who broke into her house and went on a rampage."

"Or not even a stranger. It could have been Hob Nixon," Kitty pointed out. "Everyone knows he's crazy. He's always talking to himself and starting fights in bars, and he was accused of sexual assault a few years ago by some woman down in Ulster County."

"Was Clover . . . sexually assaulted?" Jorey asked, her stomach turning over with a sickening thud at the thought.

"Nobody's saying. They wouldn't say anything the first time, either, with that Latimer woman."

"Well, maybe it was Hob Nixon," Adrienne said, "and maybe they'll get him this time."

"Maybe it wasn't," Gretchen said quietly. "Maybe it was a total stranger, just a random thing."

"Well, if that's the case," Kitty said, "if some crazed maniac is on the loose in Blizzard Bay, then it could happen again. To anyone."

"I don't think it was a crazed maniac who killed Clover," Adrienne said, toying with the buttons on her cashmere cardigan. "If it wasn't Hob Nixon, then I'll bet it was Sheryl Frampton."

"Her business partner?" Jorey asked. "I saw her out in front of the house with the police when I drove by yesterday, and she looked distraught."

"She could have been acting," Adrienne said. "She wanted to buy out Clover's half of the store, and Clover refused to sell it to her. But now, with Clover dead, the business will probably be all hers."

"Have you ever met Sheryl, though?" Kitty wanted to know. "She doesn't seem like the kind of person who could kill someone. Then again, neither does Johnny, and the police spent hours questioning him last night, like they thought he knew something he wasn't telling."

"Does he know anything at all?" Gretchen asked. "Was Clover with anyone at the store, or did she say anything about her plans for the evening?"

"She was alone, as usual," Kitty said. "All she said was that she wanted to get home to feed her cats. That's what she was buying. Cat food. She said she had run out."

"She also talked about Jorey and Sawyer Howland," Adrienne reminded her. "Don't forget that."

Jorey shifted on the uncomfortable antique couch, wanting to swat the catty look off Adrienne's pretty face.

She snuck a glance at Gretchen and saw an expression that was impossible to read. She wondered, as she had all morning, whether Gretchen had figured out where she had spent the night.

She had been up, in the kitchen, when Jorey got home this morning, and though Jorey swept up the stairs to take a shower before greeting her she figured Gretchen was aware that she had been gone overnight.

It was obvious from the way she acted—more reserved than usual, and somewhat ill at ease in Jorey's presence.

When she said that Kitty and Adrienne would be coming over, Jorey was relieved. It wasn't that she was eager to face them, knowing they'd been gossiping and speculating about her and Sawyer, but she wasn't entirely comfortable being alone with Gretchen.

After all, here she was, staying under Gretchen's roof, even prying into Gretchen's relationship with Karl, yet sneaking around behind her back with a man Gretchen had warned her to stay away from.

But she isn't my mother, Jorey thought with a flicker of resentment, glancing at Gretchen's stoic face. *I don't owe her anything. Why do I feel like I'm letting her down?*

Because shy, upstanding Gretchen had always been the most decent, the most moral, of her friends. She was the one who, growing up, made her want to do the right thing.

Jorey knew that Gretchen wouldn't see sleeping with Sawyer Howland as doing the right thing. Especially when a second woman had been found dead, and Gretchen had considered Sawyer a likely suspect in the first murder.

So why did you do it? Jorey asked herself, not for the first time since she had guiltily crept home from Sawyer's apartment.

Because I couldn't stop myself.

And I didn't believe he could do something like that—kill someone. Kill two people.

What about now? Did she believe in his innocence as strongly as she had before?

Yes, came the firm reply.

Then why did you run away this morning, as if you were running for your life?

Because the experience of making love with Sawyer Howland had left her more vulnerable than she'd ever realized she was capable of feeling. And she had known that he was a man she could fall in love with, if he'd just let her.

If she'd just let herself.

"Where was Sawyer the night of the murder, Jorey?" Adrienne asked, startling her.

Jorey looked at her, and then at the others. They were all watching her, waiting for a reply.

"I don't know," she admitted finally, truthfully. "He wasn't with me."

"Have you seen him since you found out about Clover?" Kitty wanted to know.

Jorey didn't want to lie. She shouldn't *have* to lie, she thought defensively. But she heard herself telling them, "No. No, I haven't seen him."

She could feel Gretchen's pale blue gaze on her, and she was certain then that Gretchen knew where she had spent the night. She even knew what Gretchen was thinking.

How could you, Jorey?

She was wondering the same thing herself.

Sawyer stood, concealed by the full, low branches of the evergreen trees at the edge of the woods, watching as the pickup truck drove away, rattling down the rutted, snow-covered lane leading to the road.

The moment the sound had faded in the distance he sprang into action, moving out of his hiding place toward the battered trailer several yards away.

He went around to the far side, climbed up on a

conveniently placed tree stump, and reached up with a
practiced hand to fiddle with a window.

Moments later, he was pulling himself through and
carefully climbing over the narrow countertop below
the window inside. It was cluttered with dirty dishes and
empty beer cans, and he spotted an enormous cock-
roach scurrying down the edge of the filthy sink.

Sawyer stealthily jumped to the floor and wrinkled
his nose as he looked around in disgust. The smell of
cigarette smoke, spoiled food, and garbage hung over
the small, single room, and it was even more squalid
than it had been the last time he'd been here.

That had been two months ago, in early September,
not long after he'd arrived in town.

He stepped around a pile of *Soldier of Fortune* maga-
zines on the floor and went to the far side of the trailer,
where a rumpled bed and low dresser were wedged
beneath the window. He began with the dresser drawers,
most of which were already ajar and spilling over with
clothing. Searching them took only a few moments, and
he came up with nothing except a small handgun. It
had been here before, and the murder victims had been
stabbed, not shot. He put it back.

He lifted the mattress of the bed, saw that the space
beneath was empty, and felt along the crack between
the frame and the wall. Nothing.

He bent to look beneath the bed, heard something
rustling and scampering away, and shuddered before
turning on the flashlight he'd brought with him. The
space under the bed was jammed with dirty clothes and
garbage and odds and ends, as it had been before, and
it took him a long time to rummage through it. Still
nothing.

Sawyer moved methodically through the trailer, covering every inch. When he was finished, he had uncovered no evidence that Hob Nixon had killed Clover Hartdale. Just as he had found nothing here two months ago to indicate that he had killed Rebecca Latimer.

That didn't mean he hadn't done it. It was easy to imagine that the scruffy loner was responsible for slaughtering two innocent women in their homes.

Maybe too easy.

But Sawyer didn't know where else to turn. Three months in Blizzard Bay, and the only likely suspect he could come up with had already been cleared by the police in the first murder, when they could find no evidence against him.

Sawyer knew they hadn't had probable cause to obtain a search warrant for Nixon's trailer, and that Nixon hadn't consented to let them search it. Either he had something to hide, or he was simply disgruntled that the police were focusing any attention on him. Sawyer had taken it upon himself to do a little private investigating, both in September and now.

What had he been expecting to find?

A bloodied knife, its wooden handle monogrammed with Clover Hartdale's initials?

All right, maybe nothing so obvious, but something, *something* that would offer a solid lead.

If Hob Nixon was guilty of the two murders, Sawyer thought grimly, looking around the cluttered trailer, he had done a good job of covering it up.

And if he hadn't done it . . .

Then who had?

Karl showed up just as Jorey and Gretchen were sitting down to a pizza that had just been delivered.

Jorey, seated in the dining room, heard him say "I'm sorry I couldn't come last night," in the front hall as soon as Gretchen opened the door. "I've been thinking about you all day. Are you all right?"

"I'm just upset," Gretchen told him, and Jorey heard her voice waver. "I'm still having a hard time believing it happened."

There was a moment of silence, and Jorey assumed Gretchen was in Karl's arms.

Then she heard her say, "Come in, Karl. Jorey and I were just about to eat dinner."

"Then I won't interrupt you."

"No, it's fine. It's just pizza we ordered from Domino's. Have you eaten?"

"Actually, I stopped to get take-out on the way home from Saratoga. It's in the car. I just wanted to stop in and make sure that you were all right. I haven't heard anything all day. Have the police caught whoever did this to Clover?"

"Not as far as I know."

"Do you know if there are any suspects yet?"

"I have no idea."

"I read in this morning's paper that it might have been linked to the murder in August."

"I read that, too. Why don't you come in?" Gretchen said again. "Even if you can't stay long."

There was a long moment. Jorey knew Karl was hesitating, and then she heard him say, "All right. But just for a few minutes."

Jorey pretended to be surprised when Gretchen reentered the dining room with Karl in tow. She couldn't help noticing that her friend seemed pleased and almost smug when she announced the obvious.

"Karl's here, Jorey. He wanted to make sure that I was all right."

Her tone seemed to say, *See? He does care about me, no matter what you were trying to imply with all your questions about our relationship.*

"That was sweet. Hi, Karl."

"How are you, Jorey?"

She shrugged. "I've been better."

She noticed that he was wearing a dress shirt and outdated style of tie underneath his long, wool overcoat, which was frayed around the cuffs. And that he could use a haircut.

Gretchen had mentioned that he didn't have much money; he was paying alimony to his wife and she had gotten their house in the divorce. That was why he had to live year-round in a small cabin that hadn't even been winterized.

Jorey found herself feeling sorry for the man, and even more sorry for Gretchen. There was something vaguely sad about both of them, as though they were needy, searching souls who couldn't quite get it together.

What about you? You're needy and searching, too, Jorey reminded herself. Wasn't that why she had come here in the first place?

Now she found herself in the midst of a double murder scene and romantically entangled with a man who was all wrong for her, a man who might even be dangerous.

What was it that had triggered the nagging doubts that had darted in and out of her mind ever since she'd awakened in her old bed in her old room? Why couldn't she put her finger on whatever it was that was bothering her?

Did it even have anything to do with Sawyer?

She couldn't be sure. She only knew that there was something dark and oppressive hanging over her, something that she needed to remember.

"Would you like a slice of pizza, Karl?" Gretchen was asking.

"No, thanks. I told you, I have my supper waiting in the car. So I guess I should be going, now. I have to let the dog out, and I should get home."

"Are you sure?" Gretchen looked crestfallen.

He nodded. "I'll be home all night, though. Call me if you need anything, all right?"

"I might do that," she said. "I was a little worried about staying alone in the house last night with a murderer on the loose."

"Well, you're not exactly alone," Karl pointed out. "Jorey's here, and your Uncle Roland."

"Actually, Jorey wasn't here," Gretchen said a little pointedly, not looking at Jorey, who squirmed in her chair, wondering if Gretchen was going to tell Karl she'd been seeing Sawyer Howland.

But all Gretchen said was, "She was out. And Uncle Roland wouldn't provide much defense against a murderer—he wouldn't hear if I screamed, or even be able to call the police. Besides . . ."

"What?" Karl asked, when she didn't go on.

"Nothing. It's just . . . I'm a little concerned about my uncle. I'm afraid he's getting a little senile."

Jorey raised her eyebrows, wondering if this was what Gretchen had started to say last night.

"What do you mean, Gretchen?" she asked.

"It's just . . ." Gretchen looked from Karl to Jorey. "Please don't say anything to anyone. But I've been missing things around the house lately . . . loose change, and jewelry—nothing worth much, but still.''

"You think that your uncle has been stealing it?'' Jorey asked.

Gretchen shrugged. "I'm not sure. I just wonder sometimes if he's all there. He's always been in his own little world because of his condition, but lately he just seems . . . different. Like he's not all there.''

"Maybe you should take him to see someone, then,'' Karl suggested.

"Do you mean a psychiatrist?''

"Maybe.''

"But he can't hear and he can't speak. That wouldn't do him any good,'' Gretchen pointed out.

"I'm sure there are doctors who can help people like him,'' Jorey said. "Maybe in New York.''

"Maybe,'' Gretchen agreed. "But it's probably nothing. Forget I said anything. I'm probably just letting my imagination get carried away, and I've been so upset about Clover and everything . . .''

"That's understandable. Wait until some time has passed, and then you can deal with your uncle's problems,'' Karl suggested, jingling his car keys in his coat pocket. "I should really be on my way.''

"I'll walk you to the door,'' Gretchen said, putting her hand on Karl's arm.

He turned to Jorey, who sat with the still untouched slice of pizza on her plate. For one of the first times in her life, she had no appetite.

"It was nice seeing you again, Jorey.''

"You too, Karl.''

"How long are you staying in town?''

She hesitated. "I'm not sure. I'll probably head back

to New York after Clover's funeral, which should be tomorrow or the day after."

Gretchen looked surprised. "You're planning to leave so soon, Jorey?"

"I should. I hate to put you out—"

"You aren't putting me out. There's plenty of room, Jorey. You can stay as long as you like."

"Thank you," she said. "But . . ."

But the longer I stay, the better the chance that I'll dig myself in deeper with Sawyer.

"I do have things I need to get back to," she said lamely.

"But not a job," Karl said, "isn't that right? Gretchen told me that you're unemployed at the moment."

"She did?" Jorey glanced at her friend, who looked apologetic.

"I told Karl that you're in between careers right now," Gretchen clarified hastily. "I figured that since you didn't have to get back to an office, you might stay up here for a while. It's just that it's . . . been so nice having you around, Jorey. This big old house gets so lonely sometimes, now that Mother and Dad are gone."

"It's been nice being here," she said, touched by her friend's words. "But I really can't stay very much longer. I'll probably head back by the end of the week."

"Well, I hope to see more of you before you leave," Karl said politely.

"Maybe the three of us can go out to dinner tomorrow night," Gretchen suggested. "Jorey and I can meet you in Saratoga—"

"I'd love to," Karl told her, "but I've got a busy day tomorrow. Can we play it by ear?"

"Sure we can," Gretchen said, looking at her shoes. Couldn't Karl see that she was crazy about him? Was he leading her on, or did he have real feelings for her? It wasn't easy to tell where he was coming from, but it was certainly clear that Gretchen was head over heels.

Jorey found herself thinking back to their teenage years, when Gretchen developed occasional crushes on some of the more popular boys in town, who never gave her a second glance. Because she was so shy and private she never mentioned her infatuations to anyone, but Jorey remembered how easy it had always been to tell what her friend was thinking, how she used to blush and get flustered and stammer whenever the latest object of her affections came around.

Oh, Gretchen, Jorey thought, *you deserve to be happy. You deserve, for a change, to have someone care about you the way that you care about him. You deserve to be in love, and to be loved back.*

And so do I.

As Gretchen and Karl went back to the front hallway, Jorey's thoughts drifted to Sawyer.

Should she leave town without saying good-bye? Would he even bother to come looking for her?

He hadn't when he'd emerged from the shower to find her gone this morning. All day, she had found herself expecting the phone to ring, or to see his old car pull up at the curb out front. But he hadn't contacted her.

For all she knew, he was relieved that she had left the way she had, so that there would be no awkward morning-after encounters between them. No stilted conversations in which they both struggled to pretend that last night hadn't happened.

Now, almost twenty-four hours later, she was almost finding it difficult to believe that it had.

If it weren't for the aching muscles in unusual spots

on her body, muscles she hadn't even known existed, there would be no proof that she and Sawyer Howland had made passionate love to each other.

Had it been just this morning that Sawyer had awakened to find Jorey, naked and sleeping, beside him in his bed?

He stood before it now, staring at the rumpled sheets he hadn't bothered to change, and he wondered whether he would be cloaked in her scent when he climbed between them tonight.

He didn't want that to happen; he should change the sheets right now so that it wouldn't.

Yet . . .

Maybe he did want it, that last tangible reminder of what had happened between them.

All day, he had struggled to keep her from his mind. It had been easier than he expected, because he was consumed by the most recent murder, obsessed by the details and his own burning need to uncover the truth.

Now, in the quiet confines of his apartment, he could no longer escape.

He stood staring at the bed and he let the thoughts come. He saw Jorey lying there, her nude body as exquisitely seductive as he'd known it would be, her eyes closed. He heard her moaning softly, panting in his ear, and he felt her writhing beneath him, felt her damp skin against his own.

"Dammit," he said, turning away from the bed and squeezing his eyes shut. "Dammit. Go away . . . can't you just go away?"

Chapter Eleven

The Hudson Funeral Home was located on Nelson Avenue in Saratoga Springs, a few blocks from the famed racetrack. It was a quiet, tree-shaded residential neighborhood of large two and three story Victorian homes, some converted to inns and apartments, but many still private residences.

Jorey couldn't help wondering as she and Gretchen walked along the sidewalk toward the funeral home what it would be like to live in a place like this—in one of these big old homes with a tricycle and picnic table in the yard, bright-colored, vinyl turkey and pilgrim decorations stuck to the front door glass, and oval Totfinder signs in the upper windows; all clues that announced to passersby that a family, a *real*, small-town-America family, was in residence.

Life was so different here than in the city, she mused wistfully, glancing up to see a young mother unloading bags of groceries and a snow-suited infant from a station wagon in a nearby driveway.

So peaceful. No incessant sirens, no honking traffic, no crowds.

And you're on your way to the wake of your friend, who was stabbed to death in her home.

She sighed and folded her arms, hugging herself as they reached the broad steps of the funeral home, an elegant, white brick, black-shuttered mansion fronted with neatly trimmed shrubbery and a tasteful, unobtrusive sign.

There were several news camera crews on the sidewalk across the street, filming the mourners as they entered, while security guards posted at the door kept a wary eye on them.

Jorey wasn't surprised by the presence of the press. The murder had been all over television and the papers today. Reporters had sensationally dubbed the killer the North Country Slasher, and the police still hadn't named any suspects.

Gretchen had brought Uncle Roland to the police station for questioning this afternoon, and had told Jorey later that it hadn't gone well. He'd been bewildered and hadn't understood what anyone was asking, despite Gretchen's efforts to moderate.

A couple emerged from the funeral home, the woman sobbing loudly and leaning on the man, who spoke to her in a low, soothing voice.

"Are you holding up all right?" Gretchen asked, glancing at Jorey as they walked up to the door.

"I'm okay. Are you?"

Gretchen nodded, but she looked ashen as she opened the door and they stepped inside.

There were several people milling about the carpeted

entry hall, and a somber-faced mortician in a dark suit directed them toward a hushed, crowded room to the side.

There, the first thing Jorey saw was the casket, closed, surrounded by floral arrangements.

The second thing she saw was Sawyer Howland, standing quietly off to one side.

Despite the grim surroundings, the sight of him took her breath away. He wore a well-cut, charcoal wool suit; the jacket was double-breasted and the trousers draped stylishly above his polished, black dress shoes. His blond hair was conservatively combed back from his ruggedly handsome face, and it occurred to Jorey that he looked like a male model in a European designer ad.

He stood apart from the crowd, alone and idle, yet somehow not appearing awkward.

Looking at him, the way he was dressed, the casual confidence he exuded, Jorey was more certain than ever that he wasn't what he claimed to be. He might own an auto body shop; he might even have expertly repaired her Range Rover, but Sawyer Howland was no small town mechanic.

What, she wondered, was he hiding? And why?

A chill slid down her spine as she stared at him.

"What is he doing here?" Gretchen whispered, following Jorey's gaze.

She bristled. "Paying his respects like everybody else, I suppose."

"He didn't even know Clover."

"You don't know that."

"She would have mentioned it."

Kitty and Johnny walked up to them then. Kitty's eyes were red and rimmed with smudged mascara, and

Johnny looked distinctly ill at ease in his snug gray blazer and navy dress slacks that were an inch too short.

"Have you seen Clover's mother?" Kitty asked, sniffling.

"We just got here," Gretchen replied.

"Well, she's a wreck. She flew in from Florida last night. When she saw me she grabbed me and started crying, asking me why this happened. This is so horrible, I just—"

"Take it easy, Babe," Johnny said, putting a hand on her back. "Don't get all worked up again. It's not good for the baby."

"I can't help it."

"You should sit down," Gretchen told Kitty. "Let's go over to those folding chairs."

"Did you see who's here?" Johnny asked Jorey as they followed behind.

"Hob Nixon," she said, spotting him in the doorway, looking out of place in dirty jeans and an army camouflage jacket. His hair was greasy and uncombed, and he glanced around warily.

"What's he doing here?" Jorey wondered.

Johnny glanced that way and shrugged. "I have no idea, but he wasn't who I meant."

"Who did you mean?" she asked reluctantly.

"Sawyer Howland. Over there. He's looking right at you."

Jorey didn't turn her head, unwilling to confront his piercing blue gaze. She felt it, and it rattled her.

"What's going on between the two of you?" Johnny asked. "You're not really going out with him, are you, Jorey? Because Kitty said—"

"This isn't high school, Johnny," Jorey snapped. "I don't really want to discuss my private life. Will you please tell Gretchen and Kitty that I went to find the ladies' room? I'll be back."

She turned and walked away before he could say another word, ducking back into the lobby.

She realized that the viewing room had been too warm and crowded, and that the smell of flowers had been overpowering. She leaned on the banister at the foot of a sweeping staircase and took a deep breath, and then another.

"Are you all right, Jorey?"

Startled, she looked up to see Sawyer standing beside her.

She hadn't expected to come face-to-face with him this way; hadn't wanted to. But now that he was in front of her, she found herself relieved to see him.

She didn't want to discuss what had happened between them, or the fact that she was going to leave in another day or two. If he brought it up, she would tell him so.

But this was hardly the setting for him to dredge things up, and she felt safe speaking to him. Here, they could carry on a casual, polite conversation like any two acquaintances running into each other under such circumstances.

"I'm fine," she told him. "Just a little—"

"You look pale."

"I'm all right. Really."

"It isn't easy to lose someone close to you," he said, putting a hand on her arm.

And she realized, guiltily, that he thought she had been overcome by grief in there. He hadn't a clue that *he* was the reason she'd had to flee the room. That she had been thrown by his unexpected presence, and the incessant gossip about the two of them.

"Clover and I—we weren't that close. Not anymore. I hadn't seen her in years before my visit in August."

He shrugged. "Still, she was a friend when you were young. And the way that she died—"

"I know." She suppressed a shudder. "The whole thing feels so unreal. I keep having to remind myself—"

"Do you have any idea who would have done this to her?"

Jorey shook her head. "I didn't know much about her life these days, other than that she ran a New Age boutique of some sort here in Saratoga. It could have just been one of those random things, I guess, or—"

"Jorey, there you are!"

She looked up to see Adrienne sweeping in from the next room. Clad in a chic, black silk suit, hat, and gloves, she looked every inch the sophisticated mourner. A cloud of expensive perfume clung to her, and though she clutched a white linen handkerchief Jorey saw that her eye makeup hadn't been marred by tears.

"You must be Sawyer Howland," Adrienne said, looking him over appreciatively yet somehow with a hint of disdain. "I've heard so much about you."

He raised an eyebrow at that and looked at Jorey, who scowled.

"I was just speaking with Kitty and Gretchen," Adrienne went on, "and I invited them back to my house after the service for coffee. I don't think any of us wants to be alone tonight."

"Where's your friend the senator?" Jorey asked a bit snidely. "Isn't he here with you?"

Adrienne didn't look the least bit flustered as she said, "He couldn't make it. He's a busy man, you know."

And, being married, he can't exactly show up at such a public event, with all the news cameras outside.

"Aren't you going to introduce me, Jorey?" Adrienne asked, looking Sawyer over with a shrewd expression.

"Adrienne Von Deegan, this is Sawyer Howland," Jorey obliged tonelessly.

"You're the mechanic at A-1 Auto Body in Blizzard Bay?" Adrienne asked incredulously as if that were news to her, as her gaze swept over his expensive suit.

Sawyer nodded.

"Pardon my saying so, but you don't look like a mechanic," Adrienne crooned.

Sawyer's gaze narrowed as though he'd been insulted, and he responded, "I couldn't exactly show up here in my greasy coveralls, could I?"

"No, I don't suppose you could. If you don't mind my asking, why *are* you here?" Adrienne asked.

Her question was bold and completely uncalled for, but Jorey had been wondering the same thing herself.

"I didn't know your friend personally," Sawyer said. "But I've been reading about her in the papers, and the horrible way she died, and it seemed fitting to come and pay my respects."

Adrienne nodded, but there was a gleam in her eye that told Jorey she didn't entirely buy his answer.

Jorey found that as much as she wanted to trust him, she didn't entirely believe him, either.

"Ooh, look," Adrienne suddenly said, turning her blond head and nudging Jorey. "There's Hob Nixon. What's *he* doing here?"

Jorey saw the scruffy loner sidling through the doorway from the next room. His gaze was focused on his feet, clad in muddy work boots, but then he glanced up and looked directly at her.

"Oh, ugh," Adrienne said in a stage whisper, and made a face. "He's so . . . repulsive."

Jorey wanted to tell her to shut up, that her voice had undoubtedly carried to Hob Nixon's ears. She saw the hard expression in his dark eyes that narrowed in their direction before he turned and disappeared around a corner.

"Anyway, I would love it if you came with Jorey to my house afterward," Adrienne said conversationally, turning back to Sawyer. "Can I expect you?"

"I don't think so," Sawyer told her. "But thank you for the invitation."

Adrienne shrugged and said, "You can always change your mind," before drifting back to the next room.

Jorey met Sawyer's gaze.

"She doesn't seem like your kind of person," he told Jorey in a straightforward tone.

"Actually, she isn't. There was a time when we were good friends, but things change. I used to think that I had so much in common with Adrienne—the others, too. But we've all gone in different directions."

"That happens."

"I know . . . but I guess I wasn't expecting it," Jorey said. "When I came up here, I kind of pictured everything the same as it always had been. I thought, I guess, that I could pick up where I left off. The funny thing is . . ."

"What?" he prompted when she trailed off.

"I don't really remember where I left off. That last summer I spent here was a blur. My parents had just told me they were splitting up, and I was completely traumatized by it. I just don't remember much that happened during those weeks while I was here. It's as if everything was erased from my mind when Papa May died, and . . ."

Sawyer was watching her carefully. "What is it, Jorey?"

She looked at him. "It's just . . . I have a strange feeling. As if there's something I should be remembering about that summer. For the life of me, I can't seem to catch whatever it is."

"Something important?"

"I don't know—"

"Hello, Jorey," a voice interrupted, and she saw that Karl had just walked in the door. He wore the same worn overcoat from the night before, and his graying hair was slightly mussed from the wind. He was eyeing Sawyer suspiciously.

"Hi, Karl," Jorey said, deciding not to bother introducing the two men. She knew what Karl thought about Sawyer.

Instead she said, "Gretchen said she didn't know if you'd be able to make it."

"I had a late meeting, but my office isn't far from here, and I hurried over."

"Gretchen's in there," Jorey said, gesturing, hoping he would take the hint and leave.

There was a rumbling from the next room just then; the scraping of chairs and an announcement that the service was about to begin.

"Are you coming in?" Karl asked Jorey, again glancing at Sawyer, who showed no sign of recognition.

"In a minute. You go ahead," Jorey told him.

Karl nodded and slipped out of his coat, then made his way into the room.

Jorey turned to Sawyer. "That was—"

"Karl Andersen. I know."

"You know him? Why didn't you say anything?"

"We've never met. I just know who he is. And I'm sure he knows who I am."

"He does."

"He's one of the people who warned you to stay away from me—that I'm dangerous."

"How did you know that?"

"It isn't hard to tell what people think about you in this town, Jorey," Sawyer told her.

"I thought you didn't care that people are afraid of you."

"I don't." He paused. "Is that why you left the way you did yesterday morning? Because you were afraid?"

So there it was. He had brought it up, after all.

She looked him in the eye, lifting her chin. "I'm not afraid of you, Sawyer."

"Why did you leave?"

"Because I had to. Because there was nothing for us to say to each other."

"Not even good-bye?"

"I hate good-byes."

"So do I," he said in a low voice, and tilted his head toward the next room, where the service was beginning. "Should we go in?"

"We should—"

"But you don't really want to," he told her, watching her.

"No," Jorey admitted. "I really don't."

She loathed the thought of walking into that room with Sawyer Howland in front of all those curious people, people who would nudge each other and speculate; people who actually thought he might have had something to do with Clover's death.

Jorey didn't believe that. No matter what she tried to tell herself when she wasn't with him, she was convinced

now that there was nothing dangerous about Sawyer—
not in the way people thought.

She didn't want to trust him; she didn't want to believe
that he was a decent human being, because that would
mean that she could fall in love with him.

She didn't want to do that.

No, she couldn't go and do that.

Nor could she keep telling herself, though, that he
was someone to fear. Not when it was becoming more
and more clear that only when she was with him did
she instinctively feel . . .

Safe.

The thought caught her off guard, and she wondered,
safe from . . . what?

From loneliness? Or the past?

It didn't make sense, and yet . . .

"Come on, Jorey," he whispered, "let's get out of
here."

"I should tell Gretchen."

But she couldn't go in there. She would leave a note
on Gretchen's car, she decided. She knew Gretchen
wouldn't approve, but suddenly she thought, *To hell with
her. To hell with all of them.*

"Let's go," she told Sawyer abruptly.

When Sawyer had heard on the radio this morning
that Clover's wake would be held tonight at The Hudson
Funeral Home, he'd known he had to go, though his
presence would undoubtedly arouse suspicion.

There was no telling what he could learn by watching
the crowds who came to mourn her. Somewhere among
the sorrow-stricken family and friends there might be

a clue. Maybe the murderer would even be among them, pretending to grieve with the others.

Now, as he left the white brick mansion behind, Sawyer was no closer to knowing who had killed Clover Hartdale and Rebecca Latimer.

He had been startled to see Hob Nixon there, and wondered why he had come. Had he actually been acquainted with Clover? He was from town, and didn't live far from her house. Still, he didn't seem the type who would show up at a wake out of some sense of neighborly duty.

Sawyer remembered how he had seen him at the crime scene, too, and wondered again if he was the one who had killed Clover. The man was definitely a suspect, but there was no way to tell if he was guilty.

All that had been clear to Sawyer inside the funeral home was that he had to get Jorey out of there. If she stayed, if he even let her out of his sight tonight, she would be in danger.

That knowledge had come to him the moment he'd spotted her standing there, looking lovely in a simple black dress, her curls tamed in a black bow at the nape of her neck.

He couldn't keep from watching her, and when she left the room, looking disturbed about something, he had known he had to follow her.

The last thing he wanted to do was spend a tortured night in her company, fighting the powerful attraction between them. But he had sworn to himself that he would protect her, and he was certain that her life depended on him tonight.

"Where are we going?" she asked him as they walked along the sidewalk toward Gretchen's car.

"Where do you want to go?"

"I don't know." She looked up at him. "I shouldn't be leaving with you. I should be in there, listening to the service for Clover."

"It's all right, Jorey. You said yourself that you weren't very close to her these days."

"But she was murdered," she said, her voice shaking. "My friend was murdered. Sawyer, what's going on in Blizzard Bay? Things like this aren't supposed to happen around here."

"Things like this can happen anywhere, Jorey."

"I know that. I guess it's just that they're not supposed to happen to people I know."

He gave a short, bitter laugh. "Now you sound like the sheltered princess I thought you were when I met you."

"Maybe I was, when you met me."

"But that was less than a week ago."

"I know." She stopped in front of a dark, midsized sedan and pulled a pen and a scrap of paper out of her purse, poised to write a note to Gretchen. "Where should I tell her I'm going?"

"That's up to you."

She thought for a minute, then slowly put the pen and paper back into her bag.

"What are you doing?" he asked, worried that she had changed her mind about coming with him, that she would turn around and walk back into that funeral home, where she wouldn't be safe.

"Forget it," she told him, turning away from the car. "I don't need to leave a note. Why do I keep feeling as if I'm a teenager again—as if I owe everyone an explanation for every move I make? I'm a grown woman. I've always made my own decisions, and I've never felt compelled to account to anyone for what I do. I guess it's just . . . being back here."

"Being back with your old friends, maybe." He started walking across the street, toward his car, and she fell into step beside him.

"I guess. We used to be so close. But I guess that's how it is when you're a kid. You're close to your friends. You care what they think."

"Do you have a lot of friends now, back in New York?" he asked, curious, suddenly, about her world.

"In a way. But it's different. They're more like . . . social acquaintances."

"What about your family?"

She made a face. "What about them?"

"Are you close to them?"

"To my father. I was his favorite, a real daddy's girl."

"What about your mother?"

"She couldn't stand me," Jorey told him bluntly.

"She couldn't *stand* you?"

"I reminded her too much of him."

"I take it they didn't have a wonderful marriage?"

"They were divorced, as I said, when I was seventeen. Neither of them was particularly sad to see it end, and my sisters weren't, either. I guess I was the only one who was surprised . . . and upset."

"Why is that?"

"Because I always had an idea of what we should be— our family. I always wanted things to be normal—to live in one home, the same home, and do normal family things. But it wasn't like that. We were always moving from one apartment to another, and my father was wrapped up in running his business, and my mother was wrapped up in money, and my sisters . . ."

The wistful note in her voice touched him, and he fought the urge to reach out and take her hand in his.

"What about your sisters?" he asked. "You aren't close to them now?"

"No. They're so different. Both of them are married, and they have children."

"You don't want to get married?" he heard himself ask. "Or have children?"

He found himself holding his breath for her answer.

"I do," she said, and again he heard that wistful tone. It touched something deep inside of him, some part of him he had sworn he wouldn't let her, wouldn't let anyone, touch. Not after all that he'd lost.

"But I don't want to do it their way," she went on. "My sisters have nannies who raise their children, and their relationships with their husbands seem more like business arrangements than marriages."

"And you want more," he said softly, glad he couldn't see her face, afraid of what he might find there.

"I want more," she echoed. "I want . . ."

She trailed off, and he couldn't bring himself to ask what she had intended to say.

Instead, he walked along beside her, and they were both silent until they reached the Chevy.

"Where are we going?" she asked again, as he reached past her to unlock the passenger's side door.

"I have no idea where we're going, Jorey," he replied. "I'll leave that up to you."

For a moment, she seemed lost in thought. Then she said slowly, "I know a place."

* * *

"It looks the same," Jorey said, standing in the middle of the clearing, turning around slowly, taking in the sight before her.

The pine forest had given way to a sheltered pond surrounded by evergreens and jutting boulders. Rising in the distance, beyond the rim of the trees, the snow-covered ridges of the Adirondacks were just visible.

"It looks the same," she said again, "except that everything is white. And dark."

"You were never up here in the dark?" Sawyer asked, leaning against a tall rock nearby, his arms folded across his chest as he watched her.

"Sometimes we got here just before the sun rose—me, and Papa May," she told him. "The sky would be all pink and light, and we sat right over there"—she pointed to a flat boulder by the water's edge—"and he smoked his pipe and watched the sunrise while I baited our hooks. Papa May liked to get an early start to every day. But you know what? I don't know if I've seen a sunrise since that summer."

Sawyer was silent, and she turned to look at him. Shadows hid his face, but she sensed that he was deep in thought.

Who are you? she wondered, gazing at the man who seemed even more of a stranger dressed in that suit, the overcoat that looked like cashmere.

His attire was preposterously out of place in this setting, as was her own, but they hadn't stopped to change before hiking up here. She hadn't wanted to, afraid that if they delayed, even momentarily, she wouldn't get here at all.

She needed to be here.

She turned back to the pond, hugging herself as she stared at the murky black water. Something flitted at the edge of her mind, a thought that vanished before it had formed, and she frowned, frustrated, certain that there was something she should be remembering.

What had triggered it?

Being in this particular spot after all these years?

She concentrated, but nothing came to her. Nothing but a memory that had haunted her for years, a memory of the last time she had ever been to this secluded pond.

It was so fuzzy, really. All she recalled was chattering to Papa May, and realizing that he hadn't responded in some time. Then she turned to him, and she heard the horrible gasping sound, and she knew . . .

He was gone seconds later, and she was alone.

She closed her eyes and allowed the memory to wash over her, shivering as if it were a splash of icy water.

She saw him lying there, lifeless; heard her own voice echoing in the quiet solitude, screaming, "Papa May? Papa May, please wake up. Papa May . . ."

She felt warm arms closing around her from behind and a sob escaped her.

"It's all right, Jorey."

"No," she said, turning toward Sawyer, burying her face in his broad, warm chest. "It isn't all right. I needed him."

"Your grandfather." It wasn't a question.

"I needed him, and he left me. I was all alone. I've always been all alone."

"No," he whispered.

His arms tightened around her, and she lifted her head to look at him. As her face came up, his came down to meet it, and his lips singed hers in a sweeping kiss. She reached up to touch his shoulders and her hands encountered the soft folds of his coat.

So it *was* cashmere, she thought, letting her fingertips wander over the soft fabric as his lips moved over hers.

"Jorey," he murmured against her mouth, holding her to him. "Oh, Jorey . . ."

It's happening again, she realized, *and I can't stop it. I can't.*

Not with him.

She was lost, every logical thought she'd ever had sailing out of her head, replaced by pure heated sensation.

She was barely conscious of him pulling away momentarily to remove his coat and spread it on the ground behind her. Then he pulled her down and she sank to her knees in the powdery dusting of snow. She felt the wet chill of ice crystals against her bare legs as he gently leaned her back against the soft cashmere, fumbling with the front of her coat.

His suit jacket was open and she tugged at his dress shirt, first trying to unbutton it, then, frustrated, untucking it from his waistband, wanting only to touch him. She felt her way through the layers of clothing until her hands found his bare back and shoulders. She could feel the muscles rippling beneath his warm, smooth skin as he pushed her coat aside and began working on her silk dress.

They were both breathing hard, and as he shifted his weight she gasped, feeling his arousal against her lower stomach. She wriggled so that he was pressed against the most intimate spot between her legs, and heard him groan as his breathing grew more labored.

Still, he labored on the pearl buttons of her dress slipping them open one by one, then expertly unfastening the front clasp of her lace bra, baring her breasts to the cold night air and his heated mouth. She trembled as his tongue gently licked first one pebbly nipple, then the other, and when he lifted his head and kissed her again she could no longer stand it.

"Please," she heard herself moan as her hips strained upward, locked against his. "Please, now . . ."

He needed no further urging. She heard the zipping sound of his trousers being lowered, felt him raising her skirt up to her hips and tugging the flimsy scrap of her lace panties down over her thighs and knees.

She opened her legs to him and reached down to guide him into her, gasping with pleasure as he filled her and began to move. She moved with him, clinging to his bare shoulders, her cheek against his hair as he panted hot into her neck. The rhythm built to a mighty crescendo. He erupted into her as a thousand rainbows exploded before her closed eyes, and afterward he held her, still inside her.

She lay staring up at the night sky, noticing the full moon and a million glittering stars. His weight shifted, and she felt him withdraw, and then he lay beside her, the length of his body against the length of hers, his fingers reaching out to intertwine with hers. Slowly, she drifted back to reality.

"Sawyer?" she whispered, "can you tell me? Please? I need to know."

He was silent for a moment, and when he did speak she half-expected him to play dumb, to say, *Tell you what?* though she was certain that he knew what she meant.

But he didn't say that.

He raised his head and he looked down at her and he said, quietly, "All right. I can tell you."

He paused, took a deep breath, and let it out slowly.

Then he said, "She was my sister. Rebecca Latimer. My kid sister."

Confused, she asked, "Who?"

"The woman tourist who was murdered here in August."

As she grasped the startling news, a strange combination of horror and relief settled over her. Horror that he had lost someone so close in an unsolved, violent murder, and relief that he hadn't committed it.

Because no matter how many times she had tried to convince herself that he was innocent, that the rumors about him were unfounded, there had always been, in the back of her mind, the slightest disconcerting doubt.

"Sawyer," she said softly, looking into his tortured blue eyes, "I'm so sorry. My God . . ."

"She was so sweet, Jorey. Growing up. She was naive and trusting and always believed the best of people. That's why she got tangled up with Warren Latimer. I knew he was a loser from the moment I met him, but I had problems of my own, then. I didn't look out for her the way I should have. She married him. He divorced her a year later, and it was ugly. The messiest divorce I've ever seen. Rebecca was completely devastated. That was why she came here.

"It was an impulse, really. A friend of a friend had a cottage to rent for the summer, and she had to get away. So she came here, alone, to get her thoughts together. I should have stopped her . . ."

Those last words were so ragged, so plaintive, that Jorey reached out to touch his shoulder, startled by the haunted expression in his eyes.

"Why would you have stopped her?" she asked, shaking her head. "You didn't know what was going to happen to her here, Sawyer. It wasn't your fault."

He opened his mouth as if about to say something else, then seemed to catch himself and closed it again.

"What is it, Sawyer?" Jorey asked, watching him, concerned by the ravaged look on his face.

"Nothing. It's . . . nothing." He inhaled deeply, then sighed heavily. "Anyway, that's why I'm here. I swore I would find out who did this to my sister. I swore I would make them pay."

"But why the need for secrecy? Why make everyone in town think that you're up to something?"

"It's nobody's business what I'm doing here," Sawyer told her. "I don't want the police involved, and I don't want the media involved. I want to accomplish this on my own. It's . . . I owe it to her."

Jorey absorbed that, struck by the conviction in his voice and the anguish in his eyes. And she realized that there was something else.

Guilt.

He blamed himself for his sister's death; that much was obvious.

There was something else, something he wasn't telling her. She wanted to come right out and ask him what it was, but she couldn't bring herself to pry. His pain was too raw; he had already bared his soul to her.

"Sawyer," she said quietly, lightly touching his cheek to remind him that she was here. "Have you found anything to—any clues?"

He shook his head. "Nothing. When the police couldn't solve the case I told myself that it was just because they weren't trying hard enough. She was an outsider here, and maybe it didn't matter as much to them as it would if the victim had been a local. But I couldn't find anything, either. All these months living here, watching the people in this town, visiting the place where it happened, and I've come up with nothing but a dead end."

"Sawyer . . . do you think that whoever killed your sister killed Clover?"

He seemed to contemplate that, and slowly nodded. "I do. I think there's a serial killer in Blizzard Bay . . . and that this is only the beginning."

Something in his eyes, in the way he was looking at her, sent a chill down Jorey's spine.

"That's why I want you to go, Jorey," he said then. "I want you to get the hell out of here, go back to New York, and never look back."

Get the hell out of here.

Not because he didn't want her near him; not because he didn't feel anything for her.

Because he was trying to save her life.

And why?

Was it because he cared about her? Because he . . . *loved* her?

She wanted to believe that.

But in her heart she knew the truth. He needed to save her life, because he hadn't been able to save his sister's.

"Let me help you, Sawyer," she said, needing to ease his pain. "I can help you. We can look into this together, and—"

"No, Jorey. Aren't you listening to me? I told you . . . you *have* to leave."

"But I'll be careful. What makes you think this killer's going to come after me?"

He hesitated, then shrugged. "I just don't think there's any reason to stay here. You came because you wanted to reconnect with your childhood, to make peace with your past. Now you've done it. You've visited this spot where your grandfather died, you've seen the old house, your old room, and you've realized that you have nothing in common with the friends you once had. It's time to go, Jorey. Just . . . *go.*"

She sat up abruptly and the icy mountain wind struck her, making her realize, for the first time, how cold it was out there; how underdressed she was. She shivered and began buttoning her dress with suddenly numb fingers.

"If I leave," she said to Sawyer, "you and I will never see each other again. Is that the idea?"

"It's not what I want, Jorey. Believe me. I wish it could be some other way. But . . . I can't get involved with you."

"Not even when this is all over? After you've caught the killer and avenged your sister's death, or whatever it is that you feel you have to do?"

"Don't you dare belittle what I'm trying to do, Jorey." His voice was as brittle as the ice shards in the murky pond. "And don't ask me for something I'll never be able to give. There are things about me that you don't know."

"Then *tell* me, Sawyer," she said. "Don't be so secretive. Don't shut me out. Tell me the rest."

"No!" The word was a bitter roar.

She stared at him. Then, in silence, she turned away. She finished dressing and got to her feet.

"Jorey," he called as she picked her way over the uneven, snowy ground in boots that were hardly made for hiking. "Wait. I'll walk back to the house with you."

"It's okay. I know the way," she told him.

"But—"

"Don't worry, I don't need your protection. Believe

me, I can take care of myself, Sawyer. I've been doing it my whole life.''

She made her way back through the woods, grateful for the bright moonlight reflecting off the snow. A few times she caught the heels of her boots on roots and rocks buried beneath the drifts, causing her to nearly fall. She remembered how different it had been hiking up here with Sawyer at her side, his hand on her elbow to help her along.

It wasn't until she reached the house that she remembered he had driven her here. She was stranded.

There was nothing to do but wait for him to come back so that he could give her a ride back to town.

She sat glumly on the familiar stone steps leading up to the front porch, gradually growing conscious of the vast emptiness surrounding her—the open fields and the deep forest and the towering mountains in the distance.

Here in this place where she had always felt so safe, she realized that she was more vulnerable than ever before.

It's all his fault, she thought angrily. *Sawyer, with his talk of serial killers and my being in danger.*

But she knew it was more than that. She didn't just fear the nameless, faceless killer who was lurking out there somewhere. She didn't just fear the palpable presence of death.

She feared *life*—her life. A life that seemed more barren and hollow than ever now that she had sampled a fleeting taste of what she had always dreamed of; what she had come here searching for.

And there was something else. Something that had happened back at the pond, when she had found herself momentarily haunted by an elusive thought. What was it that she should be remembering about that last summer here?

Footsteps crunching in the distance made her look up to see Sawyer trudging toward her, his shoulders straight and broad, his head held high despite the chilling wind that whipped across the wide open lawn.

She stared at him and felt his eyes on her, and she willed herself to not look away. She didn't dare reveal any hint of her sudden vulnerability.

She said nothing as he drew within earshot, reluctant to ask him for anything, even the obvious.

He didn't make her do that.

"I'll drive you back," he told her when he arrived in front of her. It was impossible to read his tone or the expression on his chiseled features as he spoke.

She nodded and walked with him to the car.

They were silent all the way into town, and when he finally pulled to a stop in front of the bed & breakfast and she put her hand on the door handle to get out, she uttered a single, final word.

"Good-bye."

Chapter Twelve

The 1890 House was dark and felt empty when Jorey
returned. She hesitated just inside the front door, listening to the stillness, suddenly finding herself reluctant
to be here—especially alone.

She heard a faint creak and jumped, then pressed a
hand to her racing heart.

That was nothing, she told herself. *Just the wind, or an
old house doing whatever it is that old houses do. Settling—
isn't that what they call it?*

Sawyer's warnings about the serial killer really had
gotten to her, dammit. Irritated with him and with herself, she forced herself to move forward and up the
stairs, turning on lights as she went.

In the second floor hall she saw that the sconces were
already lit, the low-watt bulbs casting an almost eerie
glow along the corridor.

She rounded the corner toward her room and

stopped short as she heard footsteps on the steps at the end of the hall.

Her heart began to pound again, and she hurried toward her door even as she told herself that it was probably just Gretchen's uncle.

But how do I know he's not the killer? she wondered, reaching her room and grabbing the knob as the footsteps reached the hallway.

She heard a strange sound behind her; a guttural grunt that chilled her blood. Terrified, she turned and saw that Uncle Roland was standing a few yards away, at the foot of the stairs leading to the third floor.

He came toward her, gesturing wildly with his hands, making that sound again, a feral sound that came from deep in his throat. Panic seized Jorey. She jerked the door open just as the old man reached her.

His gnarled, bony hand shot out and grabbed her arm. His grip was strong, and his face, only inches from hers, revealed an urgent, almost savage expression.

"No! Let go of me!" she yelled, wrenching herself from his grasp.

She leapt into the room and pulled the door closed behind her, both hands clenched around the knob and her feet braced where the door met the floor. She waited for him to try to open it, to try to break in, but nothing happened.

Then, stunned, she heard his footsteps retreating along the hallway, and back up the stairs. Moments later, a door closed somewhere above.

For a long time, Jorey stood by the door, holding it, half-expecting another attack. But nothing happened.

Gradually, she realized that he had retreated.

Shaken, she fought the urge to bolt from the room and leave the house.

She couldn't just leave. It was well past midnight, and she had no place to go.

You could go back to Sawyer and tell him what happened, she told herself, but quickly pushed the thought away.

She wouldn't go back to Sawyer. He had made it clear that he felt nothing for her, nothing more than concern, and that that wouldn't change. He didn't love her, he only wanted to protect her because of his own complicated guilt complex.

You don't need his protection. You can protect yourself, just as you told him.

Jorey lifted her jaw stubbornly and looked around the room. Then she dragged the chair over to the door and piled luggage on top of it, as she had several nights ago.

The barricade in place, she stepped back and perched on the edge of the bed, wondering what to do next.

She could hardly believe Gretchen's uncle had actually attacked her.

But was it an attack? she found herself questioning. *He didn't actually hurt you. And when you pulled away he didn't break down the door and kill you.*

She remembered the wild look in his eyes and the frenzied sounds and frustrated gestures he had made. The more she replayed the scene in her mind, the more convinced she became that he hadn't meant to harm her, after all.

It was almost as though he was trying to communicate something to her.

The old man was locked in a silent world, unable to speak, unable to read or write.

If he *did* want to reach out and tell her something, how else would he do it?

Well, he didn't have to frighten me to death, Jorey told herself.

She would wait up, and when Gretchen came home she would tell her that Uncle Roland seemed upset about something. Maybe, she and Gretchen could go up and figure out what it was that he needed.

Jorey settled back against the pillows to wait and then, after a moment, pulled a blanket around her. The room was drafty and she was still wearing her dark silk dress. She couldn't help remembering how Sawyer's hands had roamed over her clothes and burrowed beneath them.

She longed to change into something warmer and more comfortable, something that didn't remind her of what had just happened between her and Sawyer, but she didn't dare.

If she was warm and comfortable, she might fall asleep, and she couldn't do that.

What if she'd been wrong about Uncle Roland?

What if, the moment she drifted off he came sneaking back down and attacked her?

No, she thought with a yawn, she didn't dare risk falling asleep.

So he had gone and done the one thing he had sworn he wouldn't do.

He had told Jorey his secret.

Sawyer stared darkly at the cold, empty hearth of the fireplace in front of the couch, seeing not the smoke-darkened brick, but Jorey's face before his eyes.

Why did you tell her, dammit?

After months of solitary silence, what had made him

open up to a woman he had sworn he would put out of his life?

What had made him pull her close when he knew he should be pushing her away?

At least you didn't tell her all of it, the whole story, he reminded himself. *At least she doesn't know everything.*

But it had been tempting, so tempting, to simply lift the floodgate and pour it all out to her. He didn't trust himself not to do just that the next time they were together.

That's why there can be no next time, he realized. *You told her to leave town and go back to New York. If she's smart, she'll take your advice.*

If she doesn't . . .

He swallowed hard and stared bleakly off into space.

Jorey awakened to sun streaming in the windows and a loud knock at her door.

For a moment, she couldn't move, wondering where she was and why she was so uncomfortable.

Then it all came rushing back at her.

Last night.

Clover's wake.

Sawyer.

Uncle Roland.

"Jorey?" Gretchen's voice came through the door. "Are you in there?"

"I'm here." Her voice came out as a croak, and she cleared her throat, straightening her stiff legs and stretching her aching back. She had apparently slept all night sitting up against the headboard, wearing the uncomfortable dress and even her high-heeled leather boots.

"Jorey?" Gretchen rattled the knob, sounding impatient. "Are you there?"

"I said *yes.*" It came out loud and clear this time, and a touch cranky.

Well, who could blame her? She felt mentally and physically exhausted, as though she hadn't slept a wink.

She got off the bed and went to the door, trying to be quiet about disassembling the elaborate booby trap she'd arranged there with the chair and luggage.

"Jorey? What are you doing? Are you all right?" Gretchen asked as she inadvertently thumped a suitcase against the wall.

"I'm *fine.*" Jorey shoved the chair aside and opened the door, belatedly running a hand through her tangled mass of curls.

"My God, what happened to you?"

"What do you mean?" Jorey glanced over her shoulder and caught a glance of herself in the mirror across the room.

She looked as horrible as she felt; dazed and rumpled and stale and drawn.

"Where were you last night?" Gretchen asked, and Jorey noticed that her eyes were devoid of their usual warmth. She looked clean and well-scrubbed and pulled together, making Jorey even more aware of her own unkempt, unwashed state.

"I was here. Where were you?"

"You came straight home from the funeral parlor?" Gretchen tossed her head, her perfect blond braid swinging over one shoulder. "How did you get here?"

"I . . ." She closed her mouth and looked at Gretchen, suddenly resenting the pointed questions.

"He drove you, didn't he?"

"Who?"

"Sawyer Howland. Karl said he saw you with him when he got to the funeral home just before the service started. He said the two of you were obviously involved in some kind of deep conversation, and that you made him feel out of place."

Fury tore through Jorey, as well as a sudden, intense dislike for Karl, but she forced herself to keep her mouth shut. She turned away from Gretchen and walked over to the dresser, picking up a hairbrush and beginning to yank it through her snarled mass of hair.

"You left with him, Jorey, didn't you? You didn't even bother to stay for the service for Clover. I just can't—what kind of friend are you?"

Jorey whirled around. "What kind of friend are *you*, judging me this way? And judging Sawyer, when you don't even know him. You and everyone else in this town—Karl, and Kitty, and Johnny, and even Clover. All of you think you can go around accusing him of murder when you have no idea who he is or why he's here. If you only knew—"

She cut herself short, realizing she had been about to spill Sawyer's secret. Angry as she was at him, she couldn't bring herself to betray his trust that way. So she closed her mouth and turned away from Gretchen, though she saw her friend's face reflected in the mirror, behind her. Gretchen looked startled, then curious.

"Then tell me. Who is he, Jorey?" she asked quietly. "Why is he here?"

"That's none of your business. Just as it's none of your business whether I'm involved with him, or anyone else. If you want my advice, you should spend more time worrying about your own relationship."

She saw Gretchen's mouth drop open. "What's that supposed to mean?"

"I just mean that it's obvious that you and Karl aren't exactly sailing blithely along in paradise, Gretchen. Anyone can see that you're falling all over the man—although God knows why—and he barely gives you the time of day."

As soon as the words were out of her mouth Jorey wished she could take them back. She didn't dare look at Gretchen's face, knowing exactly what she would see there.

She closed her eyes briefly and winced when she saw her friend's expression anyway, reflected in her memory of the vulnerable child and painfully insecure teenage girl Gretchen had once been.

She remembered how susceptible Gretchen had always been to the teasing of the others; how quickly she looked wounded when somebody made a teasing yet stinging joke, or criticized her her old-fashioned parents, or her ramshackle home.

But it was the others who did most of the teasing—*especially Adrienne,* Jorey reminded herself.

Meanwhile, *she* had been the one to stand up for Gretchen, to change the subject or speak up on her behalf.

So what had gotten into her now?

Poor Gretchen. She's your friend. How could you say something so cruel to her?

Jorey opened her eyes and turned to look at Gretchen. She saw that her head was bent, and she was staring at her sneakers, intently dragging one toe along the edge of a floorboard.

"I'm sorry, Gretchen," Jorey said quietly. "I didn't mean to pry into your relationship with Karl."

Gretchen looked up. She shrugged, but Jorey could see something hard and angry in her expression as she said, "It's okay, Jorey. You just don't know Karl the way I do."

"And you just don't know Sawyer," Jorey heard herself responding.

Mentally, she added, *Maybe I don't, either.*

She took a deep breath, then said, "I'm going to leave town today, Gretchen. I think it's time for me to go back home to New York."

"You don't have to do that, Jorey," Gretchen protested, and she looked and sounded genuinely dismayed. "It's been so good having you here. Look, I'm sorry for the things I said. You were right. It was unfair of me to judge you and Sawyer. I didn't mean anything by it. I was just worried about you, especially after what happened to Clover."

"I know." Jorey set her hairbrush down and turned away from the mirror. "But I really have to get back to my life. I can't hide away up here forever. It's time for me to make some decisions and figure out where I'm headed. I don't even have a career, remember?" she said with a brittle laugh.

"Maybe it's easier for you to see things clearly while you're up here in Blizzard Bay, though," Gretchen pointed out. "The more time you spend away from home, the better perspective you might have."

"That's what I thought at one point," Jorey said. "But now I'm realizing that being up here is just an escape."

And being too close to Sawyer will only remind me of things I'll never have.

Gretchen was silent for a moment, then said quietly, "If you really feel like you have to go, Jorey, then you should go. But I want you to know that you'll always be welcome here, if you want to come back to visit."

Jorey smiled at her. "Thank you. You've been a good friend, Gretchen. Maybe . . . the only true friend I've ever had."

Gretchen looked pleased, though she frowned slightly and asked, "What about the others? Kitty, and Adrienne, and . . ."

Clover.

"It's not that I—I don't know. I guess that being here has made me realize that they're a part of another lifetime," Jorey told her. "Things were so different back then. We were just kids. So carefree . . . until that last summer I spent here. I wish I could remember—"

"What?"

Jorey shook her head. "I don't know," she repeated. "I just know that last summer here was a turning point for me. I realize that my parents' divorce and my grandfather's death triggered it, but everything that happened in between is a blur. I can't help feeling as if there are other things I'm not remembering, and I should be."

"That's why you don't remember Hob Nixon being your secret admirer?" Gretchen asked. "Or that Johnny was head over heels for you? You think you have some kind of . . . amnesia?"

"I don't know."

"Well, maybe you should stay around a while longer. I can help refresh your memory. Maybe then everything will come back to you."

"Maybe if I stayed it would. But maybe it wouldn't. How long can I put my life on hold? Anyway, what's the point? What will filling in the blanks do for me? No," she said conclusively, shaking her head. "I have to go. And I should go today. The sun is shining and the snow is melting, so there's no chance of my being caught in a blizzard the way I was the last time."

"You never know around here," Gretchen said. "Storms sometimes come up out of nowhere."

Jorey pondered her words, finding them oddly ominous. But she forced away a sudden sense of uneasiness and said, "Well, I'd better start packing."

Gretchen nodded. "I'll go make breakfast for us. You can at least eat some pancakes before you get on the road."

Jorey smiled. She was going to miss Gretchen's quiet friendship. "Thank you. You know, you're going to have to visit me in New York sometime so that I can return the hospitality. I can't promise pancakes, but do you like blueberry muffins?"

"Sure. I'll take you up on it sometime," Gretchen said before leaving the room.

Jorey picked up her hairbrush again and lost herself in the memory of that long-ago morning in the cozy kitchen with Papa May, eating blueberry muffins hot out of the oven, talking about fishing at the pond.

The pond.

What about the pond?

Jorey closed her eyes and tried again to grab the evasive memory that darted in and out of her mind. She couldn't retrieve it, could remember nothing but . . .

A scream.

A shrill, high-pitched scream echoed through her mind, echoed over the years that had passed since that summer. . . .

She saw, in her mind's eye, the still, murky pond and the dense evergreens that circled the clearing. And the terrible scream erupted into another, and then another . . . relentless, chilling, pitiful screams that filled her mind so that she had to clap her hands over her ears to shut them out.

Then there was silence, and she was back in the quiet bedroom, alone and shaken.

Her subconscious mind was trying to tell her something, dammit, she just couldn't grasp it.

What on earth had happened that summer?

Why couldn't she recall it?

What did it have to do with the pond in the woods?

There's been another one.

Sawyer sat straight up in bed and blinked, having gone from being sound asleep to wide awake in the space of seconds.

There's been another murder.

The knowledge chilled him to the core, spurred him to get out of bed and stride across the room. He came to a stop in front of the bookcase, and his gaze fell on the stuffed dog sitting on the top shelf. The dog he had found tucked into the secret cupboard beside the fireplace.

He stared at it for a moment, then picked it up. As his fingers closed over the worn, stiff fur he shivered, then lifted it to his cheek.

This was Jorey's, he told himself, resting his head against the old stuffed toy. He was certain of it, as certain as he was that there had been another murder; that somewhere in Blizzard Bay, a body lay lifeless and cold, perhaps yet undiscovered.

"Jorey," he said aloud, stroking the little dog and shaking his head.

Was she safe?

He told himself that she was, yet he couldn't know

for certain. Maybe he only wanted her to be safe; maybe he couldn't face the knowledge that something might have happened to her as he slept.

There was only one way to find out.

He carefully set the stuffed animal back on the bookshelf and strode grimly across the room to get dressed.

At the bed & breakfast Jorey pushed back her plate, which was empty except for a few stray crumbs embedded in a sticky drizzle of maple syrup.

"That was delicious," she told Gretchen. "Thanks for going to so much trouble."

"It's no problem."

"I forgot to ask," Jorey said suddenly, remembering something, "did you go to Adrienne's last night after the funeral home?"

As soon as the question was out, she wished she hadn't brought it up.

While they were eating, they had chatted about the weather and old times and the remodeling projects Gretchen had planned, both of them consciously, carefully, avoiding the subject of the night before.

The last thing Jorey wanted to do was stir up any more hard feelings, or launch another discussion about Gretchen's relationship with Karl or her own involvement with Sawyer.

"I did go, yes," Gretchen answered. "But only for a little while."

"Who was there?"

"Just Adrienne, and Kitty and Johnny, and Karl. Nobody stayed long. Kitty was having some cramps that she thought might be the beginning of labor, so she and Johnny wanted to get back home. We left right after they did."

"I should probably call Kitty and see how she is," Jorey said. "And tell her that I'm leaving."

"You can use the phone if you want to," Gretchen told her. "I've actually been wondering about her myself. Maybe by now she's had the baby."

"We'll find out," Jorey said, and went to the telephone on the wall. She dialed the number, then waited as the phone rang several times.

"There's no answer," she told Gretchen finally, hanging up. "Maybe I should ride by on my way out of town."

"That's a good idea. But if you don't get a hold of her, I'll be sure to tell her that you went back to New York. And I'll let you know when she has the baby."

"Thanks." Jorey hesitated, standing there in the kitchen, knowing that there was one more thing she should tell Gretchen before she left.

But she was reluctant to bring up the subject of her Uncle Roland. The last thing she wanted was to offend Gretchen by implying that the old man had been up to something when he'd approached her last night.

She had been pretty sure, when she had fallen asleep, that he had simply been trying to communicate with her. Now, though, she found herself wondering all over again.

"Do you want some help washing the dishes?" she asked, as Gretchen busied herself clearing the table.

"No, it's fine. I can get them, and then I'm going to run over to the dry cleaner with some things I need sent out today. I have to get them in before ten, or they won't be back until next week. You should go get packed if you're going to stop by Kitty's on your way. You don't want to get too late a start. It's a long trip, and it gets dark early these days."

Jorey left the kitchen and made her way upstairs without saying anything about Uncle Roland. But as she began transferring her folded clothing from the bureau drawer to the open suitcase on the bed, she found herself brooding about it.

If he'd meant her no harm, then what had the old man been trying to say?

She had no way of knowing.

Or did she?

Jorey paused over her packing, an idea slowly forming in her mind.

Then, abruptly, she left the room and made her way down the hall. She could faintly hear running water and dishes clattering in the kitchen downstairs. The sound was reassuring, boosting her courage to mount the steps at the end of the hall. If anything happened, she could just yell for help and Gretchen would come running.

As she slowly made her way up to the third floor, she realized that she hadn't been up there in years. It looked the same as it always had—a smaller, more compact version of the second floor corridor, with the yellowing, original floral wallpaper, lower ceilings, and fewer closed doors.

Which one belonged to Uncle Roland?

She made her way slowly along, searching for some clue.

Then, from behind the last door, she heard the sound of bedsprings squeaking slightly.

He's probably asleep, she realized, hesitating in the hallway outside the door. *I shouldn't disturb him.*

But if she didn't, she would have to leave without ever knowing why he had approached her last night.

What if he knew something about Clover's murder? Something he had tried, and somehow failed, to tell Gretchen and the police?

Jorey reached out, intending to knock on the door. Then she remembered that he wouldn't hear her.

Feeling slightly guilty for just barging into the old man's room but aware that she had no other choice, she turned the doorknob and pushed the door open just an inch.

It creaked, and she leaned forward to peer inside the shadowy room, expecting to see the old man curled up in bed, soundly asleep.

That wasn't what she saw.

There was Uncle Roland, clearly awake, his back to her as he sat on the bed in the middle of the small room.

There was no indication that he was aware of her presence; he didn't flinch or move as he sat there, his head bent over something in his lap.

Jorey wasn't sure what to do.

As she paused in the doorway the old man shifted his weight slightly, and the sun shining in the window glinted off something metallic in his hand.

Jorey gasped as she realized what it was.

She clapped a hand over her mouth in horror as she swiftly closed the door.

She backed away slowly, trembling, then raced down the stairs to her room.

Uncle Roland had been holding a long-handled kitchen knife.

Chapter Thirteen

Sawyer pulled up in front of The 1890 House and sat staring at it for a moment before turning off the motor and opening the car door. He was about to get out when he heard an engine roaring to life someplace nearby.

A moment later, he saw a familiar red Range Rover come tearing out of the driveway that ran alongside the house. As it turned sharply into the street, he glimpsed Jorey at the wheel.

He jumped out of the car and waved her down, but either she didn't see him or she didn't care. The Range Rover kept going, roaring down the street and tearing around the corner with a squeal of tires.

Sawyer slammed his door closed and turned the key in the ignition.

The engine stalled.

"Damn!" he cursed, and turned the key again. "Come on, come on."

It started this time, and he shifted into gear and drove off after Jorey.

Where was she going in such a hurry? Why was she so distracted?

That's obvious, he realized. *She must have already heard the news.*

He himself had only found out moments earlier, when a news bulletin came over the local AM radio station as he was driving into town.

"We interrupt regular programming to bring you this special report," the announcer said after cutting into Mariah Carey's latest single. "A third brutal murder has been discovered early this morning in Blizzard Bay . . ."

He spotted the Range Rover up ahead, stopped at the intersection with Main Street. He caught up with her just as the light changed and Jorey shot through, heading out of town.

Sawyer stayed on her tail, noticing that she was driving a good twenty miles an hour above the speed limit. She never glanced in her rearview mirror, as far as he could tell, and he decided she didn't know she was being followed.

He waited until they were past the city limits and heading out onto the two-lane highway that led to the Northway before he sped up and drove closer to her tail, then laid on his horn.

He saw her turn her head and look into the mirror. For a moment, she didn't react—didn't slow down, but didn't speed up, either.

He honked again and waved at her, gesturing for her to pull over.

Again, no reaction. He had just concluded that she was going to try to outrun him when she suddenly flicked on her right turn signal and hit her brakes.

She slowed the Range Rover and pulled onto the slushy shoulder of the deserted road.

He pulled up right behind her, opening his door and jumping out the moment he came to a stop. He found himself racing along through the melting snow at the roadside to her window, praying she wouldn't suddenly take off on him.

She didn't.

Nor did she open her door and get out.

When he reached the driver's side of the Range Rover, he saw that she had lowered her window halfway and was watching him warily.

"What do you want?" she demanded as soon as he was within earshot.

"I wanted to make sure you were all right."

"Why?"

He heard the chill in her voice, saw the suspicion in her eyes, and he wondered if he'd made a mistake. Maybe he should have just left it alone, let her go off to wherever it was that she was going.

But it was too late for that. He was here, and she was waiting, and he had to reply.

"I've been worried about you ever since I dropped you off last night, Jorey," he told her in a low voice.

"Well, don't worry," she replied tartly. "You'll be thrilled to know that I'm leaving town, just like you suggested."

Her tone was sarcastic, almost flippant, but he saw that her eyes were haunted and her hands were clenched and white on the steering wheel.

"You heard," he said, fighting the urge to reach out and touch her. "Are you all right?"

"Heard what?"

Her expression was truly puzzled.

If she didn't know then why was she hell-bent on getting out of there? She'd been driving as if the devil himself were chasing her.

"Heard *what*, Sawyer?" she repeated.

"About the murder. It happened sometime last night or early this morning."

"What? Who—"

"I'm sorry, Jorey," Sawyer said, and this time he did reach out and lay a hand on the sleeve of her black leather coat. "I know you were friends—"

"Who?" she demanded hoarsely. "Who's dead?"

"Adrienne Von Deegan."

Jorey stared at Sawyer in disbelief.

Adrienne?

Dead?

It couldn't be.

"I saw her just last night," she protested, her mind reeling. "At the funeral home."

"I know. It happened afterward, apparently. A maid found her body this morning, at her home. She had been stabbed to death."

"Stabbed?" Jorey squeezed her eyes tightly shut, seeing the image of Gretchen's Uncle Roland sitting alone in his room, holding that knife. "Stabbed with what?"

"I don't know. I heard about it on the radio. They didn't say. The news was just released. I thought you knew—I figured that was why you were obviously trying to get the hell out of here."

"No," Jorey said, trying to pull her thoughts together. "I didn't know. Christ. Adrienne. I can't believe it. Clover, and Adrienne. And . . ."

She opened her eyes and looked at him. "And your sister," she concluded softly.

Sawyer nodded, stark pain vivid on his handsome features. "I told you, Jorey. There's some kind of maniac on the loose in this town. I told you . . . it could have been you."

"I know." The words barely came out. She clamped her mouth shut and realized she was shivering all over.

"Why were you leaving?" Sawyer asked. "If you didn't know about Adrienne, what happened to make you tear out of here that way?"

"I didn't tear out of here," she lied, wondering how long he had been behind her.

"Yes, you did. I saw how fast you pulled out of the driveway. You didn't even look before you turned onto the road. You're running from something, Jorey."

"Did you ever think maybe I'm running from you?" she asked, looking him in the eye. "Maybe I can't wait to get away from you, Sawyer."

He shrugged, watching her, not believing her, she realized. Then she found herself telling him the truth.

"It was Gretchen's uncle," she blurted impulsively. "Her uncle Roland. I saw him a little while ago, in his room . . . and he was holding a knife."

"A knife?" Sawyer echoed. "Are you sure?"

"I'm positive." She told him the whole story, then. About how Uncle Roland had been at Clover's house the night of her murder, and how the police had tried without success to question him. And about the way he'd confronted her in the hallway outside her room last night, making strange sounds and gesturing frantically.

"I don't know what his intentions were," she told Sawyer. "I don't know if he was trying to harm me, or just trying to tell me something. But when I saw him with that knife—"

"You haven't told anyone about it?"

She shook her head. "It happened right before I left. Gretchen was out. I guess I just . . . panicked. I grabbed my things and I left the house."

"Weren't you planning to let the police know what you saw?"

She contemplated that. "Actually, I didn't think that far ahead. I just wanted to get out of there, Sawyer. Out of that house, and out of that town."

"Jorey, you may have witnessed something that could help solve these murders. You have an obligation to—"

"I *know*, Sawyer," she cut in harshly. "Don't you think I don't know that? But I told you, I panicked. I just wanted to get away. I wasn't thinking straight. I'm just so . . . *exhausted*."

She inhaled deeply, then let out a shuddering breath. She was suddenly weary of everything—everything about Blizzard Bay. Including Sawyer Howland.

She realized that if he hadn't stopped her she might very well have left town and never looked back. Once she got home to New York she might have put the entire incident behind her, and revealed to no one that she had seen Uncle Roland with a knife.

Because, after all, what did that prove?

Oh, come on, Jorey, an inner voice piped up. *The man was holding a knife. A kitchen knife. In his bedroom.*

But it wasn't as if she'd seen him use it. It wasn't as if he'd threatened her with it.

Still, Clover . . .

And now Adrienne.

She pictured her friend, always impeccably dressed

and made-up, never a hair out of place. It was impossible to imagine Adrienne lying there, waxy and cold, covered in blood.

Oh, Christ.

She looked up at Sawyer's face, expecting to see him watching her with a harsh expression. But in the depths of his blue eyes, she glimpsed a flicker of something unexpected.

"Jorey," he said softly. "You've been through so much. I haven't helped matters, have I?"

"Don't worry about it, Sawyer. I'm fine. Just let me get out of here, and I'll sort things out. I'll call the police and I'll tell them about Uncle Roland. Or I'll call Gretchen, and I'll tell her first. I just can't do it now. I just have to get out of here now. I need some time . . ." She let out a shaky breath and was horrified to find that tears had sprung to her eyes.

Don't cry, Jorey. You can't cry.

But she couldn't help it. She couldn't seem to stop the tears from spilling over. She was drained, an emotional wreck.

"You're in no condition to drive," Sawyer said, eyeing her with concern as she sniffled and wiped at her eyes with the back of her hand.

"I have to. I have to get out of here. I can't go back there, Sawyer."

"You don't have to. Come on. Come home with me for a little while. You can pull yourself together, and we can talk about this thing with Gretchen's uncle."

"I don't want to talk about it right now," she said, shaking her head. "I can't deal with all of this. Adrienne is dead. My God. Two of my friends. What's going on in this town?"

"Jorey, come home with me," Sawyer repeated, reaching up and opening her door. "I'll drive you in your car. We can leave mine here. It'll be fine for a little while."

She looked at him, fully intending to protest.

But for some reason, she didn't. For some reason, she got out of the car and went around to the passenger's side, and she allowed him to drive her back to his house.

The house she had once thought of as *her* own.

As they pulled into the driveway she turned her head and she looked out over the field, toward the woods that concealed the pond where she used to fish with her grandfather. The pond where he had died. The pond her grandmother used to warn her about . . .

Suddenly, she heard a scream.

It echoed shrilly through her head, and for a moment she thought she had actually heard it.

Startled, she turned toward Sawyer and saw that he didn't appear to have noticed anything.

It had been her imagination, she realized. Just her imagination.

Again.

Narrowing her eyes, she turned back to the woods.

Had something happened there that long ago summer? Something besides her grandfather's sudden, tragic death? Something that her subconscious mind had swallowed up for all these years?

"Are you all right, Jorey?" Sawyer asked, pulling the Range Rover up beside the porch steps and turning off the ignition.

"Can we just go inside?" she asked, uneasily shifting her gaze away from the distant thicket of evergreens.

* * *

"There's something I want to show you," Sawyer told Jorey as he held open the door to his apartment.

"What is it?"

"Just something I found."

She stepped into the room ahead of him, her hands stuffed into the front pockets of her faded jeans. He tried not to notice how the threadbare denim clung to the curves of her hips and thighs. The straight-legged jeans bagged around her ankles, above her scuffed white sneakers, and when she took off her leather coat, he saw that she wore an oversized red sweatshirt.

He had never seen her dressed this casually, and she wasn't wearing heels. She was more petite in stature than he remembered. For some reason he found her even more appealing this way.

Her face was bare of makeup, making her look even younger and more vulnerable than usual, and her curls were pulled carelessly back by a red headband. He found himself longing to reach out and tuck in a stray ringlet that kept brushing against her cheek.

"What did you want to show me?" she asked, her jacket dangling over one arm as she stood in the middle of the room, looking around.

Sawyer crossed to the bookcase and picked up the stuffed dog he'd found stashed in the secret nook by the fireplace.

As he held it up for Jorey to see, she gasped.

"Oh, my God. It's been years since I . . . where *was* that?" she asked, coming to him and reaching out for the ragged toy.

"In that cupboard," he said, pointing. "There's a shelf up against the brick, and—"

"I know," she cut in. "That was my secret hiding place. I used to keep my diary there, when I kept one."

He watched as she brought the dog's fur up to her cheek and stroked its head lovingly. "This is Rudy," she informed Sawyer. "Papa May gave him to me when I was really little. I couldn't figure out whatever happened to him. I guess I forgot him here after my grandfather died . . . things were so confusing at the time, with the funeral, and my grandmother selling the house . . ."

Sawyer nodded, thinking that she was almost child-like, conveying a sweet innocence as she stood there cuddling her stuffed animal. She made him want to take her into his arms and just hold her the way she was holding Rudy—protectively, lovingly.

"How did you know this was mine?" Jorey asked.

He hesitated, wanting to tell her the truth. About everything. Instead, he just shrugged and said, "Lucky guess."

"Well, I'm glad you found Rudy," she told him. "I'll bring him back to New York with me and keep him. Maybe someday I can give him to my—"

When she cut herself off abruptly he asked curiously, "To your what?"

She shook her head. "Nothing. I was just going to say that maybe someday I'll have a child to give him to. That's all."

"Oh . . . I'm sure you will," he told her.

He found himself envisioning Jorey with a child . . . a beautiful child who looked just like her, with flashing green eyes and a dark head of curls.

And it struck him then that he wanted it to be *his*

child. He wanted that, suddenly, more than he had ever wanted anything in his life.

The realization filled him with a yearning so strong that he had to fight to keep his expression passive, to keep his distance from Jorey, who stood so tantalizingly close to him that if he just reached out he would be able to touch her soft skin. . . .

She sighed, and lowered the stuffed dog away from her cheek, and looked at Sawyer.

He met her gaze and searched for something to say.

"I should call Gretchen," she told him after a moment. "I should tell her about Adrienne. And about her uncle. It's her responsibility to go to the police, don't you think?"

"You were the one who saw him with the knife, Jorey," Sawyer told her. "Not Gretchen."

"But there might be a perfectly rational explanation for it," Jorey pointed out. "Maybe he was using it to— I don't know. To cut a piece of fruit."

"Did you see a piece of fruit?"

She shook her head. "But that doesn't mean—"

"No," he agreed. "It doesn't."

He thought about Roland Eckhard. He had seen the old man once or twice around town, and had always felt sorry for him. He'd seen the way the local kids made fun of him, imitating his gestures and his grunts and groans.

Could Roland Eckhard be a murderer?

Had he—oh, Lord, had he killed Rebecca?

Somehow, Sawyer didn't want to believe it. Just because the man was different, just because Jorey had seen him with a knife, didn't mean that he was the one behind Rebecca's murder, or anyone else's.

But what other leads were there?

Sawyer had come up against one dead end after another, and so, apparently, had the police. There had been no suspects named in Clover's murder, and the radio announcer who had announced Adrienne's death had said that the police had no suspects there, either.

Maybe you should just give up, Sawyer told himself. *Maybe you should get out of this godforsaken town and go back to the real world, get on with your life.*

If he did that, he wouldn't necessarily have to give up Jorey. He might be able to—

No. You swore you would never get involved again. Not with anyone. Not after . . .

Susan.

Susan Boggier.

She had been beautiful, too, as beautiful as Jorey was, but in a different way. Susan had been tall and slender, with honey-colored hair and brown eyes.

Like Jorey, she had been born into affluence, the youngest daughter of one of Sawyer's Grosse Pointe neighbors. She was several years younger than Sawyer; a child, really, when he met her.

Unlike Jorey, who wore her wealth as casually as she did her fringed leather jacket, Susan had the regal bearing and sophistication that came with her station in life. But she was different from the other women in her social circle; she wasn't pretentious and she didn't put on airs.

He had fallen in love with her shortly after her twenty-first birthday; had proposed to her on her twenty-second, while they were watching the sunset from his yacht just off Mackinac Island. She had accepted, and they had celebrated with a candlelit dinner at the Grand Hotel and a chilled bottle of vintage Dom Perignon.

Her family had thrown a lavish engagement party; his

parents had bought them a sprawling home on the shore. Susan graduated from Northwestern and decided to put off the teaching career she had planned. They wanted a big family, and they wanted to start it right after the wedding.

Everything was perfect, Sawyer remembered bitterly. Until the day he had glanced at Susan and seen a shadow hanging over her.

She's going to die, he had realized, stunned. *If you marry her, she'll die.*

He had tried to tell himself that he was being ridiculous, that it was just his imagination.

But in his heart, he knew that it wasn't.

Ever since he had been a little boy, Sawyer had known things. He had known that Seattle Slew was going to win the Kentucky Derby in 1977 and that Michigan would lose the Rose Bowl three years in a row. He had known that a freak blizzard would close school for a week one April, and the moment she announced that she was pregnant with Rebecca he had known that his mother would have a girl.

The family got a kick out of his predictions, and he never saw anything dire. Things had just come to him spontaneously, and he blurted them out. His mother said he had inherited his special talent from her grandfather, who had always had a way of knowing things he couldn't possibly know.

As he grew older and more wrapped up in school in Ann Arbor, and then the family business, Sawyer's visions became few and far between. He was still occasionally struck by an image or thought that came out of nowhere, but he learned, as an adult, to keep them to himself—sometimes, even to ignore them. After all, the visions were never particularly relevant.

Until the one about Susan.

If you marry Susan, she will die.

He couldn't shake the thought, or keep from seeing shadows across her face whenever he looked at her, no matter how he tried in the months before the wedding.

But what was he supposed to do about it? Not marry her? Give up his soul mate, the woman he planned to spend the rest of his life with? For what?

He loved her desperately, and he wasn't prepared to give her up.

Still, as the wedding date drew near the shadows grew more ominous, and he was aware that time was running out. He grew more and more troubled until finally, Susan demanded to know what was wrong.

He told her.

Rather, he tried. In a roundabout way. He told her that he was worried about marrying her, worried that if he did something would go wrong.

At first, she had laughed it off, telling him he had cold feet, and that every groom felt that way.

But he had vehemently denied that was the case.

She had gotten upset right away then, thinking he was having doubts about loving her, that he was trying to back out of the engagement.

"It's not that," he had protested. "I love you more than anything, Susan. I want to marry you. I do."

"Then what is it?"

So he had blurted it out to her, right then and there. He had told her he'd seen a vision; that if they went through with the wedding, she would die.

At first she had stared at him. She had never heard about his special "gift," and the more he tried to explain it to her, the more incredulous she looked. Finally, she told him that if he didn't want to get married, he should just tell her. That he didn't have to go and make up some ridiculous story about having ESP. That she deserved the truth.

"But the truth is that I want to marry you, Susan," he had said again, realizing it was hopeless. She couldn't possibly understand, and he couldn't blame her.

And so, he had married her. As he stood waiting at the front of the chapel watching her walk down the aisle looking like an angel in white silk, he had seen the unmistakable shadow cast over her face. In the moments before she reached him, he had frantically realized that he couldn't marry her, no matter what she would think of him; that if he did, her fate would be sealed,

Then her father was placing her hand in his, and she was gazing at him with so much love and devotion that he could do nothing but swallow hard and say, "I do."

He told himself, after the ceremony, that the vision was merely a subconscious manifestation of the cold feet suffered by every groom, just as Susan had said. He did his best to believe that, even though he had never doubted for a moment that he was ready for marriage, or that Susan was the right woman.

Less than a week after their wedding, when they were crossing a Paris street while on their European honeymoon, a taxi went out of control and careened toward them.

In the split second before it struck Susan, Sawyer had realized that this was it. His prediction was coming true.

A moment later, his beautiful young bride lay crumpled on the cold, hard sidewalk, her skull shattered beneath her golden hair, her blood warm and wet on his hands.

And it was his fault.

If he hadn't married her, she wouldn't have been in Paris. She wouldn't have died.

He had returned to Michigan and sold the Grosse Point mansion that was to be their happy home, where a carefully decorated nursery waited for the babies who would never be born.

He had thrown himself into his work after that, and when his father retired a few years later he became CEO of the family's automotive company. The business consumed him; he shut out everything else.

Including the disturbing vision that came to him the night before his sister left for Blizzard Bay.

He had struggled to ignore the shadows that surrounded Rebecca's image in his mind; the same shadows that had shrouded Susan before he married her. He refused to listen to the voice that nagged at the edge of his consciousness.

He was still numb from Susan's death.

And now your sister is dead because you didn't react to the warnings, he reminded himself, as he did every day of his life.

So. It was his duty to stay here until he found out what had happened to Rebecca. If he never found out, he would never go back to his privileged existence, to the financial empire he had honed or the business he loved. He would spend the rest of his life in this remote mountain town, where he would always be an outsider; where he would be forced to face, every day, the haunting memory of his sister's death.

That would be his penance.

Chapter Fourteen

Jorey realized that Sawyer wasn't even aware she was watching him as he stood motionless, obviously lost in thought. His eyes had a faraway expression, and he was clearly troubled, yet she couldn't bring herself to ask him what was wrong. She was too afraid that she would want to comfort him, and that if she did reach out, it would lead to something she wasn't prepared to face.

They couldn't make love again, not even one last time. She was leaving; in fact, she *should* leave. What was she doing here?

Adrienne.

I have to call Gretchen. I have to tell her about Adrienne, and about her uncle. Then she can go to the police, and I'll be free to go.

"Do you have a phone?" she asked Sawyer, shattering the silence.

He looked up, startled, and it took a moment for him to answer. "Over there," he said slowly, pointing to a low table by the fireplace. "Are you going to call the police?"

"I'll call Gretchen. I need to talk to her, and she can take it from there."

He shrugged.

She went over to the phone, picked up the receiver, and dialed. It rang only once before being snatched up by Gretchen, who uttered a breathless, "Hello, 1890 House—"

"It's Jorey."

"Jorey! Where are you?"

"I'm . . . it's a long story," she said, glancing at Sawyer, who had moved to the window and was staring out, his back to her. "I just wanted to . . . have you heard the news?"

"About Adrienne? I found out while I was in town. The radio was on at the dry cleaner's, and they had a special bulletin. Jorey . . . I can't believe it. I was just with her last night, and—" Gretchen broke off.

"I know," Jorey said. "It's horrible. Are you all right?"

"I'm just stunned, I guess. Adrienne and I were never the closest of friends—we didn't have a lot in common—but I never wanted to see anything happen to her, Jorey. I was just with her last night." Gretchen's voice wavered. "I can't believe this is happening. First Clover, and now—"

"Do they think the same person did it?"

"Who knows? I've had the radio on since I got home, but they haven't given any new information. All they said was that she was found in her home by the maid this morning, stabbed to death."

Jorey winced, wanting to shut out the terrible image the words brought to mind.

"Are you coming back, Jorey?" Gretchen asked.

She hesitated before answering with a resolute, "No. I'm not coming back. I'm heading home, Gretchen."

"But, Jorey—"

"I can't. I have to go, as soon as I get off the phone." She glanced at Sawyer and saw that he had turned his head, as though he was listening.

"Even after what's happened with Adrienne?"

"I have to go," Jorey repeated firmly. "But first, I needed to tell you something. It's about . . . your uncle."

"Uncle Roland? What is it?"

Jorey paused, not knowing how to bring it up. Finally, she took a deep breath and said, "I saw him this morning in his room with—"

"In his room?" Gretchen interrupted. "What were you doing in his room?"

"He came up to me last night in the hallway and tried to tell me something . . . I think. He was gesturing, and making sounds."

She waited for Gretchen to say something, but there was silence.

"Anyway, I got scared and went into my room. I didn't know what he wanted, what he was doing. Then, this morning, I realized that maybe that was wrong of me. I thought that I should give him a chance to tell me whatever it was that he wanted to say. So I went up to the third floor, and I saw him. He had a knife, Gretchen. A kitchen knife. He was holding it. He didn't know I was there . . ."

Again, she paused for a response, but there was none.

"So I left," Jorey concluded hesitantly. "I ran downstairs, and I grabbed my bags, and I left. I was in a panic, I guess."

Silence on the other end of the line.

Jorey went on, "Now I realize that it might not mean anything, but all I could think about at the time was Clover. He was at her house that night, and she was stabbed with a kitchen knife, and ... Gretchen, you need to find out what's going on."

She heard Gretchen draw a deep breath before saying, "Jorey, you don't think that my uncle—"

"I don't know. I don't know. All I know is that I saw him with a knife."

"What am I supposed to do? Go up there and confront him? Alone? What if you're right? What if he's the murderer?"

"Don't do anything stupid, Gretchen. I think that you should tell the police."

"But Uncle Roland can't defend himself. If he's innocent. Jorey, you know that. He can't communicate."

"I know. Gretchen, you need to tell the police."

She waited for Gretchen to tell her that *she* wasn't the one who had seen him with the knife. That it was her duty to go to the police.

But Gretchen said quietly, "I know. You're right. You're right. I need to tell the police. My God, two of my friends are dead. If Uncle Roland is responsible—" Her voice cracked, and Jorey knew that she was crying.

Guilt darted through her, and for a moment she considered going back to the bed & breakfast to be with Gretchen.

But then she looked at Sawyer, and she knew that she had to leave town. Staying would only prolong her good-bye to him. She had tried to get out of Blizzard Bay without having to confront him again, but that hadn't worked. Now she had no choice but to tell him good-bye, and go before it was too late.

Too late for what? she found herself asking, but she had no answer.

"I can't believe that all of this is really happening," Gretchen said, jarring her back to reality.

"Maybe your uncle is innocent, Gretchen," she pointed out, trying to sound comforting.

"Maybe he is. But if he isn't . . ."

"Are you going to be all right?"

"I'll be fine," Gretchen said. "I'll go to Karl. He'll help me with this. He'll go to the police with me, and he'll stay with me."

Again, Jorey felt a pang of guilt. She shouldn't be abandoning her friend at a time like this. There was no guarantee that Karl would be there for Gretchen.

But surely, even if he weren't as serious about their relationship as she was, he wouldn't turn his back on her now. He would simply have to help her through this, as a friend if nothing else.

And what about you? What kind of friend are you?

Jorey pushed the thought away. She *had* to leave Blizzard Bay. And it had to be now.

Besides, Gretchen would be all right. She was stronger than Jorey had ever believed. She had survived the deaths of her parents, and she had built a business of her own.

Which was more than Jorey had ever done.

It's time for you to get your life together, Jorey told herself. *Time to go back to New York and figure out what your purpose is. You need a career. Something that will help you to forget about Sawyer and your crazy dreams of marrying him and having his babies.*

She must have been completely out of her mind to have ever imagined that a man like Sawyer Howland could ever settle down and be a husband and father.

"Listen, Jorey," Gretchen said, "I'll let you go. I'm sorry we didn't get to say good-bye, but it's okay. We'll stay in touch."

"Call me and tell me what happens with your uncle and the police," Jorey told her.

"I will."

"And with Kitty . . . have you talked to Kitty? Does she know what's going on?"

"I tried her house again, thinking you might have gone over there, and there was still no answer. Jorey, I hope she's all right. You don't think anything's happened to her, do you?"

"No!" Jorey said quickly. "Just because Clover and Adrienne—I mean, I'm positive it was a coincidence that they were both killed, and that they were friends. I'm sure Kitty's fine. She's probably in the hospital giving birth, right?"

"I guess . . ."

"Gretchen," Jorey said, suddenly worried, "be careful, okay? Don't stay alone in that house at night. Not even with your uncle there."

Especially not with your uncle there.

"I'll be okay, Jorey. Don't worry."

"But what if—?"

"What if what?"

"I don't know. It's just that . . . never mind, okay? Never mind. I'll talk to you soon."

She hung up, wondering if she should have told Gretchen what was on her mind. What if it weren't a coincidence that Clover and Adrienne were dead? What if Kitty weren't in the hospital having her baby? What if something had happened to her, too? What if someone had targeted the five of them because . . .

Because why? What could we have done to anyone to turn him into a savage killer?

Again, she had the uneasy feeling that there was something she should be remembering. Something about that last summer. Something she had blocked out of her mind.

And it had something to do with the pond in the woods. She knew that, somehow. Something had happened there. Something terrible.

If she could just remember, she might be able to unlock the mystery behind the murders of her friends.

But where does Rebecca fit in? she found herself wondering. *She was an outsider, not one of us. Could her murder be unrelated to Clover's and Adrienne's?*

Or, could it be a coincidence that both Clover and Adrienne had both been killed? Had they even been murdered by the same person?

What if Clover's partner, Sheryl, really had been behind her death? And what if Adrienne had been killed by someone else, by . . .

The senator, Jorey realized. *It could have been the senator. Maybe he thought she was getting too sloppy with their affair. Maybe he was worried that his wife would find out, or maybe Adrienne threatened to tell her, so he killed Adrienne to silence her.*

"Jorey?"

She looked up to see Sawyer watching her. He had turned away from the window and was standing with his arms folded across his chest, his blue eyes focused on her face.

"I need to go," she said, hastily slipping into her coat. She would just go outside and, before driving away, return to the pond. Maybe something there would trigger her memory.

Sawyer just watched her.

She zipped her coat and met his gaze, trying her hardest not to flinch or show emotion.

She cleared her throat. "If you can just give me my keys so that I can get on the road—"

He shook his head. "I can't."

Her heart skipped a beat. What was he trying to pull? Did he think he could keep her here?

"Because we have to go back and get my car. Remember? I left it out on the highway earlier. So I'll have to come with you, Jorey."

"Oh."

Why had she agreed to let him drive her back here? Why hadn't she just made her escape while she could, without complications?

"Before we go, then," she said slowly, "I have to see something."

"What is it?"

"It's . . . personal."

"Where is it?"

"On this estate. It's just . . . there's something I want to do before I go. I might never be back here. Look, can you just give me some time alone? Maybe an hour? And then I'll come back up here and we'll go."

He shrugged. "Fine. Go ahead, Jorey. I'll be waiting for you. But be careful, all right?"

"I'm always careful, Sawyer."

That's why I'm leaving town. That's why I'm going to say good-bye to you and never look back.

The woods were silent except for the sound of Jorey's footsteps and the steady dripping of melting snow from the branches overhead. The sun was shining warm on her face as she made her way over the mucky ground, where only scattered, dirty patches of white remained. The temperature today had to be in the sixties, she realized.

It almost feels as if spring is coming, she realized as a balmy breeze stirred the trees and ruffled her hair.

How deceptive. She could almost believe, on a day like today, that winter was over.

In reality, it hadn't even begun yet. Not officially. The season of storms and darkness and bitter cold still lay ominously ahead.

Suddenly, Jorey heard something rustling in the trees behind her. She stopped short and listened, her heart beginning to pound. Someone was there. She could feel the presence.

A twig snapped and she tensed, prepared to scream, to run for her life.

Then there was a thrashing in the brush, and a fawn emerged from behind a stand of evergreens.

Jorey heaved a silent sigh of relief.

The creature didn't appear to see her, but Jorey watched, fascinated, as it bent its head to nibble on a low-hanging branch. She noticed that there were nubs on its head where its antlers would form one day, when it was grown.

More rustling of the branches, and another fawn emerged, and then a larger deer, and finally, a buck, with a magnificent rack of antlers.

Jorey was absolutely still as the deer grazed not more than a few yards from where she stood.

Then, all at once, the buck froze and cocked its head, as if it had sensed something. It didn't look in Jorey's direction, but into the thick forest behind her.

Suddenly, as if triggered by pure instinct, all four

animals turned and galloped away, disappearing into the woods in a matter of moments.

Jorey clenched her hands in her pockets but remained absolutely still, listening. She heard nothing.

Yet it was obvious that something had frightened the deer away.

Perhaps a stealthy predator lay in wait nearby—a coyote, maybe, Jorey thought, remembering the stories her grandfather had told her about the natural order of animals in this mountain wilderness.

Or maybe the predator wasn't an animal, after all. Maybe it was human. Maybe its prey was human, too. . . .

A chill slipped down Jorey's spine despite the warm, November sunshine peeking down through the trees.

Was someone there, watching her?

Panic sliced through her as she thought of the women who had been attacked so mercilessly, murdered by an unknown hand. Whoever had killed Adrienne and Clover and Rebecca was still at large.

What if he was hiding in these woods, stalking her?

Calm down, Jorey commanded herself. *Why would the killer be here, of all places?*

Growing up, she had spent a lot of time exploring her grandparents' property, and she had never come across another human being in the forest. Except, of course, for Hob Nixon, whose trailer was located on property not far from here. He and his father used to hunt and fish there, although her grandfather had threatened several times to have them arrested for trespassing on his land.

Hob Nixon.

She remembered seeing him at Clover's funeral, remembered how edgy he had seemed and how his gaze had darkened when he'd overheard Adrienne's insensitive remarks. What had she said about him?

He's so repulsive.

Jorey heard her friend's comment echoing in her head, and saw once again the distasteful expression on Adrienne's pretty face. Had she angered him enough to make him . . .

Was Hob Nixon the murderer?

Was he hiding in these woods at this very moment, watching Jorey?

A shiver slithered down her spine, and she began walking abruptly, pushing her way forward again, toward the pond. She wondered momentarily if she should be heading in the opposite direction, back toward the house.

But then she lifted her head stubbornly and told herself that this was her one last chance to visit the secluded spot before she left town. This was her last effort to try to remember whatever it was that had escaped her over the years.

Besides, she didn't really believe that Hob Nixon or anybody else was hiding in the forest, watching her . . . did she?

Of course not.

It had probably just been a coyote lurking there to frighten the deer away. A coyote, or maybe just a squirrel or a possum, some harmless creature that had triggered the defensive instincts of the deer.

Yes, Jorey decided. That was exactly what had happened.

She couldn't let her imagination start getting the best of her now.

She continued to make her way forward, until at last she reached the clearing that surrounded the pond.

It looked so different today, in the sunshine. Last night when she was here with Sawyer, surrounded by shadows, the spot had seemed ominous. But as she looked out over the sparkling water that reflected the piercing blue sky overhead, Jorey was carried back to the innocent, happy childhood days she had spent here with Papa May.

She remembered how he'd helped her bait her hook in the beginning, though she insisted that she didn't mind touching worms.

"I know you don't mind the worms. But I don't want you to pinch yourself on the hook, Munch," he would say. "It's sharp and you could get hurt."

He had always looked out for her, tried to keep her safe. So did grandmother, in her own stern way. That was why she had warned Jorey away from the pond.

But . . . had she known something Jorey hadn't? Had Grandmother believed that there were dangers in the woods that had nothing to do with deep, cold water?

Jorey shivered and closed her eyes, hugging herself as if the weather had suddenly changed. It hadn't, but she became aware of goosebumps rising on her skin, and her heart rate seemed to be picking up speed.

Something happened here, she told herself. *What happened? What was it?*

She heard a scream again, in her mind. A woman's scream, or that of a young girl. The voice was familiar . . .

Who? Who is it? Who's screaming that way, sounding so desperate?

She heard a frantic splashing, too, and her eyes snapped open to stare at the pond.

The water was still, undisturbed except for the small

rings of ripples around a water bug that had just landed on the surface nearby.

The splashing had been in her mind, like the scream. The sounds had been locked in her memory all these years, but now they echoed back clearly to her.

Screaming.

Splashing.

Cries for help.

No! Don't leave me! Don't leave me here alone! Please . . .

Those were Jorey's own words, she realized. Words she had wailed to her grandfather as he lay still on the ground before her, his life ebbing away.

What happened?

What happened?

She *had* to remember.

Her heart pounded; she could almost hear the blood rushing through her veins.

Splashing.

Screaming.

No, don't leave me! Don't leave me here alone . . .

Was she remembering her grandfather's death and her own reaction? Or was it something else, something else. . . .

Oh, God, what had happened?

Jorey struggled to concentrate, to uncover the secrets that were locked in her mind. She was close, so close . . .

And then a sound behind her snapped her out of her reverie—just as she was about to grab onto an image that had suddenly flitted at the edge of her consciousness like a white flag of surrender.

At the sound, Jorey jerked her head around and cried out, startled.

She saw nothing but the jutting gray rocks and trees surrounding the pond.

But something was there, in the woods.

Something . . .

Or someone.

This time, she realized, it wasn't a coyote, or a squirrel, or deer. She could feel eyes on her, human eyes, watching her.

"Who's there?" she called, wary, trying not to show her fear. "Who's there?"

There was no reply.

She tried to tell herself, as she had before, that it was her imagination. But this time she knew that it wasn't. This time she was positive that she wasn't alone, that someone was concealed in the branches or behind a tall rock, watching her, perhaps sensing the terror that gripped her.

"I know you're there," she called, her voice high-pitched and echoing off the water. "Come out."

Nothing.

Silence.

She started to tell herself that she was losing her mind, nobody was there.

Then she heard it.

The unmistakable sound of footsteps rustling the fallen leaves that carpeted the forest floor.

Jorey was filled with panic, yet remained motionless as she waited.

Another footstep.

Then a figure emerged from the trees, and she gasped at the sight of the familiar face.

Sawyer saw that Jorey's face had gone pale, and her eyes widened at the sight of him.

"It's all right," he said, striding quickly toward her. "It's only me."

"You followed me?" she asked incredulously, taking a step backward as he approached. "How could you follow me? I asked for some time alone."

"I know you did, Jorey, but I couldn't . . . when I saw you heading into the woods, I couldn't let you go alone. Three women are dead in this town because somebody killed them, and whoever did it is still on the loose. You would be foolish to take any kind of chance under the circumstances."

"So you followed me," she said coldly, shaking her head. "You thought it was your duty to keep me safe. Is that it?"

He shrugged. "You're not thinking clearly right now. You've lost two friends in the space of a few days, Jorey—"

"And you lost your sister," she cut in grimly. "You're the one who's not thinking clearly. You think because of what happened to her that it's your duty to protect me, for some reason."

He let her words sink in, then nodded. He couldn't deny it. She spoke the truth, and they both knew it.

"I care about you, Jorey," he said, taking another step toward her.

He expected her to move back again, but she didn't. She stood her ground and she looked at him with those big eyes of hers, eyes that were the deep green shade of the moss growing on the stones surrounding the pond.

"If you care about me," she said, low, "then you'll leave me alone. You'll let me go."

"I'm not keeping you here."

"You are!" she protested instantly, her eyes flashing. "Every time I try to leave you behind, you follow me."

"I was worried—"

"It's not your place to be worried about me. We barely know each other, Sawyer."

But he could see that she didn't believe that. She looked away from him, focusing on the woods over his shoulder, and he took another step toward her.

"We do know each other, Jorey."

She didn't reply.

"You say that you don't need me, that you can take care of yourself," he went on. "And maybe you don't, and maybe you can. But *I* need to do this. I need to see that you're safe. For whatever reason."

"What are you going to do when I'm back in New York?" she demanded. "Call me every hour to make sure I haven't gotten myself into trouble?"

"Once you're back in New York, you'll be fine," he informed her.

Then suddenly, he found himself wondering if that was true.

He had assumed, all along, that the danger was waiting for her here, in Blizzard Bay. But now he realized that he envisioned the shadows still hanging over her, even when she left, returning to the city, to her home, where she belonged.

He swallowed hard, reached out, and put his hands on her shoulders. She flinched but didn't pull away.

"Jorey," he said, looking intently at her, "you *have* to listen to me. You're in danger. I can't tell you how I know, but I do."

"Why can't you tell me?"

Why can't I? he wondered fleetingly. Why not just confess the truth—all of it?

Why not tell her his real name, and about the life he had left behind in Michigan?

Why not tell her about the visions that had plagued him, visions about her, and Rebecca, and Susan?

Because she won't believe me, he reminded himself. *Susan didn't believe me, and she was in love with me. So why should Jorey?*

Jorey wasn't in love with him, he told himself. Just as he wasn't in love with her.

What had happened between them, what was *still* happening between them, was lust. Pure physical attraction, nothing more. It could never *be* anything more.

As long as he kept that in mind, he would be fine.

"I can't tell you anything else, Jorey," he heard himself say. "That's all there is to it. Just . . . trust me."

She snorted, and her eyes flashed. "Trust you," she echoed. "Why should I trust someone who sneaks around, following me, spewing dire warnings without giving me reasons to listen? Why should I trust someone who's making love to me one minute, then turns his back the next and tells me to get out of his life? Why should I trust someone who is obviously incapable of feeling anything, someone so selfish—"

"Selfish? Incapable of feeling? Is that what you think?" He stared at her, incredulous. "You think I used you, is that it? That I used you for my own pleasure, then cast you aside because I don't care?"

"What else could I think?"

"I'm sending you away *because* I care, Jorey. I'm doing now what I should have done before, with . . ."

Susan.

He closed his eyes against the pain and tried to swallow the enormous lump that had risen in his throat. It wouldn't go away, and he knew that if he opened his eyes again tears would spill from them.

"Jorey," he whispered, shaking his head. "Just go. Now."

"But your car—"

"Just go. I'll get it later. I can't . . ."

He couldn't look at her again. It would be better if he didn't have to watch her walk away. Easier.

"Go," he repeated hoarsely.

Then he felt something graze his cheek. Her fingertips, he realized. Her touch was gentle; she was stroking his skin.

His eyes flew open and he saw her standing there, looking up at him, her hand against his cheek. He caught her fingers in his own and moved them away, wanting to let go of her, but unable to do it.

"Sawyer," she said softly, "you're in so much pain. It isn't just because of your sister's death. There was somebody else, wasn't there? Somebody you loved. And you lost her."

"How do you know that?"

"It's why you won't let me in. Not because you don't care. I was wrong about you, wasn't I?"

He swallowed hard, nodded.

She reached out, caught his other hand, pried open his clenched fist as he struggled to maintain control. "Sawyer," she said gently, "it's all right. I understand now—"

"No. You couldn't possibly."

"Then help me."

"Don't do this, Jorey."

"I deserve answers."

"Why? Why can't you just leave it alone? Just leave me alone," he said raggedly.

"I will. I promise. I'll go. But first, just tell me."

He shook his head.

She stepped closer, the length of her body against his. Suddenly, despite his resolution not to lower his guard, he found himself stirring to life. He was aroused by her nearness, by her hands warm in his.

"No," he whispered, unable to take his eyes off hers. "Go, Jorey. Go now."

She tilted her head, looking up at him. He closed his eyes, trying to summon strength, then felt her releasing his hands from her grasp.

She's going to go, he realized, relieved even as a bitter bolt of disappointment shot through him. *It's best if she just goes.*

Then he felt her hands again, on his neck, in his hair. She was pulling his face downward and before he knew what was happening her lips were on his. Her kiss was more sweet and tender than it was passionate, but it ignited the embers that had been smoldering inside him.

He groaned and deepened the kiss as desperately as a thirsty, dying man gulping icy water. He wrapped his arms around her and he crushed her against his chest, thinking that if he could just hold her like this, if he could just keep her here with him, if time could just stand still, then everything would be all right.

He tore his lips from hers long enough to murmur, "I want to make love to you, Jorey . . . please . . ."

"Yes," she whispered, her breath hot against his ear. "One last time, Sawyer . . . But then I have to—"

"One last time," he repeated, shushing her by claiming her mouth again. He didn't want to think about what would happen afterward; he didn't want to think at all.

His hands were already stripping her of her jacket; her fingers had slipped inside his coat, probing beneath his flannel shirt to caress his bare chest.

They undressed each other swiftly, their clothes tumbling carelessly around them until they were both naked in the dappled sunshine filtering through the trees. He took her hands in his and raised them against his shoulders, and for a long time, they just stood that way and kissed.

Then, at last, taking her into his strong arms, he lowered her to the ground. He lay her gently on her back on a bed of moss and pine needles.

"Are you all right?" he asked, positioning himself between her parted knees.

She nodded.

He looked deeply into her eyes and felt her reach down to take him into her hand. He felt himself throbbing, springing in her fingers as she guided him to the moist folds between her legs.

He tried to prolong it, wanting to memorize this moment, the way the sun had turned her eyes as translucent as the smooth, green bottle glass that washed up along the beach; the way the breeze had lifted a stray curl so that it fell wantonly across one arched brow.

Finally, he entered her with a hushed sigh of pleasure, embedding himself in her silky heat. Their gazes locked and he began to thrust, slowly, rhythmically, taking his time, wanting to make it last.

She followed his lead, wrapping her legs around his hips, moving perfectly with him. Even their breathing was synchronized, and he realized, for the first time, what it truly meant to make love, to join together so that two bodies became one, so that two beings became one.

Oh, Jorey, I don't want this to be over, he thought, even as he felt the telltale pressure building within him. *I don't want to be alone again.*

He studied her eyes as they searched his own, feeling as if she were reading his thoughts; as though she shared them. As though she needed him as much as he needed her. She shifted her weight beneath him and the slight change in angle heightened the sensations shooting through him.

Hold back, he commanded himself, managing to curb his thrusts though his instinct was to do the opposite. He longed to increase the delicate friction of his hard masculinity against her pliable, welcoming flesh, to drive them both toward release.

No. You can't. Don't let it end.

As if sensing his intense need to prolong the inevitable, Jorey slowed her movements just as he did, and for a moment they were both utterly motionless.

Then he lifted himself on his elbows, nearly withdrawing, poised over her, breathless, quietly frantic. It was exquisite agony to allow only the tip of his manhood to remain inside of her when the rest of him pulsated with fiery need.

He held back for as long as he could.

Then he sank into her again, slowly, and they sighed in unison. The breeze rustled the trees and fluttered her hair against his shoulder. He dipped his head and kissed her deeply, swirling his tongue into her mouth, tasting her, aware of the length of his body against hers, feeling himself wrapped snugly in her intimate core.

Oh, Jorey. Oh, Jorey . . . if only this didn't have to end.

He held back as long as he could and then, finally, he lifted his mouth from hers, and he lifted his hips again. It took every ounce of strength he possessed to hover above her once more, just once more, before he could no longer stand it.

Then, knowing it was time, he plunged into her once more until he was buried to the hilt. Instantly, he felt her begin quivering around him. Her mouth parted and she cried out softly, tangling her fingers in his hair, and he felt himself start to shudder.

This time he had reached the point of no return, and there was no holding back. He was coming, and so was she. His body took up the rhythmic movements again and he felt himself turning molten, gushing into her with every thrust, her name spilling helplessly from his lips.

"Jorey . . ."

"I know." She stroked his head and let out a shaky breath. "I know."

Spent and sated, he collapsed against her, letting his head fall against her shoulder. He ran his hand tenderly along the taut flesh of her hip and thigh, feeling himself growing soft inside her. Suddenly, he was overwhelmed by exhaustion. He wanted more than anything to close his eyes and sleep.

It was as though, for a few fleeting moments, he had discovered the tranquility that had been missing from his life these past few years. Throwing himself first into his work, and then into finding his sister's killer, he had been caught up in a tense, lonely existence with no reprieve.

Now, at long last, here was Jorey, sweet Jorey, here beneath him.

And here was peace.

Chapter Fifteen

Jorey opened her eyes and blinked, disoriented.

Where . . . ?

What . . . ?

It came back to her in a rush, then, and she remembered that she was at the pond in the woods, and that she and Sawyer had made love and then fallen asleep. He lay next to her on his side with his face toward hers, his head against her shoulder, his eyes closed. He was sleeping, and she was startled to see that he looked young—almost like a boy, a golden boy, with his hair streaming around him and his features at rest.

She realized that the hard lines of anxiety around his eyes and mouth had softened in his slumber, and it was all she could do not to reach out and gently touch the skin that was marred by worry when he was awake.

She didn't want to wake him, though. She wasn't yet ready to face him, or what had happened between them.

One last time, she reminded herself, her own earlier words echoing through her mind. *It was the last time.*

It was what they had both wanted. Neither of them expected anything more. Anything more would be impossible.

But I'm not ready to say good-bye, Jorey thought, gazing at Sawyer. *I know it's coming, but I'm not ready.*

She sat up carefully, quietly, and the chilly air hit her as soon as she rose away from his body heat. The sun was warm for November but she was naked, and she quickly reached for her red sweatshirt, which lay in a heap on the ground nearby.

She brushed a flurry of soft pine needles from the fabric and then pulled it on, huddling in the warmth and wondering what she should do.

She could wait for him to wake up.

Or she could get dressed and leave him here asleep.

That way, there would be no good-bye. It would be easier on both of them.

It was the right thing to do, she knew, as she reached for her jeans, with her white silk panties still bunched inside the waistband. He would probably be relieved when he awakened and found her gone.

What about his car out on the highway? she asked herself, though she knew she was just looking for an excuse.

That wasn't a good reason to stay. He could find someone to give him a ride out there to pick it up.

But who? He doesn't have a friend in this town.

Besides, should you really leave him alone here in the woods, asleep and naked?

She found herself gazing down at his magnificent body, noting the contours of his flawlessly sculpted flesh. She admired the bulges of the muscles in his upper arms and his rippling washboard stomach, and her eyes traced the line of golden hair that led provocatively downward toward the apex of his legs.

She remembered how he had felt, firm and pulsing inside of her, and she turned her head away, swallowing hard.

It was more, so much more, than the physical sensations of their passion that had left a mark on her. She knew that what had happened between them was about pure emotion—that for that all too brief interlude their bodies, their minds, and hearts had been in perfect harmony.

And Jorey had almost been able to believe that it could last.

Almost.

She abruptly pulled on her panties and then her jeans, and then she got to her knees and reached for one of her socks. She put it on. The other was nowhere to be seen, and she stood quietly and began to hunt for it.

Sawyer stirred slightly on the ground and sighed, murmuring something in his sleep.

Her name.

He was murmuring her name.

She froze and looked at him, waiting for him to awaken and stare at her with those probing eyes. She knew she couldn't bear it if his gaze had grown icy blue again, and she wasn't ready to hear him tell her in that no-nonsense tone that it was time for her to leave.

She *knew* it was time. But that didn't stop her from trying to prolong the moment when she would leave him behind forever.

She waited until she was certain he wasn't going to awaken, and then she resumed the hunt for her other sock. A splashing sound nearby made her look up just as a fat, brown duck plopped into the pond, seemingly unaware of her presence.

She watched it swim away, and as she stared out over the rippling water she struggled once more to find a hold on the murky past.

Slowly, the images before her blurred, and she drifted back . . . back. . . .

In her mind's eye Jorey found herself looking at the pond—not from this pine-needle and moss-carpeted spot in the clearing where she stood, but from the trees that rimmed the edge of the water.

She was crouched behind a low evergreen, peering at the pond through the branches, spying on something.

She was no longer wearing jeans and a fleecy sweatshirt; it was June, and she had on cut-off shorts and a bikini top. She became conscious of mosquito bites on her bare legs, and of the telltale heat on her shoulders and back, and knew that meant she was sunburnt. She had always been sunburnt during the first few days of the season, when she took little care to protect her city-white skin from the country summer sun.

The air was close and warm around her and abuzz with insects; it was late afternoon and the shadows were lengthening across the water.

She inhaled and her lungs filled with the heady scents of honeysuckle and pine, damp earth, and algae from the pond. She felt a tickle in her nose and realized that she was going to sneeze. But she held it back. She knew that she needed to be very quiet and still, so that she wouldn't be heard, because—

All at once, her mind snapped back to the present.

No! she screamed inwardly, trying to recapture the images and sensations that had been so vivid. *Come back!*

But they were gone; she was in the here and now, and utterly confused.

What was that all about? she wondered, frowning, turning to look at the thick wall of trees behind her. *Why would I have been hiding back in there, watching the pond?*

Puzzled and frustrated, she tried again to bring the elusive memory back, but it had dissolved completely.

She struggled to go over what little she had captured, unwilling to let it, too, fade.

All she knew was that there had been a time, in her past, when she had been concealed in the trees, spying on something, or someone.

And she hadn't been alone.

She seized that bit of knowledge, and with it came a dark, uneasy feeling.

Why?

Who had been there with her, hiding in the woods?

Jorey clenched her fists and narrowed her eyes in concentration, but nothing more would come. She fought back bitter tears of frustration, realizing that she had been close, so close, to remembering.

She felt as though she had been pushed out a door that had been slammed closed and firmly locked behind her, and it wouldn't budge no matter how she tried to get back in.

Finally, she turned away from the pond and her gaze fell on Sawyer, still sleeping on the ground nearby.

She walked quietly over to him and stood for a moment, watching his chest rise and fall.

Then she caught sight of the sock she had been missing. It was poking out from beneath Sawyer's jacket that had been so hastily discarded earlier.

Jorey stealthily grabbed the sock and pulled it over her bare foot, then grabbed her shoes and jacket. She didn't dare pause to get them on; the longer she lingered, the more likely it was that he would awaken. And she didn't want that.

She only wanted to go . . . *now*. To get away from this place and the cryptic half-memories it inspired; to flee this man whose heart she knew would never belong to her.

She turned her back on him and began to steal away. She had almost reached the edge of the woods when she heard his voice behind her.

"Jorey? Where are you going?"

She stopped, cursed softly, and turned to look at him. He had, of course, awakened, and was sitting up, his gaze focused on her. There was nothing groggy about his expression; he appeared fully alert—and fully aware of what she was up to.

"I was going back to the house," she told him, and was dismayed that her tone seemed uncertain. She did her best to sound more forceful as she added, "It's getting late, and I wanted to leave before dark."

He was pulling on his clothes before she finished speaking, moving so hastily that mere moments later he was on his feet and striding toward her.

"Aren't you going to put on your shoes?" he asked, eyeing the sneakers she clutched, with her leather jacket, in her now trembling hand.

"I . . . I forgot," she said lamely, and bent to pull first one, and then the other, onto her feet. She swiftly tied the laces, then stood again and faced Sawyer.

"Ready to go?" he asked, apparently choosing not to address the fact that she had so obviously intended to leave him behind without saying good-bye.

There was nothing for her to do but nod and follow him back to the path that led toward the house.

* * *

Jorey insisted on driving back out to the highway. That didn't surprise Sawyer; he had expected her to, and didn't argue when she told him to get into the passenger's seat.

His mind was reeling as she headed the Range Rover down the long, winding drive away from the stone mansion. He wanted to say something meaningful, but he didn't know what it could possibly be.

Making love to her that last time had changed everything. Until now, he had been able to pretend that she could walk out of his life and he could forget about her. That what he felt for her was lust, and a fierce protective instinct, and nothing more.

But something profound had passed between them as they looked into each other's eyes, their bodies intimately joined. Something stronger, even, than what he had felt for his lost bride—stronger, perhaps, than the rage and guilt he had carried since his sister's murder.

But it couldn't change anything . . . could it? She was going to leave, and he was going to let her go.

He longed to know what Jorey was thinking.

Her gaze was focused straight ahead, through the windshield, as if she were concentrating intently on her driving. As though there was something tricky about steering a vehicle along a paved driveway at twenty miles an hour.

He cleared his throat and opened his mouth to say something, anything, then closed it again when nothing at all would come to mind.

Had it been only an hour or so ago that they had lain naked and asleep, entwined in each other's arms? He had awakened from a dream about her—nothing concrete, just images of her, and she was laughing and she was looking at him with love in her eyes, and she was his.

But now the dream had evaporated, replaced by the harsh reality of her leaving.

The spell had been broken too easily, he thought, wanting to turn his head and look over at her, to study her face and see if he could tell what she was thinking.

He didn't dare.

If he looked at her he might speak to her, and if he spoke to her he might say something he would regret. Something he didn't mean. Something like . . .

Please don't go.

Or . . .

I love you.

The words rushed into his mind without warning, slamming into him and snatching his breath away like an icy blizzard wind.

I love you?

But he didn't.

I love you.

He couldn't.

He had sworn that he would never love anyone again.

His love for Susan had gotten her killed.

His love for his sister had deafened him to the warnings that she was in danger.

He refused to helplessly love another woman who would only be lost to him. If Jorey didn't leave Blizzard Bay, she would die.

Even if she leaves, she might die, anyway.

Again, the thought occurred to him, and this time he tried not to dismiss it as willingly as he had before. He pondered the notion that the danger might follow her back to New York. He imagined her there, and there was nothing as concrete as the shadows he saw surrounding her in Blizzard Bay, but he couldn't shake his apprehension about her safety.

What if something happened to her in New York? He wouldn't be there to protect her.

He couldn't go with her. He belonged here, in Blizzard Bay. He had sworn that he would find out who had killed his sister if it took him the rest of his life. Now that the killer had apparently struck again—twice—his chances were better than ever. Clover's and Adrienne's deaths might provide the clues that had been missing in Rebecca's.

But what about Jorey?

What about her? a voice protested in his mind. He wondered whether his attraction for her had clouded his perception of the warnings that had come to him regarding her. Maybe he was conjuring images of danger waiting in New York simply because he didn't want her to leave.

It made sense.

Just as it had made sense to attribute his visions about Susan to his own subconscious fears about being married.

"There's your car."

Jorey's words startled him out of his reverie, and he glanced up to see that she was slowing the Range Rover and pulling onto the shoulder of the highway. His Chevy waited just ahead, where he had abandoned it earlier.

He realized that the sun was sinking fast in the west, casting long shadows over the deserted road. He didn't like the thought of her driving all the way to New York alone, in the dark.

He noticed that she didn't put the car into park when she came to a stop at the side of the road, just kept her foot on the brake and her hands positioned on the wheel.

"Jorey," he said, "it's getting late—"

"I know it is. That's why I need to get going as soon as possible," she said pointedly.

"Maybe you should wait until tomorrow morn—"

"No," she cut in. "I'm going now. I can't stay another night. I don't want to go back to the bed and breakfast now. And I can't . . ."

She trailed off, but he knew what she meant.

I can't stay with you.

If she stayed, they would spend the night in each other's arms. God only knew whether he would ever be able to let her go after that.

It was now or never.

He knew it, and so, apparently, did she.

He turned to look at her, memorizing her profile as she stared straight ahead. He saw that her jaw was clenched and knew that she was doing her best to remain stoic.

There were so many things he wanted to tell her.

That he would treasure the memory of what they had shared together.

That if she ever needed anything, anything at all, he would be there for her.

That if things were different, he would never be able to let her go like this.

He swallowed hard and put his hand on the door handle, mustering every bit of strength he possessed to keep his voice from quavering as he said, "Jorey, take care of yourself."

She nodded, not looking at him.

He desperately wanted to reach for her, to haul her into his arms and just hang on.

Instead, he opened the car door, stepped out into the dusk, and began walking toward his car.

She drove past him, picking up speed and disappearing around a curve in the highway before he had reached the Chevy.

But he noticed that she glanced into her rearview mirror just before she vanished, and when she did, he lifted an arm to wave a final good-bye.

The tears hadn't come when Sawyer closed the car door behind him with a resolute slam, or when he walked away. They didn't even come when she caught a last look at him in the rearview mirror and saw that he was waving.

No, she managed to stay calm until she was back on the Northway, heading south.

Then, without warning, she found herself sobbing so hard that she had to pull onto the shoulder and bury her head in her arms against the steering wheel. She didn't know how long she sat that way, crying bitter tears. When she finally pulled herself together and got back on the road, darkness had fallen.

She turned on her headlights and then the radio, but thought better of that. Instead, she put in a Rolling Stones CD and pushed PLAY.

She certainly didn't want to chance hearing any news bulletins about Adrienne's death. Now that she had left Blizzard Bay, she intended to put everything behind her.

The murders, Sawyer, her own fragmented, disturbing memories of the past . . . all of it.

There was nothing else she could do.

She had almost believed, in the emotionally charged

moments before he got out of the car, that Sawyer was going to ask her to stay.

She knew now that if he had, she would have fallen into his arms and told him yes.

Thank God he hadn't asked.

She heaved a heavy sigh and turned the Stones CD louder, hoping it would drown out her own thoughts. But her mind kept going, and she kept rehashing the strange day.

She came to the conclusion that she had done the right thing by leaving. She didn't belong in Blizzard Bay.

But did she belong in New York?

What was waiting for her there?

You have a life there, she reminded herself. *You have family there, and an apartment, and friends.*

Yes, it was time to go home.

The only thing was, when she thought about New York it no longer seemed like home, and she knew that it never would.

But Blizzard Bay didn't feel like home anymore, either—not the way it once had. Not with Papa May gone and the big stone house filled with strangers.

And Sawyer.

She realized that the only times she had felt at home since Papa May had died were when she was lying in Sawyer Howland's arms. And that would never happen again.

You need to move on, Jorey told herself. *You need to figure out what to do with your life, and where to be.*

She decided that as soon as she got back to New York she would start making plans. She would decide on a career, and she would concentrate on building a future for herself.

But for the next few hours, as she drove through the night, leaving Sawyer and Blizzard Bay farther behind with every mile, she couldn't help thinking of the past . . . and what might have been.

Chapter Sixteen

The first thing Jorey did when she walked into her apartment late that night was check her answering machine on a low table in a corner of the vast living room.

The red light was flashing furiously, and she discovered that she had several new messages. Most were from her friends; one was from her mother, who couldn't remember when Jorey was returning from her vacation, but when she did could she please call and let her know whether she'd be visiting for Christmas this year?

The last message was from Gretchen. She informed Jorey that she had finally reached Kitty's mother, who had told her that Kitty had gone into labor early that morning and was in the hospital. The baby was breech, and it looked as if they were going to have to do a C-section. Gretchen promised to keep Jorey informed, and added that there was no news on Adrienne's murder, and that she had arranged to meet with the police first thing in the morning regarding Uncle Roland.

Sawyer Howland hadn't called.

Well, what did you expect? Jorey asked herself, hanging up the receiver and crossing the room to stand before the floor-to-ceiling window. The city was sprawled before her, thousands of lights twinkling beyond the glass, but all she saw was Sawyer's face before her.

She closed her eyes to shut it out, wanting only to forget him now that she was back here.

Abruptly, she returned to the telephone, needing to reconnect with the world she had left behind.

She dialed her father's number first. His housekeeper answered and told her that he was out for the evening. He wouldn't be back until late. Would Ms. Maddock like him to return the call in the morning?

"Just tell him that I'm back in New York," Jorey said hollowly, before hanging up.

She wasn't in the mood to call any of her friends back, knowing they would want to make plans to get together. That could wait. Her social calendar would start filling up soon enough now that she was home. It always did.

She didn't return the call to her mother, either, knowing that it was four o'clock in the morning over there.

She hesitated only briefly before dialing Gretchen's number in Blizzard Bay. She knew that she probably shouldn't be doing it. After all, she had sworn to leave behind everything about the place. But she told herself that she was only concerned about Kitty, and whether the baby had been born all right.

Gretchen answered on the first ring.

"Jorey!" she said, sounding pleased to hear her voice. "You made it home all right. I tried to get a hold of you earlier, but you weren't there. I was worried. How long did it take you to get back?"

"Just a few hours," Jorey said. "I had a few stops to make before I got back to my apartment, though," she added, unwilling to tell Gretchen that she hadn't left Blizzard Bay until early evening. Gretchen would want to know why, and she wasn't about to reveal those stolen moments she and Sawyer had shared.

"Did you get my message about Kitty?" Gretchen asked.

"I did. Has the baby been born yet?"

"I just called the hospital, and she's in surgery. I don't expect to hear anything else for a while."

"Will you let me know what happens? I'd like to send her a gift for the baby," Jorey said.

"I'll call as soon as I hear."

"What about Adrienne? Have they uncovered anything new?"

There was a pause before Gretchen answered, "Nothing yet. But like I said, I'm going to talk to the detectives about Uncle Roland."

"You haven't let your uncle know what I saw?"

"I haven't seen him. I'm assuming he's still asleep upstairs, and when he gets up, I don't plan to reveal anything to him. Just in case . . ."

"I know this is hard for you, Gretchen. Listen, just please be careful while you're alone there with him."

"I will. Karl promised to come over and spend the night with me."

"Is he there?"

Gretchen was silent for a moment, then said, "Not yet. He must have gotten caught up in paperwork at the office. I'm sure he'll be here any minute."

Jorey bit back a comment, reminding herself that

Gretchen's relationship with Karl was none of her business.

"Listen, Gretchen, I'm going to hang up now," she said, suddenly weary. "I'll talk to you soon. Please call me if you need me, okay?"

"I will," Gretchen promised, and Jorey wondered what she would do if Gretchen did call, if she asked her to come back to Blizzard Bay. Would she do it?

I can't, she told herself, replacing the cordless telephone in the base. *I'm never going back there again.*

Yawning, she turned and made her way to the master suite. There, she undressed swiftly, washed her face, and fell into her king-size bed, where she immediately, gratefully, fell into a dreamless slumber.

Sawyer finished mounting the newspaper article in the scrapbook and sat back to read the headline.

"Blizzard Bay Socialite Murdered"

According to the article, Adrienne Van Deegan had been found brutally stabbed to death in the living room of her home. There were no signs of forced entry, and the weapon had not been recovered. However, a maid reported after an extensive inventory of the dining room that a silver-plated ice pick was missing from the home, and the wounds were consistent with those found on the victim.

The police were reportedly as baffled by this case as by the previous two, and had come up with no suspects. However, detectives were pursuing several leads.

Sawyer wondered about Gretchen's uncle. Was it possible that the man was a deranged killer?

He had been at Clover's home the night she was

killed. But what about Rebecca? What connection could he possibly have had to her?

Sawyer reminded himself that there didn't need to be a personal connection. Serial killers often targeted strangers as their victims. Anyway, Rebecca was so sweet, so naive and trusting. She would have felt sorry for an elderly deaf-mute. She would have befriended him if she'd met him.

Oh, Rebecca, what happened to you? Sawyer wondered desperately.

He wouldn't rest until he knew.

And he couldn't rely on the police to find the murderer. The local force was small and more experienced in handing out traffic tickets and rounding up bears that had gotten into residential garbage cans than they were in catching a serial killer.

Besides, they had to rely on regulations like search warrants and rules about questioning suspects.

Sawyer didn't.

He decided that the first thing tomorrow he would take it upon himself to do a little investigating into Gretchen's Uncle Roland.

He closed the scrapbook and stood, stretching. Then he carried it over to the secret cupboard beside the fireplace and tucked it into its hiding place.

As he did, he was reminded of something. He turned and saw that Jorey's stuffed dog was sitting on the table where she had left it.

Rudy, she had called him.

I'll bring him back to New York with me.

But she had left the little dog behind once again. Sawyer crossed the room and picked it up thoughtfully, wondering if Jorey had missed it yet.

What about him?

Did she miss him?

Or had she forgotten all about him the minute she'd gotten back to New York?

He wondered if he would ever get her out of his mind. Not likely while he was stuck here in Blizzard Bay. Every time he turned around, he knew, he would see something that would remind him of her.

That was how it had been with Susan. After she was gone, he had been haunted by her memory. He had even considered leaving Grosse Pointe for good, but had realized he didn't want to. It was the only home he had ever known, and besides, there was the business. He couldn't run the Detroit-based business if he left the area. And running the business was all he had left.

Until Rebecca was killed.

Now he was as consumed by the need to solve her murder as he once had been by the need to make his father's company an unparalleled success. He had achieved that goal. Would he achieve this one?

What would he do once he found the killer?

Would it be enough just to know what had happened?

Or did he need more?

Did he need vengeance?

He sighed, and his thoughts slipped back to Jorey. If he accomplished what he had come here to do, he would be free. Free to go back to Grosse Pointe and return to his job; free to follow his instincts wherever they led.

What if they led him to her?

Would she give him a second chance?

Somehow, he didn't think so. He had hurt her too deeply. And he came with far too much baggage for any woman, even Jorey, to understand.

Then again, she hadn't turned her back on him when

he made it clear that he wasn't emotionally available. She had asked him for explanations; he was the one who was reluctant to give them.

Maybe she would be able to understand what he had been through; why he was so afraid to let himself love again. Maybe she was the one woman who was capable of bringing him back to life after everything he had lost.

Then again, maybe she wouldn't be around to do that.

A chill slithered down his spine as he thought about Jorey and the danger that surrounded her.

He hadn't been able to shake the troubling notion that something was going to happen to her, even now that she was back in New York, two hundred miles from Blizzard Bay. Rather than lessening in the hours since she had left, the notion had only grown stronger.

Now, thinking about her—and realizing that he could no longer protect her if she needed him—he fought back a prickle of panic.

It's out of your hands, he reminded himself. *And she's out of your life. Let her go. Just let her go.*

The ringing telephone woke Jorey from a sound sleep, and it took her a moment to realize where she was.

She pushed back the goose down comforter and reached blindly toward the polished Stickley table by the bed, feeling around for the phone. She finally found the receiver and lifted it, noticing that the light filtering in the window was a gloomy gray. It was still early morning . . . who would call her this early?

"Jorey?"

"Gretchen?" Her eyes widened and she sat up, clutching the receiver.

"Did I wake you?"

"Actually . . . yes. But it's okay. What's the matter? Is everything all right with Kitty?"

"Kitty? I haven't heard anything yet. That's not why I'm calling."

Jorey noticed that her friend's voice sounded grim. Something had happened, she realized.

"What is it, Gretchen? What's wrong?"

"I'm so scared, Jorey. I'm just so scared . . . " Gretchen's voice trailed off.

"What happened? Are you in some kind of trouble?"

"I woke up this morning and found a note pinned to my pillow, Jorey."

"My God."

"Right next to my head. It was right next to my head." Gretchen's voice rose in pitch, as if she were on the verge of hysteria. "Jorey, somebody was in my room while I was sleeping. Somebody snuck in there and left this note—"

"What did it say?"

"It said . . ." Gretchen paused and drew a shaky breath. "It said, 'You're next.' "

Jorey gasped, understanding immediately what it meant.

"Did you go to the police?" she asked Gretchen.

"Not yet. I'm too afraid to, Jorey. I'm too afraid that something's going to happen to me if I stay here another minute. I have to get away."

"Maybe it was just a prank of some sort," Jorey told her, trying to sound convincing.

"No way. Nobody I know would have done something like that. It had to be whoever killed Adrienne and

Clover," Gretchen said resolutely. "Now he's after me, too. I can't just stay here and wait for him to get me, Jorey."

"No, you can't. But . . . who was with you last night? Was Karl there?"

"No. He never showed. He called and said he was stuck at work, and for me to just go to bed."

Suspicion twisted in Jorey's gut. "What about Uncle Roland?"

"He was here, I guess. I assume he was still asleep when I went up to bed because I didn't see him. But he's illiterate, Jorey. He couldn't have written that note."

"How do you know that?" A chilling thought struck Jorey. "How do you even know that he's deaf and mute, Gretchen?"

Her friend was silent for a moment.

Then she said in an oddly little girl voice, "I'm scared, Jorey. I'm so scared. I have to get out of here. Please . . . can I come there?"

"Here?" Startled, Jorey asked, "Why do you want to come here, of all places, Gretchen? I mean, isn't there someplace else where you'd feel safer?"

"There's no place else. There's no one else. You're the only person I know who doesn't live in Blizzard Bay, Jorey. But if you'd rather I didn't—"

"No," Jorey cut her off hastily, as guilt came over her. Of course she wanted to help her friend.

"It's okay, I can just—"

"No, come here, Gretchen. You can stay here with me, for as long as you want. You'll be safe here. Just please don't tell anyone where you're going. Not even Karl."

"Not even Karl?" Gretchen echoed, sounding incredulous. "Jorey, you can't possibly think that Karl—"

"He has the keys to your house, doesn't he, Gretchen?"

"Yes, but—"

"Don't trust anyone, Gretchen. *Not even Karl,*" she repeated. "I mean it. I know you're in love with him, but you might not know him as well as you think you do."

"You're wrong about that, Jorey." Gretchen's voice was flat. "But I'll do whatever you think is best. I can't think straight right now. Hang on, will you? I've got someone on call-waiting beeping in."

There was a click, and Jorey rubbed the sleep from her eyes as she waited for Gretchen to come back on the line. She wondered how long her friend would want to stay with her, and whether she would mind playing hostess to her after vowing to leave everything about Blizzard Bay behind for good.

This is different, she told herself. *You're helping a friend in need. This has nothing to do with Sawyer, and Gretchen's presence doesn't need to be a reminder of him.*

A moment later Gretchen was back on the line, saying, "It was Johnny. He told me that Kitty had the baby a few hours ago. Another girl."

"Is everything all right?"

"I don't know. He sounds exhausted. He's still on the other line. I told him to hang on so that I can talk to him again. I said I was on long distance with you, but that I would hang up."

"You told him you were talking to me? Gretchen, remember what I just said. Don't tell anyone that you're leaving town, or where you're going."

"Not even *Johnny?*"

Jorey rolled her eyes skyward and counted to three

before answering calmly, "Not even *anyone*. You have to be careful. Promise?"

"Promise," Gretchen said, sounding reluctant. "I'll talk to Johnny quickly, then I'll pack and leave right away. I thought I'd take the train from Albany. There's one leaving in about two hours. It gets in to Penn Station at one fifteen."

"I'll meet you there," Jorey told her. "At the top of the escalator leading up from the track."

"I'll look for you. I really hope I'm not interrupting any plans you had for today, Jorey," Gretchen said worriedly. "You know that I wouldn't have called you at all if I had anywhere else to turn."

"I know you wouldn't have. I'm glad you called me. Don't worry, you aren't interrupting anything."

All I had planned was to figure out what I'm going to do with the rest of my life. God knows I don't have the first clue where to start.

Hearing the back door open, Sawyer flattened himself against the wall of the house, concealed behind a rhododendron that was taller than he was. He peered through a cluster of oval leaves and saw that Gretchen Eckhard had emerged from the back door of the house.

She was carrying a suitcase, which she set down on the step beside her as she turned to lock the back door with a key.

Sawyer watched her pick up the suitcase again and go down the steps, then walk briskly across the driveway to the car that was parked in front of the rundown detached garage. She got in, started the engine, and drove away without ever seeming to sense that she was being watched.

Where was she going?

Why was she leaving town now, in the midst of the murder investigation?

He waited a long time in his spot behind the tall plant, in case Gretchen came back home for some reason. Finally, he decided it was safe and went back to what he'd been doing before she had come outside.

He crouched near the cracked concrete foundation of the old house and continued to work on the ancient lock of a narrow window that sat close to the ground. He worked swiftly and silently, though he realized that his mission would be far simpler now that Gretchen was out of the house.

He had planned to slip in and see what he could find even if she were around, figuring it wouldn't be hard to avoid being discovered in a place as big as this old house. But now Gretchen was gone, presumably for some length of time, judging by the suitcase.

The only person he would have to steer clear of was Uncle Roland. According to Jorey, the old man slept days and was deaf, so he wouldn't even have to be guarded about his footsteps.

Finally the lock broke and Sawyer stealthily pushed the window open a crack. He saw that the basement was dark and assumed it was empty, though he was careful to be quiet as he crept through the window and closed it behind him.

He would start on the bottom and work his way up, he decided, glancing around at the immense, shadowy basement. There were built-in cupboards and shelves, as well as several cobweb shrouded doorways leading to other rooms. Plenty of places for a killer to hide the evidence.

This search is going to take a long time, Sawyer realized with a sigh of resignation. *Maybe even all day.*

There was nothing to do but get started.

Jorey surveyed the throng of baggage-laden people heading toward her on the escalator, looking for Gretchen's familiar face. She spotted it and began to wave, but Gretchen didn't appear to see her yet.

She was struck by how out of place her friend looked in Manhattan. She was wearing an unzipped, red nylon ski jacket over a pair of denim overalls while nearly everyone around her was dressed in a black, gray or navy business suit. And her white-blond hair was plaited in two braids that hung down either side of her round, scrubbed face.

Jorey saw the woman standing next to her—an impeccably madeup, hair-sprayed, middle-aged matron in a fur coat—glance at Gretchen, then smirk, obviously amused, and poke her well-heeled male companion.

Anger welled up in Jorey, along with an almost forgotten protective instinct. She wanted to turn to the smirking woman and say, "Hey, don't you dare make fun of my friend," to stick up for Gretchen as she always had.

But that had been a long time ago, and they were no longer kids on a playground.

Besides, she couldn't help feeling a little disconcerted at the mere sight of Gretchen. It brought back everything she had left behind, and Jorey found herself wondering about Sawyer.

She had almost managed to avoid thinking about him this morning as she busied herself with unpacking her bags and running down to D'Agostino's to get some food.

But every once in a while a mental image of him caught her off-guard. Like now.

Instead of Gretchen's face, she was seeing Sawyer riding toward her up the escalator.

When Gretchen threw herself into Jorey's arms, exclaiming, "Jorey, I've missed you!" it was Sawyer's voice she heard uttering those words.

"How can you miss me? I only left yesterday," she protested, trying to force away the unwelcome thoughts of the man she was supposed to have forgotten.

"I know, but it seems as though so much has happened since then," Gretchen told her. "None of it good."

"What about Kitty and the baby?"

"She's in rough shape. There was some complication with the anesthesia during the C-section, and Johnny said she's pretty out of it. She won't be out of the hospital for a while. But the baby's fine."

"Good." Someone jostled Jorey from behind, and she banged her leg on Gretchen's suitcase. "Listen, let's get out of here, okay? Stay right with me." She began pushing her way through the crowd toward the escalators leading to the taxi stand upstairs.

There was a long line waiting for cabs.

"Looks like it's going to be a while," she told Gretchen, who shrugged. "You must be exhausted from travelling. Your train was over an hour late."

"I'm just happy to be out of Blizzard Bay," she said, fingering the tip of one of her braids. "That note scared the hell out of me, Jorey."

"You didn't tell Karl where you were going, did you?" Jorey asked her.

"I didn't talk to him before I left. I didn't see Uncle

Roland, either. He must have been sleeping. So nobody saw me leave."

"Good. You'll be safe here," Jorey said with a confidence she didn't feel.

She couldn't help wondering why the killer had targeted Gretchen—and whether he had somehow managed to follow her to New York.

She found herself looking over her shoulder at the crowd of people waiting for cabs, almost expecting to see a sinister face watching her. But there were only the blank gazes of detached strangers, and she told herself not to be paranoid.

There was no real reason to believe that the killer had trailed Gretchen all the way here on the train—or that they were both in danger.

Still, Jorey felt a growing sense of trepidation, and remembered Sawyer's warnings to be careful.

I'm trying, she told him silently, turning around again and staring off into space. *I'm trying, but I can't help wondering if I needed your protection, after all.*

It was nearly five o'clock when Sawyer finally reached the top floor of the old house. Nobody had disturbed him in all the hours he had spent rummaging through closets and under beds and beneath couch cushions, and he was beginning to wonder if he was the only person in the house. There was no sign of the mysterious Uncle Roland, nor any evidence that the old man was the killer.

The search had been entirely uneventful, until he had seen the room where Jorey had stayed while she was here. He had known it had been hers the moment he had pushed the door open downstairs; her presence remained though there wasn't a physical trace that she had been there.

He had sat on the bed for a long time, thinking about her, wondering whether she was all right. He had a growing feeling of uneasiness about her, and it had become stronger and stronger as the day passed.

Maybe it was just the house, he told himself now, pushing open the door to the first third floor bedroom at the top of the stairs. There was something cold and foreboding about the place; something that made him want to finish his search as quickly as he could and just get the hell out of here.

Still, he took his time searching the third floor, moving slowly from room to room until there was only one closed door left, at the end of the hall.

He hesitated, knowing that if Uncle Roland were in the house, he had to be in that room. There was no other place where he could be.

As he placed his hand on the knob Sawyer felt an odd sensation pass through him. It was so unsettling that for a moment he removed his hand.

What was on the other side of the door?

Was he about to unlock the key to the murders?

Or was he walking into a trap?

He steeled his nerves and reached for the knob again. This time he fought back his misgivings and made himself turn the knob. He pushed the door open a tiny crack and saw that the room was dark.

That was a good sign.

If Uncle Roland were awake in there, he would have the light turned on at this hour of the day, with twilight having already fallen outside.

So either the room was empty, or the occupant was asleep.

Or . . .

What if Uncle Roland was silently waiting for him, crouched in the shadows?

There was only one way to find out.

Sawyer braced himself as he pushed the door slowly open.

It took a moment for his eyes to adjust to the dim light filtering through the window pane.

Then he took a step into the room. . . .

And gasped in horror.

Chapter Seventeen

"Jorey, this is just . . . it's just . . ."

Jorey watched as Gretchen stood speechless in the middle of her living room, slowly pivoting around to take it all in—the designer furnishings, the Oriental carpet, the expansive view of the city beyond the glass doors leading to the terrace.

Finally, Gretchen said, "You must have been unbelievably uncomfortable staying with me for such a long time."

"Uncomfortable? Of course not, Gretchen. I loved staying with you."

"But how could you, when you're used to all this? You're really living the life of luxury."

"I guess." Jorey tried to see her home through Gretchen's eyes, knowing she was right. But to her, it suddenly seemed sterile. Empty.

This was the kind of place pictured in *Architectural Digest* or *House Beautiful,* not the kind of place where a big, rugged man could tread around in L.L. Bean boots covered with mud from a field, or throw his greasy mechanic's overalls onto the floor.

Not the kind of place where a child could sprawl on a couch watching Barney and eating a messy sandwich of peanut butter and grape jelly.

So? There's no man in your life, no child. . . .

"I really feel like a country bumpkin now," Gretchen told her, shaking her head. "You must think I'm a real hick and that my house is just a shack. I mean, even Adrienne's place is nothing compared to this, Jorey."

"Gretchen! I love your house. It has so much charm and character. This place is really just a sterile box. There's not really all that much space, and no front porch, and no yard."

"But you have a balcony," Gretchen said, walking over to the glass doors. "Can I go out?"

"Sure. I hardly ever use it," Jorey said, following her.

They stepped outside and walked across the flagstone terrace to the iron railing. Faint traffic noise drifted up from more than thirty stories below, and a light rain was falling from the overcast gray sky. Lights had started coming on in some of the buildings; it was nearly dark out now. Several hours had passed since Jorey met Gretchen at the station. They had gone for a late lunch at one of Jorey's favorite French bistros before coming back here, and the wait for a table had been lengthy despite the hour.

"What a beautiful view," Gretchen murmured, leaning on the railing and looking over.

"That's the East River," Jorey said, pointing it out. "And there's the Empire State Building. And the Chrysler building is the tall one a few blocks beyond, to the right, with all the chrome on top."

Gretchen nodded, apparently awestruck as she glanced around, then down at the street. "It sure is a long way down," she observed, then looked at Jorey. "Doesn't it make you nervous, living so high up like this?"

Jorey shrugged. "I'm pretty much used to it, I guess. It doesn't bother me. It's quieter up here."

"Mmm." Gretchen gave another glance over the railing, then shivered and held out a hand, palm up. "You know, it's starting to rain out here. Let's get back inside."

"Good idea."

Jorey followed her back to the living room, then gave a brief tour of the rest of the apartment. She was aware of Gretchen's appreciative scrutiny in every room and it made her slightly uncomfortable, just as she had felt when she had first arrived at the bed & breakfast and become aware of the vast difference between Gretchen's life-style and her own.

Gretchen commented on everything: the vintage crystal lining the shelves of the breakfront in the dining room, the state-of-the-art restaurant stove in the kitchen, the antique sword mounted over the fireplace in the den that had once belonged to a Maddock who had fought in the Civil War.

Jorey brought Gretchen last into the guest room with its private bath right down the hall from her own room and told her to make herself comfortable, unpack her suitcase, and rest for a while if she wanted to.

"Take your time. I'll wait for you in the den," she told her friend. "Then we can go out and do some sightseeing before dinner if you want."

"I don't know . . . I'm a little tired," Gretchen said.

"After everything I've been through, I might be more comfortable if we stayed in, at least for the rest of today."

"Oh . . . that's fine with me," Jorey said. "I just figured that since you'd never been to New York you might want me to show you around. I thought it would take your mind off of things."

"Just being out of Blizzard Bay helps," Gretchen told her. "Thank God I was able to count on you to be there for me, Jorey. You've always been such a good friend to me. Not like all the others."

Jorey shifted uncomfortably. "What do you mean?"

"Nothing," Gretchen said, shrugging. "Just that Adrienne always made me feel so inferior . . ."

"She's a terrible snob, Gretchen," Jorey said, then realized she was referring to Adrienne in the present tense. "I mean, she *was,*" she corrected awkwardly.

"I know . . . and I suppose I shouldn't be criticizing someone who's dead," Gretchen told her. "That's what I was telling Karl just yesterday . . . that I can't have any hard feelings toward someone who's dead. I had told him about Adrienne, and about Clover and Kitty, and how I never felt as though I fit in with them. But you were always different. I told him that, too. 'Jorey was always the one who stuck up for me.' Even before he met you, Karl said he knew he was going to like you. He looks out for me, too, Jorey. Just like you always did."

"I'm glad, Gretchen," Jorey said, wanting to ask where Karl had been last night when Gretchen needed him.

Again she thought of the note Gretchen had found on her pillow, and the fact that Karl had the keys to the house.

Don't be paranoid, she told herself. *That doesn't mean*

anything. Plenty of people have had access to that house. It's a bed & breakfast. Strangers come and go freely. Somebody could have stolen a key and had it duplicated ages ago without Gretchen ever knowing.

Even, she remembered suddenly, Hob Nixon. Hadn't Gretchen said something a while back about hiring him to do some painting? What if—

"Jorey," Gretchen said, "I know you said not to tell Karl where I went, but I just want you to know that you're worrying for no reason. I can trust him. I know I can."

Jorey's blood ran cold. "But you didn't tell him, did you, Gretchen?"

"You said not to, didn't you?" Gretchen stifled a yawn. "Maybe I do need to rest. I'll just unpack my bags and lie down for a while. Thanks for the hospitality."

"You're welcome," Jorey said with a tight smile.

As she left Gretchen in the guest room and headed to her own room, she couldn't help thinking about what Gretchen had said. *You've always been such a good friend to me.*

But had she always?

Of course you have. You never made fun of Gretchen, or made her feel inferior, or rubbed her nose in the fact that she didn't have a boyfriend like everyone else did.

Adrienne had been terrible about doing just that, Jorey remembered. And even Kitty and Clover had joined in on occasion, falling into the adolescent trap of following the ringleader. But Jorey had never done that . . . had she?

She thought back over the years, trying to remember.

The ringing telephone interrupted her thoughts.

She hurried to pick it up, wondering if it was Sawyer calling, then catching herself. Why would it be? He wouldn't be calling her here. It was over; he was a part of the past.

Still, her "Hello?" was a little breathless with anticipation.

"Jorey! You're home."

"Hi, Daddy."

"I've missed you. How was your vacation?"

Vacation was such an innocuous, unsuitable word to describe the past week of her life, but she didn't tell her father that. She simply said, "It was fine, Daddy."

"Did you get a chance to go out to the old place and have a look around?"

Yes. I even spent the night there, in the bed of a man who lives in my old room.

"Actually, I didn't bother," she heard herself telling her father. "It's been converted to apartments, and I really didn't want to see it that way. I'd rather remember it the way it was when Papa May lived there."

"I know what you mean," Mayville Maddock said with a sigh. "Seems like only yesterday that Pop was alive, sitting on that old front porch with his pipe. And Mother hollering at him that it stunk, and to put it out."

"I loved the smell of his tobacco," Jorey said, remembering. "Vanilla, wasn't it?"

"Most of the time. I liked it, too. But Mother never did. She never seemed to like anything about him, did she?"

"No, she didn't." Jorey thought of her Grandmother Maddock, who now had Alzheimer's Disease and was ensconced in a private nursing home in Westchester County. She supposed she should go visit her one of these days, even though her grandmother had no idea who she was. The last time Jorey had been there, in the spring, her grandmother kept calling her Lottie and asking whether she was prepared for the spelling bee. It has been so depressing that Jorey had left in tears.

"Now that you're home," Jorey's father said, "I thought you might be interested in a little project I have in mind for you, Jorey."

"What kind of project?"

He explained that he would be opening a store at a new mall that was being built in New Jersey, and would have to hire someone to oversee the process.

"And you want me to do it?" Jorey asked, incredulous.

"You'd be perfect," her father said. "I need someone I can trust, and you need something to do. It's time that you figured out what you want to do with your life, Jorey."

"I know," she said, wondering how her father had read her mind over these past few days. "I know I need something."

But I don't think that a career with the department store is the answer to my problems.

"Listen, Daddy, can I give this some thought? I'd like to hear more about the job first, and find out exactly what it would entail. Why don't we have lunch tomorrow?"

"That would be—wait, not tomorrow. Tomorrow I have appointments from morning till night. The day after?"

Jorey agreed, thinking Gretchen wouldn't mind occupying herself for a few hours, and they made plans to meet at a restaurant in the Village.

After hanging up, Jorey wondered if she should just take her father up on whatever he was offering. Just plunge in and get busy doing something productive, even if she didn't enjoy it. Something that would take her mind off Sawyer, and what could never be.

"Knock, knock."

Jorey looked up at the sound of the voice to see Gretchen standing in the doorway of the den. She had changed from her overalls into a pair of jeans and a flannel shirt, and her hair was hanging loose, the blond tresses crimped from the braids she had worn earlier.

"Hi," Jorey said, putting aside the newspaper she had been trying to read. "Did you get some sleep?"

Gretchen shook her head. "I couldn't. I've got too much on my mind."

"Still worried about that note? I really think you should call the police in Blizzard Bay, Gretchen." Jorey had suggested it to her several times earlier, while they were eating lunch, in fact.

But Gretchen shook her head now, as she had before. "I can't do that yet."

"But you were supposed to meet with them today, about Uncle Roland. Don't you think they want to hear from you? Don't you think they're wondering where you are?"

Gretchen shrugged and walked over to a table, picking up a framed photograph. "This must have been taken just before your grandfather died," she said, studying the image of the old man with his arm around the eighteen year-old Jorey. "I remember thinking that he looked like Colonel Sanders. His mustache had turned completely white that summer."

"It had, hadn't it?" Jorey looked over her shoulder at the picture, noticing that Papa May looked as jovial as ever but that her own face was haunted.

It was the divorce, she told herself. *I had just found out about the divorce and I was shattered.*

Looking into her own eyes, she was transported back over the years to that terrible summer, remembering the hollow emptiness she had felt when she'd arrived in Blizzard Bay. Her family had never been close; she had never had a real home; her parents had never even made a pretense of liking each other's company.

But that didn't mean she wasn't devastated when they announced that their marriage was over.

She had always dreamed of having a *real* family and a *real* home. As long as her parents were together, she could hope that it would somehow happen someday. But when they told her they were divorcing, that hope was gone.

All she had left was Papa May, and the home in Blizzard Bay . . . and that hadn't lasted more than a few weeks after she'd arrived. Two terrible blows.

The days that were sandwiched in between remained a blur.

Again, she wondered what had happened at the pond. The day that kept coming back in bits and pieces. Someone had been splashing, and screaming for help. And she had been hiding behind the trees.

"You're so quiet. What are you thinking about, Jorey?" Gretchen asked, turning to look at her.

Tell her. Maybe she can help. Maybe she knows.

She knew about Hob Nixon being your secret admirer. And about Johnny having a crush on you. She must remember other things about that summer.

Tell her.

Tell her.

"It's just . . . there's something that's been bothering

me lately, Gretchen. Ever since I went back to Blizzard Bay."

"What is it?"

"I can't remember.

"What can't you remember?"

"That's the problem. I can't remember much of anything that happened the last summer I spent there. Everything about it seems so fuzzy up until Papa May's death. But there's this one thing that's been bothering me . . ."

Gretchen was watching her carefully, as though she sensed how troubled Jorey was over this. "What?"

"I keep getting these flashes of something happening out by the pond on my grandparents' property. I know that's where my grandfather died, but it's something else. Not just that. Something else happened there, and whatever it was really disturbed me. Do you remember anything?"

"There *was* something," Gretchen said slowly. "Something that happened at the pond."

"What?"

"It was a really hot, humid afternoon, and you and I and the others—"

"Clover and Adrienne and Kitty?"

"Yes, all of us. We were sitting around on the porch at your grandparents' house, talking about how nice it would be to go swimming. But none of us had our suits, except you."

"Yeah . . ." Jorey had a sudden, vague recollection of that day. They were eating Popsicles. Hers was root beer flavored, and it kept dripping sticky, brown trails down her wrist because the blazing sun was melting it faster than she could lick it.

"And so Adrienne suggested that we go skinny-dipping at the pond. She said it while I was in the house, going to the bathroom, and by the time I came back out, everyone had decided that it was a great idea. I didn't want to go along with it, but everyone made such a big deal that I didn't want to seem like a baby, so I agreed.''

Jorey nodded, remembering this, too. She saw Gretchen's hesitant expression, and the way she slouched in her oversized sleeveless blouse and baggy khaki shorts, trying to conceal her overweight, fleshy body. She remembered thinking that if she were Gretchen she wouldn't want to take off her clothes in front of the others, either—lean, lithe Clover, wiry, athletic Kitty, and perfectly proportioned Adrienne. And of course, Jorey, with her petite frame, was as slender as the rest of them.

"I was so ashamed of the way I looked," Gretchen said in a faraway voice. "But I was more ashamed of not fitting in. I told myself it would be no big deal— that nobody would be interested in seeing what I looked like. And it was so damned hot . . . remember how hot it was, Jorey?"

She nodded, recalling now the still, heavy air that hung over the pond when they reached it, and the way the sweat was trickling down her forehead.

"Adrienne suggested that we all get undressed behind the trees, then take turns running and jumping into the water." Gretchen's voice was shaking now. "So I went behind this big pine tree that I thought would shield me, and I took off all my clothes. I folded them neatly and I put them on a stump . . ."

In her mind's eye, Jorey saw her doing that. She saw Gretchen's ample, white, dimpled folds of flesh and the way her hands shook as she folded her clothes. She saw her from behind, through the low-hanging boughs of a tree, and she heard muffled giggles beside her, and Adrienne's voice saying, "Shhh!"

Then she saw Gretchen tentatively move forward, toward the clearing and the pond, leaving her clothes behind on the stump, and saw Adrienne stealing over to them. She saw Adrienne silently gathering the folded blouse and shorts and panties and bra, even the size ten sneakers and white ankle socks.

Stop her! a voice shrieked in Jorey's mind. *Don't let her steal Gretchen's clothes. This isn't a joke . . . it's cruel. It's so cruel.*

But she watched dully, feeling powerless to do anything, powerless to even care. She was detached from the situation in the way that she was detached from everything else that summer. Her life was falling apart, and she felt completely numb, unable to act or react to anything.

"When I got to the edge of the trees," Gretchen was saying now, "I waited for someone to say something, to run and jump into the water. But there was only silence, Jorey. Nobody made a sound. I started calling names, but nobody answered. Then, something made me turn around and look for my clothes. I knew, even before I saw what had happened, that they would be gone. I knew that you had stolen them."

"*I* didn't—" Jorey protested weakly.

"All of you. Adrienne, Clover, Kitty, and even you, Jorey. You didn't stop them. You always stood up for me. When they teased me or made fun of me, you stopped them. Only, this time you didn't. And this was the one time it really counted."

"I couldn't . . ." Jorey closed her eyes, remembering how she had run through the woods with Adrienne and the others, running all the way back toward the road, where Johnny and a bunch of his friends waited. She remembered then that it had been prearranged, all of this. Adrienne's big plan.

"The ultimate practical joke," she had called it.

She remembered getting the boys, and then all of them racing back to the pond. She remembered seeing Gretchen huddled in the bushes, naked and crying, and the way she had screamed and run and jumped into the water when she heard the boys approaching.

She had wondered why. Why would Gretchen jump into the water? Why wouldn't she just hide in the bushes?

Then she had realized that the water provided a way to hide her body from probing eyes. In the water, Gretchen was safe. No one could see her.

"I was terrified," Gretchen said, her voice taut.

Jorey couldn't look at her. She stared off into space, remembering how Gretchen had sputtered and splashed in the pond, then started whimpering as the boys hid in the trees and taunted her. They called her names.

Thunder thighs.

Lard Ass.

Terrible names.

She remembered crouching at the edge of the clearing, behind some rocks, with Kitty and Adrienne and Clover. She remembered that Adrienne was hysterical with laughter and the others were giggling nervously.

Stop them! Stop them!

The words kept going through Jorey's mind, but she did nothing about them.

"I stayed in the water for hours," Gretchen said. "Long after I stopped hearing the boys, and the rest of you hiding in the bushes. I stayed until I was freezing and wrinkled and the sky was getting dark. I kept thinking that you would come back, Jorey. But you didn't.''

No, Jorey remembered. *I didn't. I left the pond when the others did, and Adrienne promised she would bring the clothes back to Gretchen in a little while. And I told myself that I should go check, make sure she had. But I never did.*

"Why didn't you come back, Jorey?"

She blinked at the plaintive note in Gretchen's voice, and slowly turned to look at her.

"Why didn't you come back? I thought you would.''

"Adrienne did. She brought your clothes back to you—''

"No. She never did.''

Jorey stared into Gretchen's pale, slate-colored eyes, and what she saw there took her breath away. It was hatred. Pure hatred.

"I . . . what did you do?" Jorey asked in a ragged whisper.

"Somebody finally came along. Hob Nixon came along, Jorey. He must have heard me screaming. I screamed until I was hoarse. And he told me he'd help me.''

"Hob Nixon helped you?"

"He went back to his trailer and he brought me some clothes. His clothes. They were smelly and ripped, but he said he would let me have them. For a price,'' she added in a brittle tone.

"Oh, Gretchen . . .''

"I paid his price, Jorey. I had no choice. I was already naked, anyway. All I had to do was lie there on the ground and let him climb on top of me and . . . I closed my eyes so I wouldn't have to see his face. And I bit my lip so I wouldn't scream. Because it hurt, Jorey. It hurt like hell. It was my first time."

Jorey closed her own eyes to keep from seeing Gretchen's ravaged face, and she bit her own lip to keep from sobbing out loud.

"It was over with finally, and Hob Nixon kept his word. He gave me his clothes to wear, and then he even drove me home. And you know what? I never forgot that he had helped me. I think that there was something about him that I related to. He was an outcast, just like me. He just did what he felt he had to do under the circumstances. I never blamed him for that. No, I never blamed *him.*"

Something in her tone made Jorey's eyes snap open. Her gaze collided with Gretchen's, and again she felt a chill. Gretchen was angry. So terribly angry, *furious*, and after all these years.

"I blamed you, Jorey."

"Me?" she asked incredulously.

And a flicker of an idea formed in her brain. An idea so outrageous, so unlikely, so utterly horrible, that she pushed it away before it could fully take shape.

"All of you. Adrienne, Clover, Kitty, and you. You were supposed to be my friends. You, most of all. How could you betray me that way?"

"I don't know," Jorey told her, hearing her own voice crack with emotion. "I don't know how I could have done something like that. I just wasn't myself, Gretchen. I don't even remember."

"Oh, you were so traumatized that you blocked the whole thing out? Is that it? Tell me, Jorey . . . why can't *I* block it out? Why does what happened haunt my every waking moment to this day? Why does it even haunt my sleep? I had nightmares about it, Jorey. Every damned night of my life. Until Karl came along.''

Her voice softened, and a faint smile touched her lips. ''When I met Karl, and he was interested in me, I finally thought I could get over the past. I thought he would love me, and we would be together, and I could shut everything out, and it wouldn't matter anymore.''

''It doesn't matter anymore, Gretchen. Just forget it.''

''I can't! *You* can forget it, Jorey. I can't. Don't you get it?'' she demanded shrilly.

A prickle of panic shot through Jorey, and again she tried to block out the disturbing idea probing at the edge of her mind.

She tried to sound calm and soothing as she told Gretchen, ''It happened a long time ago, and I'm sure nobody else remembered. You have to let go, Gretchen.''

''Nobody else remembered?'' Gretchen laughed hysterically. ''You're wrong, Jorey. I made sure they remembered. Clover remembered. Right before she died. And so did Adrienne. We talked about it. And they both agreed that it was time they paid for their sins.''

''*What?*'' Stunned, Jorey could only gape at Gretchen, truly seeing her for what seemed like the first time.

She's deranged, she realized in sheer dread. *She's out of her mind. She killed Clover and Adrienne.*

And she's going to kill me.

''It wasn't easy to convince them that they had to pay, Jorey.'' Gretchen sounded almost conversational now. As she spoke, she moved away from Jorey. Step by step. Away from the couch.

Why? Jorey wondered. *What does she have in mind?*

"But I told them that it was only fair," Gretchen went on. "After all, I had suffered for years. Now it was their turn to suffer. And they did. Believe me, they suffered."

She took another step back, toward the fireplace.

Jorey watched her, frantically wondering what she was up to. She was certain now that Gretchen had come here to kill her. To make her pay the way the others had.

"I had planned for it to be your turn before you left Blizzard Bay. I never thought I'd have to travel all the way down here just to take care of this," Gretchen said. "But you ruined my plan when you left, Jorey. Oh, well. Everything will go smoothly from here on in. First you, and then Kitty. She'll have to be last. I had to wait until she had the baby. After all, it wouldn't be fair to punish an innocent baby, would it? I mean, I'm not a *monster.*" She let out a high-pitched, hysterical laugh.

"You can't mean any of this, Gretchen," Jorey said in a low voice. "I know this isn't you. You're not the kind of person who would—"

"And you're not the kind of person who would betray a friend, Jorey. But you did it, anyway. Now it's my turn to surprise you. Are you surprised? Hmmm?"

Gretchen stood with her back to Jorey, in front of the fireplace. She was absolutely still, as though poised, and Jorey's mind whirled, wondering what she was going to do.

Then her eyes fell on the sword mounted over the fireplace, and she knew, in that terrible instant, what Gretchen had in mind. A moment later, Gretchen was reaching up and taking the weapon down, then turning to brandish it at Jorey.

"Touché," she said, and giggled crazily. *"En garde,* Jorey."

"Gretchen, put that down. You can't do this."

"I have to do this. It's your turn." Gretchen turned the blade so that it caught and reflected the lamplight. "It's time for you to be punished."

"But you'll be caught, Gretchen. Somebody will figure out sooner or later that you killed Adrienne, and Clover, and—"

"And Rebecca."

Gretchen spat the name and her eyes flared dangerously.

Startled, Jorey repeated, "Rebecca?" *Sawyer's sister.* "Why would you kill Rebecca?"

"Because I caught her with Karl. I stopped by his place one night in August to surprise him with a picnic supper in a wicker basket. I had prepared it so carefully. Fried chicken that it took me hours to make, and biscuits, and a bottle of champagne. And strawberries. Strawberries are so romantic, don't you think?"

Jorey nodded, mute.

"But then I saw him with *her.* On the beach. They were walking together, and I saw him put his arm around her and pat her on the back. Like they were lovers, Jorey. She wanted to steal him away from me, but he was mine. I told her that."

"Oh, Gretchen."

"I just meant to talk to her, Jorey. When I waited for her at her cabin later that night, I only meant to talk about it. But I got upset. I couldn't help it. I love Karl so much . . . I can't lose him."

"Karl wouldn't want you to hurt anyone, Gretchen," Jorey said rationally, conscious of the sharp blade Gretchen held aloft in front of her, rotating it slowly, thoughtfully.

"Karl doesn't know. He'll never know."

"If you . . ." Jorey swallowed hard. "If you kill me, he'll know. Because they'll put two and two together, and they'll figure it out, Gretchen."

"Not if *you* confess."

Bewildered, Jorey asked, "What are you talking about?"

"Clover and Adrienne were killed while you were in town. Isn't that a coincidence? It's perfect. I'm so glad I thought of it. You confess to killing them—"

"But I'm not going to—"

"Right before you commit suicide. You confess in a note. So start writing, Jorey."

Shocked, Jorey found her voice and protested, "What are you talking about? I'm not going to kill myself."

"Sure you are. You're going to go out to that beautiful terrace of yours, and you're going to climb over the railing, and you're going to hurl yourself down twenty-three stories until you go *splat* on the sidewalk, Jorey. But first, you have a note to write. And you'd better get started, or else . . ."

Suddenly, the blade came closer, and Jorey heard a ripping sound as it tore into the sleeve of her blouse, up near her throat.

She flinched as Gretchen held the tip of the sword there, against her skin.

"Are you going to write the note, Jorey?"

"Ye-e-s-s," Jorey breathed, trying not to shudder, trying not to move.

"Good. I'll tell you what to say. Do you have a pad and paper handy?"

"In . . . in the desk."

"Great. Get it, would you?" Suddenly, Gretchen was all business. Pleasant sounding, even. She withdrew the tip of the sword and motioned for Jorey to cross the room to the heavy oak desk that stood beside the fireplace.

As she walked on wobbly legs, Jorey desperately tried to think of a way to outwit Gretchen. There must be something she could do, something she could say. . . .

Sawyer, she thought suddenly. *Where are you? I need you.*

Tears sprang to her eyes as she thought of him, and realized that she would never see him again.

She had told herself that was the case when she was leaving Blizzard Bay . . . that it was over, and she never wanted to lay eyes on him again.

But she realized now that deep down inside she hadn't believed it. Deep in her heart, there had been hope. That was why she had been so reluctant to figure out what she was going to do with her life, to even discuss the job opportunity her father had offered.

I wanted to be with him. I believed that he would come after me, and that we would end up together somehow. . . .

"Stop dawdling!" Gretchen barked behind her. "Get that pad and start writing, Jorey!"

"I'm going," she said shakily. "I'm getting it."

She reached out and opened the drawer, wondering if there were something inside that she could use as a weapon. If she dug around, maybe . . .

"Don't you dare try anything," Gretchen said behind her.

Jorey felt something jab into her back and realized that it was the tip of the sword. Swallowing hard, she blindly grabbed a yellow legal pad that was sitting on top and fumbled for something to write with. Her fingers closed around a pen.

"Now sit," Gretchen ordered, and she pulled out the chair at the desk. "And write what I tell you to write."

"I will," Jorey promised in a whisper.

She wondered what would happen if she started screaming at the top of her lungs. Would anyone hear her?

No. There's no way. The apartment was soundproof. She had seen to that when she moved in. She had hired an expensive insulation specialist to make sure that the place was buffered against noise from the elevator and the tenants downstairs. Just one more added touch of luxury.

Now it would cost her her life.

She started writing as Gretchen dictated, slowly taking down the rambling, disjointed statement about how she had killed her old friends in a fit of rage and then found it necessary to end her life. She did her best to stall, painstakingly forming the words and letters, struggling to buy time, hoping that somehow something would happen to prevent the inevitable.

"Now say good-bye," Gretchen said. "Say good-bye to anyone you would want to say good-bye to. Your loving daddy, maybe . . ."

"And my mother . . . and sisters," Jorey said. "And their husbands, and my nieces and nephews . . ."

Anything to make the writing go on and on. Anything to stay alive another precious minute or two.

"Is that everyone?" Gretchen asked impatiently, looking over her shoulder.

"Let me think . . . Who else? Is there anyone else . . . ?"

Sawyer. I would want to say good-bye to Sawyer. I would want to tell him all the things I'll never have a chance to say. . . .

She wrote his name in a trembling hand, and paused with the pen still on the paper.

"Are you finished? Is that it?" Gretchen demanded, poking her in the back with the sword.

"No ..."

I love you.

The three words came quickly, and she scrawled them in bold, certain strokes, realizing they were true.

She loved him.

She wondered if he would somehow see this note. She wondered if he would believe that she had taken her own life; if he would believe that she had murdered Clover and Adrienne. ...

No, she thought resolutely. *He would never believe that. He would never think that of me.*

She felt tears stinging her eyes again and she blinked them back. If only she could have another chance with Sawyer ...

What would have happened between us? she wondered. *Would we have gotten married? Would we have had children? Would we have found a place to live happily ever after?*

"It's time, Jorey."

Gretchen's voice jerked her back to reality. She sat perfectly still in utter dread, unable to face what was about to happen.

This can't be it, she thought wildly. *This can't be the end. My life can't be over now. I just figured out what matters to me. What I need.*

I need Sawyer. I need to marry him and have his babies, and that's all I want to do. That's all I'll ever need.

"Let's go outside. Leave the note there."

She rose automatically, allowed Gretchen to steer her through the quiet rooms of the apartment. She heard the mantel clock ticking and their muffled footsteps on the carpet and her own shallow breathing, and she was overcome by an urgent sense of panic. She wanted to break away, to fight, to run for her life, and she knew that it would be futile. She was a trapped animal with no means of escape. There was nothing to do but accept her fate, and wait for death.

She wondered if this was what Clover, Adrienne and Rebecca had felt, knowing they were about to die.

Gretchen opened the door to the terrace and shoved Jorey out onto the wet stone floor. It was pouring now, a raging thunderstorm, with the wind lashing cold rain against her face. Nobody would hear her out here even if she dared to scream for help.

"Get up on the railing," Gretchen instructed.

Jorey turned to look at her.

Gretchen's blond hair was plastered to her round face, and her expression was hardened and determined. She was all business, consumed by the need to avenge something that had happened all those years ago.

"I never meant to hurt you, Gretchen," Jorey said. "I cared about you. I really did."

"No," Gretchen said, shaking her head and narrowing her eyes. "You didn't care. You were never my friend."

"I was. I don't know why I let it happen, Gretchen. I don't know what was wrong with me that summer. I was just so upset about my parents splitting . . . I wasn't myself."

Gretchen laughed. "You think that changes things? 'I wasn't myself,' " she mimicked. "Well, I'm not myself right now, Jorey. I haven't been myself in a while. And I'm going to make sure that you pay the way the others paid. It's only right."

"No, Gretchen . . ."

"Yes, Jorey. Get up on the railing."

Jorey gulped and stared at the low iron rail in front

of her. It was slick with rain, and would be slippery. If she climbed onto it, she might fall.

Oh, Christ, what am I thinking? I'm supposed to fall. Or she'll push me. That's the point. That's why we're out here.

The whole thing seemed so ludicrous.

"Go!" Gretchen bellowed behind her.

She took a step forward, and then another.

She reached out for the railing.

The metal surface was cold and wet.

She put one knee on it, then gingerly let her leg drop over, so that she straddled it.

"Good," Gretchen said. "Now bring the other leg over and put your back to me."

Jorey fought the urge to whimper as she did what Gretchen told her to do. She gripped the railing with both hands, sitting with her back to Gretchen.

Don't look down, she commanded herself. *Whatever you do, don't look down.*

"There. See? It won't be so bad, Jorey. You just sit there, and I'll give you a little push. You'll be flying through the air, and then it will be all over in a flash. You'll feel nothing. You're lucky, Jorey. Luckier than Adrienne, Clover and Rebecca. You're braver, too. They begged. All three of them. Begged me to stop. Even when their own blood was choking them, they begged. And do you know what I did?"

Jorey shook her head slightly, afraid to speak, but willing Gretchen to keep talking.

Every second counts, she thought, though she knew that she was only prolonging the inevitable. No one knew she was here with a madwoman. No one knew her life was in danger.

Except Sawyer.

He had tried to protect her.

How had he known?

"I laughed," Gretchen was saying. "They cried and screamed and begged, and I laughed. But Jorey, you're not crying or screaming or begging. And I'm not laughing. Because with you, it's different. With you, I actually feel kind of bad."

Jorey held her breath, sat motionless, gripping the railing. Was Gretchen going to change her mind? Was she going to let her live?

Please, please, let her change her mind.

"Oh, well," Gretchen said breezily behind her. "I'll get over it. I'll go on. Karl will be there for me. No matter what you think, Jorey, he loves me. He really does."

"I know he does," Jorey said, squeezing her eyes shut and praying. "I could see it in the way he was looking at you the last time I saw him, Gretchen. He loves you."

"You think?"

"Of course. I can't believe I didn't notice it sooner. Karl is head over heels for you. It's obvious."

"How could you tell?" Gretchen asked, sounding as eager as a twelve-year-old with a crush. "Did he say anything to you?"

"He did. But what was it? Let's see . . ."

"What did he say? Come on, Jorey."

It's working, she thought breathlessly. *Keep it up.*

"He said that he was thinking of proposing. He wanted to know what I thought you'd say if he did."

"What did you tell him? You told him you thought I'd say yes, didn't you?"

"Let me think . . ." Jorey stalled.

"Didn't you?" Gretchen asked shrilly.

Jorey tensed, gripping the railing. "I did," she said hastily. "I told him—"

"What was that?" Gretchen cut in. "Did you hear that?"

"What?"

"A thump. I heard a thump. Over there."

"I didn't hear—"

Gretchen shrieked then, a sudden, bloodcurdling sound that jolted Jorey to the core. She felt herself wobbling on the railing; felt herself tilting forward.

"No!" she screeched, frantically fumbling for a hold. One hand caught the slippery pole along the top as she was going over, and then her legs were dangling twenty-three stories above the street.

Where was Gretchen? What was going on?

She struggled to hang on, knowing that to lose her grip on the railing would mean certain death.

Above the noise of the storm, she vaguely heard the sounds of a scuffle above her. She heard Gretchen cry out, cursing at someone, and then nothing more from her.

But another voice was mingling with the wind and the rain, shouting Jorey's name.

A familiar voice.

A dear voice she had thought she'd never hear again.

"Sawyer!" she screamed. "Help me! Please!"

"I've got you, Jorey."

She felt his hand on hers, felt him pulling her up, over the railing, into the safety of his arms. She glimpsed the crumpled figure of Gretchen lying on the concrete before she blindly buried her face in his shoulder and felt him clutching her against him so tightly that she could barely breathe, and she didn't care.

She was alive.

And he was here.

Why was he . . . ?

How had he . . . ?

The questions weren't important. There would be time for answers later. Right now, all that mattered was that he had come to her.

Chapter Eighteen

"Thank you, Dr. Eisen," Jorey said as the middle-aged man with the kind, brown eyes picked up his trench coat from the chair beside her bed. "I feel better already."

"Well, take care of yourself, young lady," he said, picking up his bag. "I want you to take it easy for the next day or two. You've been through quite an ordeal."

"I'll be fine." She made a move to get off her bed. "Let me—"

"Sit. Doctor's orders. I'll see myself out."

"Thank you." She leaned back against the pillows and pulled the goose down comforter up to her chin. She heard the doctor's footsteps retreat down the hall, and the low-pitched sound of two men in discussion for a few minutes before the front door opened and closed.

Sawyer appeared in the doorway then, looking relieved. "How are you feeling?"

"Fine. My arms are sore. I guess I was out of shape."

"Not that out of shape. You managed to fight the wind and rain and hang on to a slippery railing twenty-three stories off the ground, Jorey. The thought of what could have happened makes me shudder."

"Me, too. But I'm all right now, Sawyer. The doctor just said to take it easy for a while."

"He told me. Nice man. I didn't realize doctors still made house calls these days. Especially at this hour." The bedside clock showed that it was well after midnight.

"Most don't. But Dr. Eisen has taken care of me since I was a baby and since you insisted on my seeing someone . . ."

"I was worried about you."

"Don't be, anymore. I told Dr. Eisen everything—about the memory loss, too. And he said the partial amnesia was a response to the traumas I had gone through that summer—first my parents' divorce, then the disaster with Gretchen at the pond, and Papa May's death. I tried to block it all out afterward. If I hadn't, I would have known Gretchen might be the one—"

"I don't know, Jorey," Sawyer said, crossing the room and perching on the edge of her bed. "I don't know if anyone could have imagined or believed that she was so troubled, that she had so much hatred and anger locked inside."

"Or that she was actually capable of murder." Jorey shivered despite the heavy warmth of the comforter. "I can't believe she tried to kill me. Or that she actually killed the others."

Sawyer nodded grimly, and she knew he was thinking of his sister. Poor Rebecca Latimer had simply been in the wrong place at the wrong time. Karl had said, when he was contacted by the police earlier, that nothing had been going on between him and Rebecca, and he had no inkling Gretchen had even seen him with her on the beach that night. He said that Rebecca was confiding in him about her ruined marriage, and he was trying to comfort her, having been recently divorced himself.

He also said that he had sensed that Gretchen wanted more from their relationship than he did, and had tried to tell her that he wasn't ready for anything permanent. He said Gretchen hadn't seemed to grasp what he was telling her, and that he had been trying to ease the contact between them, rather than break things off entirely. He had sensed her vulnerability and felt sorry for her, but had never imagined that she was capable of the heinous crimes she had committed.

"Do you think she'll be mentally fit to stand trial for the murders?" Jorey asked Sawyer quietly, remembering how Gretchen had ranted after she had regained consciousness and found herself in police custody. The officers had arrived moments after Sawyer had knocked her out and rescued Jorey; Sawyer had dialed 9-1-1 after breaking into Jorey's apartment and seeing what was happening out on the terrace.

"I doubt she's mentally fit," Sawyer told Jorey. "To have done what she did—and carry on a semblance of a normal life. She clearly believed that she was only doing what was right. That justice was being served."

"I know. But your sister—and Uncle Roland . . ."

Sawyer shook his head. "That old man didn't have a chance. When I walked into that room and saw him lying there covered in his own blood . . . I'll never forget the sight."

"And all because she thought he was on to her. He had found the knife she had used to kill Clover. She must have stashed it someplace in the house. And I'm sure he knew what it meant, Sawyer. That must be what he was trying so hard to tell me that night. If only I hadn't told her—"

"You did what you believed was the right thing to do, Jorey. Stop condemning yourself for it. None of this was your fault."

"I know. I know. It's just so hard to get past it. I wonder if I'll ever be able to forget."

"Probably not entirely. But time will help. Both of us."

She nodded, studying his handsome face. He was only a few feet away from her, sitting on the edge of the bed. If she wanted to, she could reach out and touch him . . . but did she dare?

"Sawyer," she said quietly, "how did you know it was Gretchen? And how did you know I was in trouble?"

He sighed and looked at her. "When I found her uncle, I just knew all at once what had happened. The way I knew where she had gone . . . and that you needed me. I knew, Jorey, because I've always had a way of knowing things I couldn't possibly know."

She stared at him, sensing that he was finally going to open up to her. And she did touch him, then. She reached out and she took one of his big hands in both of hers, and she held it tightly as he began to talk.

As his deep, dark secret spilled out she found herself awed . . . and relieved. She didn't know what she had been imagining he was hiding, but she had somehow assumed that it would be something terrible. Something she couldn't handle.

Not this revelation that he had this inexplicable power, this sixth sense, that had made his life pure hell for the past few years. Tears sprang to her eyes when he talked about Susan, the woman he had loved and married . . . and buried. And about his sister Rebecca.

When he was finished talking, she squeezed his hand and fought the urge to throw her arms around him and hold him close. She sensed that she had to tread carefully now; that he had taken an enormous emotional risk by telling her the truth.

"Sawyer," she said quietly, "you have to stop blaming yourself. None of what happened is your fault. It was fate, and you were unfortunate enough to know what it had in store for your sister and your wife."

Those last words sounded so strange. *Your wife*. He'd had a wife, a woman he loved, a woman he had planned to share his future with.

No wonder he had closed himself off to falling in love with anyone else.

That was why she had to give up her own dreams now. About marrying him, and having his children. He might have saved her life, but that didn't mean he wanted to spend the rest of it with her.

"It's funny," Sawyer said, after a long moment of silence. "Now that I know what happened to Rebecca . . . it's easier, somehow. To put all of it behind me. I know who killed Rebecca, and I know why. It's what I went to Blizzard Bay to find out, but I never really thought I'd get on with my life after I knew. I guess I never thought beyond my mission there. Now I can go back to being Scott Delaney."

She blinked. "What?"

He smiled faintly. "Scott Delaney. My real name. Ever hear of Delaney Automotive?"

"The race car manufacturer in Detroit?" She nodded incredulously. "Papa May wasn't just devoted to horse racing. He was into car racing, too. Used to talk about race cars all the time . . . You mean that *you're*—?"

"My grandfather founded it. The family business. I'm the CEO these days, although I've been an absentee ever since my sister's murder."

"But why didn't you tell me? Why weren't you using your real name?"

"Because I didn't want anyone to know who I was or why I was in Blizzard Bay, Jorey. I wanted the chance to find out who killed my sister, and I knew that it would be easier being anonymous. I had a hunch that the killer was someone local, and I wanted to be able to blend in so that I wouldn't arouse anyone's suspicions."

"Which proved to be impossible in a town that size," she pointed out ruefully.

He nodded. "But nobody ever figured out who I was. And the name Delaney would have been a dead giveaway."

"So who is Sawyer Howland? Just some name you made up?"

He shook his head. "Remember I told you that my mother always said I inherited my strange ability from her grandfather? His name was Sawyer Howland. I thought it was fitting."

"It was. And now you're back to being Scott Delaney? I don't know if I can ever get used to that."

"Well, you should start trying."

Something in his voice, something in the expression in his eyes, made her breath catch in her throat.

"Oh, yeah?" she asked slowly. "Why?"

"If you're going to be hanging around, I want you to call me by my real name."

"And why," she asked breathlessly, "would I be hanging around?"

"I just assumed ..." He paused and cleared his throat. "But I shouldn't do that, should I? I should ask."

She hardly dared to voice the question, and when she did, it was barely a whisper. "What? What should you ask?"

He stood, and for a moment she thought she'd lost him. That he was going to turn his back and walk out of there.

But he didn't.

He was getting down on one knee beside her bed, and now he was holding one of her hands in both of his big, strong ones.

"I know why I was so desperate to protect you from the moment I met you—and even before that. Because I had to make sure you had a future—and that you would share it with me. Will you be my wife, Jorey? Will you come back to Michigan with me, and will you have my children?"

She gasped, then tried to speak. She couldn't; first she would have to swallow the enormous lump that careened into her throat. Be his wife? Go to Michigan? Have his children?

This was all she needed, she realized in wonder. All she would ever need. This was what she had been searching for.

"Will you?" he asked, watching her anxiously.

Still, she was too overcome to speak. Finally, she simply nodded mutely.

He broke into a broad grin. "Is that a yes?"

This time, she found her voice. "It's a yes."

"Oh, Jorey ... Oh, how I love you."

"I love you, too, Sawyer."

"Scott," he said, laughing. "It's Scott."

"Scott. I love you, Scott."

And she realized, as he gathered her into his arms and his mouth came down over hers, that for the first time in her life Jorey Maddock had come home.